Mechanical Lumbosacral Spine Pain

This book addresses an extremely prevalent medical problem: low back pain. It is not a general anatomy book, but it relates specifically to the lumbosacral spine, encompassing anatomy, histology, histopathology, and imaging all in one volume. For students, the text incrementally introduces them to lumbosacral anatomy terms and scientific knowledge by using photographs of gross and histological sections of the spine, as well as schematic drawings and images, in preparation for clinical practice. It answers many questions about the pathogenesis of low back pain, helpful for clinicians, both for treatment decisions and for counselling patients.

Key features:

- Provides a clear explanation for many of the pain generators in low back pain and illuminates this perplexing and ubiquitous problem.
- Addresses a gap in the existing literature, as 'non-specific' or mechanical lumbosacral spine pain accounts for by far most chronic spinal pain sufferers' complaints for clinicians from general medical practitioners to spinal specialists in various fields such as sports medicine who deal with spinal pain syndromes.
- Illustrates anatomical structures that can be injured and thus become responsible for causing mechanical lumbosacral spine pain; frequently, such injuries cannot be detected on sophisticated imaging such as MRI.

Mechanical Lumbosacral Spine Pain

Anatomy, Histology, and Imaging

Lynton GF Giles DC (*Toronto*), MSc, PhD (*WAust*)

Formerly:

Clinical practice treating patients with spinal pain syndromes

Clinical Director
Multidisciplinary Spinal Pain Unit
Townsville General Hospital
Townsville, Queensland, Australia

Honorary Clinical Scientist
Townsville General Hospital

Adjunct Associate Professor (Clinical)
School of Public Health, Tropical Medicine and Rehabilitation Sciences
Faculty of Medicine, Health and Molecular Sciences
James Cook University
Townsville, Queensland, Australia

Medico–legal Consultant for Assessing Spinal Injuries

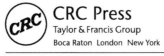

CRC Press
Taylor & Francis Group
Boca Raton London New York

CRC Press is an imprint of the
Taylor & Francis Group, an **informa** business

First edition published 2023
by CRC Press
6000 Broken Sound Parkway NW, Suite 300, Boca Raton, FL 33487–2742

and by CRC Press
4 Park Square, Milton Park, Abingdon, Oxon, OX14 4RN

CRC Press is an imprint of Taylor & Francis Group, LLC

© 2023 Lynton G.F. Giles

This book contains information obtained from authentic and highly regarded sources. While all reasonable efforts have been made to publish reliable data and information, neither the author nor the publisher can accept any legal responsibility or liability for any errors or omissions that may be made. The publishers wish to make clear that any views or opinions expressed in this book by individual editors, authors or contributors are personal to them and do not necessarily reflect the views/opinions of the publishers. The information or guidance contained in this book is intended for use by medical, scientific or health-care professionals and is provided strictly as a supplement to the medical or other professional's own judgement, their knowledge of the patient's medical history, relevant manufacturer's instructions and the appropriate best practice guidelines. Because of the rapid advances in medical science, any information or advice on dosages, procedures or diagnoses should be independently verified. The reader is strongly urged to consult the relevant national drug formulary and the drug companies' and device or material manufacturers' printed instructions, and their websites, before administering or utilizing any of the drugs, devices or materials mentioned in this book. This book does not indicate whether a particular treatment is appropriate or suitable for a particular individual. Ultimately it is the sole responsibility of the medical professional to make his or her own professional judgements, so as to advise and treat patients appropriately. The authors and publishers have also attempted to trace the copyright holders of all material reproduced in this publication and apologize to copyright holders if permission to publish in this form has not been obtained. If any copyright material has not been acknowledged please write and let us know so we may rectify in any future reprint.

Library of Congress Cataloging-in-Publication Data
Names: Giles, L. G. F., author.
Title: Mechanical lumbosacral spine pain : anatomy, histology and imaging / Lynton G.F. Giles.
Description: First edition. | Boca Raton, FL : CRC Press, 2023. | Includes bibliographical references and index. | Summary:
 "This book addresses an extremely prevalent medical problem: low back pain. It is not a general anatomy book, but it
 relates specifically to the lumbosacral spine, encompassing anatomy, histology, histopathology, and imaging all in one
 volume"— Provided by publisher.
Identifiers: LCCN 2022027063 (print) | LCCN 2022027064 (ebook) | ISBN 9781032326443 (hardback) | ISBN 9781032326436
 (paperback) | ISBN 9781003315964 (ebook)
Subjects: MESH: Low Back Pain—pathology | Lumbosacral Region—anatomy & histology | Low Back Pain—diagnostic
 imaging | Lumbosacral Region—diagnostic imaging
Classification: LCC RD771.B217 (print) | LCC RD771.B217 (ebook) | NLM WE 755 | DDC 617.5/64—dc23/eng/20220914
LC record available at https://lccn.loc.gov/2022027063
LC ebook record available at https://lccn.loc.gov/2022027064

ISBN: 978-1-032-32644-3 (hbk)
ISBN: 978-1-032-32643-6 (pbk)
ISBN: 978-1-003-31596-4 (ebk)

DOI: 10.1201/9781003315964

To Jennifer

My best friend, wife, and colleague for her unqualified support and painstaking efforts in helping to produce yet another book.

CONTENTS

Contents

PREFACE

Musculoskeletal conditions are typically characterized by persistent pain and restricted mobility (Blom et al 2021) and in the current "Findings from the Global Burden of Disease Study" (Institute for Health Metrics and Evaluation 2017), many of the top leading causes of disability in 1990 remain so in 2017, namely low back pain, headaches, and depression [in that order of ranking], reflecting a lack of progress in addressing these conditions. Thus, spinal pain syndromes are extremely common, with low back pain, in particular, being one of the leading causes of disability and chronic pain among adults and one of the most common reasons for which patients are treated with opioids (narcotics) (Waljee et al 2018). Low back pain has profound effects on the well-being of people and is often the cause of significant physical and psychological health impairments and, as the population ages over the coming decades, the number of individuals with low back pain is likely to increase substantially (Manchikanti et al 2014). There has long been a constant tension between the ability of opioids to relieve pain and suffering and the potential for severe personal and societal harm related primarily to risks of dependency and addiction (Lurie 2021). Currently, long-term prescribing of opioids for chronic non-specific, i.e. 'mechanical' or 'idiopathic' musculoskeletal pain is common in primary care (Ashaye et al 2018).

Opioids prescribed to treat persistent or severe pain attach to proteins called opioid receptors on nerve cells in the brain, spinal cord, gut, and other parts of the body, thus blocking pain messages sent from parts of the body through the spinal cord to the brain, but opioids can be highly addictive (American Society of Anesthesiologists 2019). This is because patients taking opioid medications on a daily basis over a long period of time become physiologically dependent as the body becomes adjusted to having the medication in its system, thus patients become tolerant to the medication resulting in the medications losing their effectiveness over time, but patients experience withdrawal symptoms if the medication is abruptly stopped (Institute for Chronic Pain 2019). Therefore, there is great concern regarding the overuse of opioids and the ramifications of doing so (Weeks et al 2018). For example, Australia faces a crisis regarding the use of pharmaceutical opioids (Australian Institute of Health and Welfare 2021), as is the case in many other countries.

Thus, pharmaceutical treatment of chronic non-cancer pain during the current opioid epidemic has become challenging for prescribing clinicians who are searching for safe, effective alternatives to opioids (Goodman et al 2017). Commonly prescribed opioids, for example Fentanyl—described by Professor Michael Farrell (Director of the National Drug and Alcohol Research Centre, University of New South Wales 2019) and Ramos-Matos et al (2021) as being 50–100 times more potent than Morphine, as well as the opioid Tramadol, have been reported as being associated with a significantly increased risk of mortality over one year, as compared with nonsteroidal anti-inflammatory drugs such as Naproxin, Diclofenac, Celecoxib, and Etoricoxib (Zeng et al 2019). However, Page et al (2016) cite literature suggesting that the use of nonsteroidal anti-inflammatory drugs has a role in the precipitation and exacerbation of heart failure.

As there is an opioid overdose crisis in Western societies, for example in the United States (National Institute on Drug Abuse 2019; Fatemi et al 2020), Canada (Leung 2019), Australia (Penington Institute 2021), and the United Kingdom (Ashaye et al 2018), Sleeman et al (2018) ask the question—"Why are these sometimes dangerous drugs still being given to patients?" especially as several studies have demonstrated that opioids achieve negligible improvement in pain, function, and quality of life (Ashaye et al 2018). Furthermore, given the prevalence of chronic low back pain, identifying effective nonopioid alternatives for chronic low back pain is a top healthcare priority (Waljee et al 2018), as it is for all spinal levels.

A non-opioid, paracetamol, is recommended in clinical guidelines as the first line analgesic drug for spinal pain, but the evidence base supporting this recommendation has been called into question as high-quality evidence suggests that Paracetamol is ineffective in the treatment of low back pain (Machado et al 2015). In addition, Louvet et al (2020) concluded that therapeutic doses of Paracetamol are associated with more severe liver injury than overdose in patients with excess drinking.

Furthermore, it was noted that, as opioids became less available for treating back pain patients, clinicians used off-label epidural steroid injections (Depo-Medrol) for treating back pain, so Depo-Medrol's manufacturer requested, in 2013, that epidural use be banned owing to significant risks because Depo-Medrol was approved only for injection into muscles and joints (Herman 2018). It is reported that the FDA declined to issue a ban but did strengthen the drug's label in 2014 to note the risks (Herman 2018).

It is interesting to note that Whedon et al (2021) found that, among older Medicare beneficiaries who received long-term management of chronic low back pain with opioid analgesic therapy (OAT) or spinal manipulative therapy (SMT), the adverse drug events were more than 42 times higher for initial choice of OAT versus those who initially chose SMT.

Finally, Cashin et al (2021) conducted a systematic review and meta-analysis in order to investigate the efficacy, acceptability, and safety of muscle relaxants for low back pain and concluded that considerable uncertainty exists about the clinical efficacy and safety of muscle relaxants for adults with non-specific low back pain.

It is against this background of difficulties in treating spinal pain syndromes that this book has been written in order to attempt to identify various possible causes of non-specific lumbosacral spinal pain. It is not a book on differential diagnosis, but it is a text illustrating possible mechanisms involved in lumbosacral spine pain syndromes of *mechanical* origin. The review of existing literature often dates back to the original research publications on a particular topic, in order to acknowledge the work of original authors.

Conditions causing spinal pain syndromes are many and varied and patients may present with a wide variety of symptoms and signs. Therefore, each patient needs to be thoroughly investigated before treatment commences i.e. appropriate diagnosis must be a prerequisite to treatment.

It behoves all clinicians dealing with spinal pain syndromes to note the following:

- First, do no harm (Hippocrates 400BCE, Epidemics, Bk. 1, Sect. XI). Historically, it is interesting to note that, although many arguments have been put forward to attribute this statement to various scholars, Travers (2018) finds no compelling argument denying Hippocrates' primacy.
- "If you listen carefully to the patient, he will tell you the diagnosis" (Quotation of Sir William Osler; Gandhi 2000). This statement still holds true and emphasizes the *great importance of taking a thorough history*.
- Remember that patients may present with more than one condition, so consider all possibilities for the cause(s) of a patient's presenting complaint.
- There is now general and increasing recognition of:
  - The essential *subjectivity* of the pain experience, no matter what the cause or causes;
  - The contribution of factors *other than physical lesions* to the experience of pain, to its expression and its communication and its impact on quality of life; and
  - The consequential need to *evaluate* and *respond to the subjective experience* and the other relevant factors as part of the overall treatment of patients with pain.
  - Furthermore, the person, style and *behaviour* of the examining clinician is an integral part of the total setting in which the examination takes place and can *significantly influence the patient's own behaviour* and *subsequent outcome*. In addition, the availability in a particular setting of *as full a range of treatment options as possible* seems highly desirable and care should be taken to avoid, as far as possible, the prescription of treatment based on the theoretical orientation and ideology of the clinic rather than on the need of the patient (James et al 1997).

- In my opinion, it is wise to start with non-invasive treatment to determine whether the patient will obtain relief, before progressing to invasive treatments. Inappropriate management of spinal pain syndromes, from diagnosis to treatment, causes misery for patients and adds a significant cost burden to the healthcare costs of countries around the world. In addition, adverse reactions to many prescribed medications may occur, especially when patients become addicted to drugs of dependency with the serious health and cost problems that may ensue.
- In general, appropriate care comprises the right therapy, for the right problem, for the right patient (Coulter et al 2018).
- The following Covenant has been adapted and modified from Cassel (1995):
  - Appropriate care should be tempered by the treating clinician adhering to the patient-physician Covenant bearing in mind that, at the centre of treatment, there is a moral clinical enterprise grounded in a covenant of trust; this Covenant obliges clinicians to be competent and to use their competence in the patient's best interests, as clinicians are both intellectually and morally obliged to act as advocates for the sick, wherever their welfare is threatened and for their health at all times. Clinicians should pursue their particular clinical activity with the virtues of humility, honesty, intellectual integrity, compassion, and effacement of excessive self-interest.
  - A clinician's first obligation must be to serve the good of those persons who seek our help and trust us to provide it—clinicians must never be commercial entrepreneurs.
  - In addition to the aforementioned Covenant, it is worth noting the World Medical Association Declaration of Geneva that lists the Physician's Pledge, as amended in October 2017.

Fortunately, spine-related research has evolved dramatically during the last century and significant contributions have been made by thousands of authors (Murray et al 2012), through a highly multidisciplinary process (Wilke 2016). As a result, knowledge is ever increasing on spinal anatomy and histopathology and the possible physiological mechanisms by which pain may be generated and experienced. Therefore, in this text an introductory chapter summarizes possible pain sources for *non-specific and specific lumbosacral spinal pain* syndromes due to lumbosacral spine mechanical dysfunction or failure, founded on sound basic science and known anatomical principles. Because spinal pain syndromes can be complex, there often is a tendency for clinicians to incorrectly label patients as being 'neurotic', or when patients are involved in litigation they may be considered to have litigation 'neurosis' as a motive. However, it should be remembered that it is not always possible to diagnose a patient's spinal pain condition because of many factors such as the limitations of imaging procedures and the specificity and sensitivity of laboratory tests and some clinical tests. It is important to use non-ionizing imaging procedures such as MRI where at all possible in order to protect the patient (Giles 2014).

In some cases, patients merely want reassurance, based upon a thorough evaluation leading to a likely explanation for their chronic spinal pain syndrome(s), rather than requesting treatment. The importance of providing adequate, albeit time consuming, psychological assurance should not be underestimated. Obviously, it is important to consider a particular pain syndromes' possible aetiology in great detail, while not forgetting that psychology must be taken into account for each patient, as symptoms and signs should not be isolated from the patient as a whole being. In addition, it should be remembered that the best treatment for mechanical back pain may be good old-fashioned movement and exercise (Harvard Health Publishing 2018). Drugs are not part of the latest recommendations for treating mechanical back pain because some medications carry significant risks—therefore, first-line therapy should include non-drug therapy such as superficial heat, massage, acupuncture, or spinal manipulation (Tello 2017). When spinal manipulation is well justified and when it is correctly executed, no accident occurs, or any incidents are very rare (Maigne 1972).

In addition to these therapies, patients should be encouraged to *take charge of their spinal pain syndrome(s)*, rather than allowing their pain to *control their lives*. Fortunately, using the notion of *positive health* i.e. the ability for patients to adapt and to self-manage in the face of social, physical, and emotional challenges for the treatment of back pain (Buchbinder et al 2018) is a powerful approach for patients to help themselves.

It is the responsibility of the treating clinician, relying on their independent expertise and their knowledge of the patient, to determine the best treatment and its method of application for individual patients, including referral if necessary.

No one profession has all the answers to manage challenging acute and chronic mechanical spinal pain syndrome patients. Therefore, following 47 years of clinical experience, which included some years as clinical director of the Multidisciplinary Spinal Pain Unit at Townsville General Hospital (Giles 2017) that provided acupuncture, medicine, and spinal manipulation, with access to other specialties, it is my firm opinion that multidisciplinary cooperation is essential if clinicians from different backgrounds are to best serve patients with spinal pain syndromes and the possible sequelae of such syndromes. A self-evaluation Patient Satisfaction Questionnaire, regarding the multidisciplinary team approach, was completed by 872 chronic (> 12 weeks duration) spinal pain syndrome patients at the Multidisciplinary Spinal Pain Unit, and the responses demonstrated that patient satisfaction with a multidisciplinary team approach was extremely high (Giles et al 2003).

Finally, the aim of this text is to consider issues related to non-specific and specific causes of mechanical lumbosacral spine pain syndromes by drawing together, in one text, information from numerous sources that relates to this issue, thereby getting back to the basics (Frymoyer 1997) in order to enable the reader to be conversant with the principles of lumbosacral spine anatomy, physiology, pathology, and other basic and clinical sciences.

Lynton G.F. Giles

ACKNOWLEDGEMENTS

To Anatomical Donors

I wish to express my sincere gratitude to individuals who made this work possible.

ABOUT THE AUTHOR

Dr Lynton G. F. Giles DC (Toronto) MSc, PhD (WAust) practised full time as a chiropractor for many years and, during that period, he became Honorary Clinical Scientist at Townsville General Hospital (1994–2002) and Adjunct Associate Professor (Clinical) at the School of Public Health, Tropical Medicine and Rehabilitation Sciences, James Cook University, Townsville, Queensland, Australia as well as Clinical Director of the Multidisciplinary Spinal Pain Unit that he helped to establish at the Townsville General Hospital. Prior to this he was Senior Research Fellow and Director of the Spinal Research Laboratory, Division of Science and Technology at Griffith University, Brisbane, Queensland, which he established in 1989. His clinical and research career related to spinal pain syndromes resulted in him being asked to act as a Medico-legal Consultant to assess individuals suffering from trauma related spinal pain syndromes. Dr Giles' gross anatomical and histological research of the spine led to the discovery of small diameter free ending nerves in zygapophysial ('facet') joint synovial folds in the lumbosacral spine, remote from blood vessels; using an immuno-fluorescent Substance-P antibody technique, the nerves were shown to have a putative function of nociception. During a period of 36 years Dr Giles published in multidisciplinary journals and co-edited 3 texts on the lumbar, thoracic, and cervical spines written by multidisciplinary authors. He has been a member of the Spine Society of Australia since 1992 and was a member of the British Society of Clinical Anatomists until he retired. He was honoured by the Chiropractors Association of Australia (National) Ltd in 2015 when the Giles Lecture and the Giles Medal for Outstanding Research in Health Science were established.

DISCLAIMER NOTICE

In view of the possibility of human error by the author, editors, or publisher of the work herein, neither the publisher nor the author assume any responsibility for any loss or injury and/or damage to persons arising from use of the material contained in this book. Readers should confirm information herein with other sources, and it is the responsibility of the treating clinician, relying on independent expertise and knowledge of the patient, to determine the best treatment and method of application for the patient.

Chapter 1
GENERAL INTRODUCTION TO THE LUMBOSACRAL SPINE

Abstract: This chapter discusses the prevalence of chronic low back pain syndromes and their cost to society as there is general agreement that about two-thirds of adults are affected by mechanical low back pain at some point in their lives. It sheds some light on the long-standing "medical enigma" of mechanical low back pain syndrome disorders. It discusses the possible difficulties of coming to a diagnosis for this condition and refers to some possible causes of specific and non-specific i.e. mechanical lumbosacral spine pain syndromes, with or without radicular pain. The most important step in the management of acute and chronic low back pain is for the clinician to have the ability to undertake an appropriate history and assessment and to have a good understanding of normal and abnormal spinal anatomy to enable the clinician to make an appropriate diagnosis, on which to base appropriate treatment. The important issue of erect posture plain X-ray imaging, and the limitations of supine imaging, are discussed. Weight-bearing functional/kinetic magnetic resonance imaging is also discussed.

Key Words: mechanical low back pain, medical enigma, diagnosis, radicular pain, imaging, erect posture imaging, functional/kinetic magnetic resonance imaging

Contents

Introduction

As Waddell (2004) stated, most back pain is 'ordinary backache'; this often is referred to as 'non-specific', 'mechanical', or 'idiopathic' spinal pain—serious pathology cases are infrequent: < 1% are associated with tumour/infection, < 1% rheumatological disease and < 5% nerve root pain, and Deyo et al (1992) found overall 4% of cases had overt pathology. On analysing 1,775 new patients presenting to a multidisciplinary spinal pain unit Giles et al (2003) found that, of the 949 male patients and 826 female patients (aged 10 to 91 years; average age 43 years), all of whom had some form of spinal imaging, 1% of patients had radiologically identifiable overt pathological processes, in keeping with the 1% quoted by Redberg (2013) and Traeger et al (2021). Thus, while different studies have found the percentage of overt pathology to vary within an approximate range of 1–4%, there is general agreement that about two-thirds of adults are affected by *mechanical low back pain* at some point in their lives, and only 20% can be given a precise pathoanatomic diagnosis (Perina 2020). While the pathogenesis of mechanical low back pain remains unclear, recent studies suggest that the inflammatory response may be inherent in spinal pain (Teodorczyk-Injeyan et al 2019; Gautam 2021).

Therefore, spinal pain due to *mechanical dysfunction*—or *structural failure* of the spinal components—accounts for by far the greatest number of lumbosacral spinal pain syndrome cases, so the purpose of this text is to shed some light on this long-standing 'medical enigma' of mechanical spinal disorders (Cailliet 2003; Rosatelli et al 2006; Avins 2010) that are so costly to many nations. Emphasis will be placed on some of the possible causes of such pain by including an 'atlas' section showing gross anatomy and histological sections as a basis for understanding this phenomenon and showing some of the possible anatomical causes of such pain.

Historically, it has been recognized for many years that the epidemic increase of musculoskeletal spinal pain syndromes, such as low back pain, actually threatens social welfare systems (Nachemson 1991), and their diagnosis and treatment consume a great deal of scarce healthcare resources (Ruta et al 1994). This situation still persists currently, as back pain is a massive problem that is badly treated (The Economist 2020(a)), vast sums are wasted on treatment for back pain that make it worse, and some 85% of chronic back pain sufferers have 'non-specific' back pain i.e. it has no clear physical cause (The Economist 2020(b)). For example, the annual direct cost for back pain treatment in the United States is US$100 billion, with a loss of productivity to business of US$225.8 billion (FMP Global 2018). Australia spends $4.8 billion (US$3.2 billion) per annum on management of just low back pain (Monash University 2018). In the United Kingdom back pain treatment costs

DOI: 10.1201/9781003315964-1

US$13.1 billion (Maniadakis et al 2000). Lumbosacral spine pain, with or without radiculopathy, is now the number one cause of disability (Hartvigsen et al 2018; Julin et al 2021), and low back pain is one of the most common causes of physician visits in the United States (Roudsari et al 2010). Also, spine related disorders are widespread and pose a high cost to society (Gliedt et al 2021).

The most important step in the management of acute and chronic spinal pain is appropriate assessment with the inclusion, from the outset, of an approach that acknowledges the contributions of a patient's psychological, social, and physical factors (James et al 1997).

The aim of clinical assessment is to characterize the problem, establish the cause (if possible), and assess the impact of the problem on the patient, family, and caregivers (Woolf et al 2008). We often cannot identify mechanisms to explain the major negative impact chronic low back pain has on patients' lives (Deyo et al 2014) and it is generally accepted that the diagnosis of mechanical spinal pain syndromes is often difficult, as the anatomy of the spine, including that of its neural and other adjacent soft tissue structures, is very complex; the anatomical diagnosis of low back pain is possible in approximately half of patients with chronic low back pain (Finch 2006).

Structures Associated with Spinal Pain Syndromes

In a large number of mechanical spinal pain cases, it may not be possible to identify the precise pain generator as many spinal structures are involved in nociception. *Nociceptors* are primary sensory neurons specialized to detect intense stimuli and represent, therefore, the first line of defence against any potentially threatening or damaging environmental inputs (Woolf et al 2007). Wyke (1980) described the distribution of lumbosacral nociceptive receptor systems, known at that time to be sensitive to mechanical and chemical tissue dysfunction, as being present in:

1. Fibrous capsules of zygapophysial (facet) joints and in sacroiliac joints.
2. Longitudinal spinal (anterior and posterior), interspinous, flaval, and sacroiliac ligaments.
3. Periosteum on vertebral bodies and arches (and attached fasciae, tendons and aponeuroses).
4. Dura mater and epidural fibro-adipose tissue.
5. Walls of blood vessels supplying the spinal and sacroiliac joints, and in vertebral cancellous bone.
6. Walls of epidural and paravertebral veins.
7. Walls of intramuscular arteries within lumbosacral muscles.
8. Skin, subcutaneous and adipose tissue.

In addition, more recent studies have shown that the following spinal tissues are also likely to be involved in nociception:

1. Zygapophysial joint *synovial folds* that have nerves containing substance P (Giles et al 1987(a); Grönblad et al 1991(a and b)).
2. Muscles surrounding the zygapophysial joint when its capsule—which contains small nerve fibres and free and encapsulated nerve endings, including nerves containing substance P—is injured, resulting in sensitization and excitation of nerves in the capsule and surrounding muscle (Cavanaugh et al 1996).
3. Supraspinous ligament (Yahia et al 1988).
4. The outer border of the intervertebral disc (IVD) (Yamashita et al 1993; Roberts et al 1995; Palmgren et al 1999).
5. Bone marrow cavities (Nencini et al 2016), including cancellous bone of the sacrum (Degmetich et al 2016).

Some possible causes of specific and non-specific spinal pain syndromes of *mechanical origin*—or mechanical failure—with or without radicular pain, are briefly summarized in Table 1.1; the latter provides a summary of some literature references over the years in order to give a historical background to the complex issue of specific and non-specific spinal pain of mechanical origin.

Examples of some of the conditions in Table 1.1 and others will be illustrated in the Anatomical Atlas section (Chapter 4).

This text is not a general anatomy text—it emphasizes some aspects of lumbosacral spine anatomy. For complete details of general anatomy see, for example, Moore et al (2018) *Clinically Oriented Anatomy* and von Hagens et al (1991) *The Visible Human Body: An Atlas of Sectional Anatomy* (using plastinated sectional anatomy). This text presents some important spine-related gross anatomical and histological images from cadaveric specimens—as well as schematic diagrams—and histology from surgical material to provide a current basic review for students and clinicians interested in spinal pain syndromes of *mechanical origin* or *mechanical failure*.

Pain in any structure requires the release of inflammatory agents, including bradykinin, prostaglandins, and leukotrienes, which stimulate pain receptors and generate a nociceptive response in the tissue and it is known that the spine is unique in that it has multiple structures that are innervated by pain fibres (Haldeman et al 2002). For example, stretching and distorting the articular capsule of a zygapophysial joint may result in traumatic synovitis with release of noxious neuropeptides, kinins, or other inflammatory agents (Haldeman 1999).

The neurophysiology of pain is not fully understood at this time. For example, when Slipman et al (1998) used a prospective study consisting of mechanical stimulation of cervical nerve roots C4 to C8 in patients with cervical radicular symptoms who were undergoing diagnostic selective nerve block, to document the distribution of pain and paraesthesiae that result from stimulation of specific cervical nerve roots, and to compare that distribution to documented sensory

TABLE 1.1: Some Possible Causes of Specific and *Non-Specific* Lumbosacral Spine Pain Syndromes of *Mechanical Origin* or *Mechanical Failure,* with or without Radicular Pain

Vertebral body and intervertebral disc conditions:
- Disc protrusion or herniation into the spinal canal (Mixter et al 1934).
- Intervertebral disc degeneration (Hadley 1964).
- Joint dysfunction (Schmorl et al 1971; Hooten et al 2015).
- Spondylolysis/spondylolisthesis (Schmorl et al 1971).
- Disc/dural adhesions (Parke et al 1990).
- Posterior epidural IVD migration and sequestration (Palmisciano et al 2022).
- Vertebral body burst fracture with inveterated haematoma within the injured disc (Rauschning 1997).
- Osteoarthrosis (Borenstein 2004).
- Spondylosis (Tsujimoto et al 2016).

Nerve root conditions:
- Due to IVD degeneration and fragmentation (Schiotz and Cyriax 1975), or nucleus pulposus extrusion/herniation (Mixter et al 1934, 1935; Wilkinson 1986) causing nerve root compression (Kobayashi et al 2005) or nerve root 'chemical radiculitis' (Marshall et al 1973; Goupille et al 2006; Byun et al 2012).
- Adhesions between (1) spinal nerve dural sleeves and the joint capsule, with nerve root fibrosis (Sunderland 1968; Farfan 1980; Wilkinson 1986) and (2) the medial branch of the lumbar posterior ramus and accompanying vessels as they pass through the osseofibrous tunnel of the mamillo-accessory ligament (Sunderland 1975).
- Impingement of the exiting nerve root as it crosses a hypertrophic *sublaminar ridge* (the bony, superior insertion site of ligamenta flava) immediately inferior to the mid-pedicle, lateral to the subarticular gutter, and on the medial aspect of the true intervertebral foramen (Bednar et al 2021).

Zygapophysial joint conditions:
- Joint derangement (subluxation) due to ligamentous and capsular instability (Hadley 1964; Cailliet 1968; Macnab 1977; van Norel et al 1996).
- Joint capsule tension with encroachment upon the intervertebral foramen lumen (Little et al 2005).
- Joint functional and degenerative changes, e.g. 'meniscal' incarceration (Schmorl et al 1971), traumatic synovitis due to 'pinching' of synovial folds (Giles 1986(a); Giles 1987(a); Giles et al 1987(a), synovial fold tractioning against the pain-sensitive joint capsule (Hadley 1964), osteoarthrosis (Gellhorn et al 2013) and an intraspinal synovial cyst (Hsu et al 1995; Habsi et al 2020).
- Joint effusion with capsular distension which may (a) exert pressure on a nerve root (Ghormley 1933), or (b) cause nerve root pain by direct diffusion of diffusible substances from injured tissues (Haldeman 1977).

Miscellaneous conditions:
- Leg length inequality greater than 9 mm (Rush et al 1946; Giles et al 1981) with associated postural scoliosis.
- S-I joint syndrome (Shaw 1992; Quon et al 1999).
- Spinal and intervertebral canal (foramen) stenosis (Rauschning 1987).
- Intervertebral canal (foramen) venous stasis (Sunderland 1975).
- Myofascial genesis of pain (trigger areas) (Travell et al 1952; Bonica 1957; Quon et al 1999); intrinsic muscles of the back can be a source of pain (Moore et al 2018). Piriformis syndrome may present as pain in the buttock or medial to the ischial spine with pain referral posteriorly in the lower limb (Bernard et al 1987; Quon et al 1999).
- Baastrup's syndrome (Reinhardt 1951; Bland 1987).
- Osseous vertebral anomalies e.g. hemivertebra, posterior element defects (Weis 1975).
- Idiopathic scoliosis (Ramirez et al 1997).
- Genetic influences (Tegeder et al 2009; Suri et al 2018; Zhao et al 2020(a)).

dermatomal maps, they demonstrated a distinct difference between *dynatomal* and *dermatomal* maps. (A *dynatome* is the distribution of referred symptoms from root irritation, and this is different to the sensory deficit outlined by dermatomal maps.) Therefore, Slipman et al (1998) suggest that cervical dermatomal mapping is inaccurate. Jinkins (1993) agrees that there is some overlap of sensation, and Koop et al (2021) state that the receptive field of a sensory nerve (*peripheral nerve field*) crosses over different dermatomes; therefore, the map of peripheral nerve fields over the body differs from the dermatomal distribution, since individual peripheral nerves are composed of multiple nerve roots. Thus, it is reasonable to suggest that a similar neurophysiological finding may occur at other spinal nerve root levels, including those of the lumbar spine.

Spinal pain syndromes must be viewed in the context of (i) clearly defined pathological conditions and (ii) the less well-defined—but much more prevalent—condition of *non-specific* spinal pain of *mechanical origin* (Stoddard 1969; Kenna et al 1989). It is imperative to distinguish dysfunctional mechanical causes of spinal pain from other causes, as patients with mechanical disorders of the spine are likely to respond dramatically to manual treatment (Kenna et al 1989).

Over the years there has been little consensus, either within or among specialties, on the use of diagnostic tests for patients with spinal pain syndromes, and the underlying pathology responsible for various spinal pain problems remains elusive (Videman et al 1998). Furthermore, in spite of following a thorough examination procedure, one often merely eliminates overt pathologies, and the precise cause of non-specific spinal pain syndromes of mechanical origin frequently remains obscure (Turner et al 1998).

A major difficulty involved in evaluating a patient with non-specific lumbosacral spinal pain of mechanical origin, with or without root symptoms, is that many causes of pain are possible. Because the painful structure, or structures, are not amenable to direct scrutiny, a tentative diagnosis is usually arrived at for an individual case by taking a careful case history, employing a thorough physical examination, requesting *appropriate* imaging (bearing in mind that routine imaging frequently only provides *shadows of the truth* (Giles et al 1997(a)) and can be misleading), and considering requesting *appropriate* laboratory procedures, as indicated, in order to assess any possible co-morbid condition to eliminate '*red flag*' conditions. This approach is necessary to ensure that a diagnosis of mechanical spinal pain/spinal pain syndrome may be reached with a high degree of certainty. Furthermore, there are several additional approaches that may be taken to assist in patient evaluation, for example by using subjective self-report measures to assess (i) pain severity, quality, and location and (ii) the clinically important issue of *'yellow flag'* conditions associated with *personality* disorders.

Evidence of signs and symptoms deemed excessively or inappropriately abnormal (Main et al 1982) should be recorded. However, patients should *not* be considered as malingerers unless there are very strong clinical grounds for doing so. Caution has to be exercised when making judgements on an individual's behavioural signs during examination, as *serious misuse and misinterpretation* of such signs has occurred in medicolegal contexts (Main et al 1998), and the validity of such behavioural signs has been questioned (Giles 2005).

Regarding 'malingering', it is worth noting the sobering comments of orthopaedic Professor Ruth Jackson (1956) who wrote: *"To label any condition that cannot be explained easily as psychoneurosis is indicative of diagnostic poverty and infers that those symptoms and signs which cannot be explained readily do not exist".*

Furthermore, Mennell (1960) wrote: *"A diagnosis of psychoneurosis should never be made in the absence of positive physical signs, among which the hippus reaction of a large pupil to light, hyperhidrosis of the palms of the hands, hyperreflexia in all four limbs with a negative Babinski sign, and diminished deep sensation in the Achilles tendons are a reliable tetrad".*

In addition, Teasell (1997) noted that it is not wise to label a patient as being neurotic or a malingerer, particularly as it is thought that such patients form only a small minority of cases. There has long been a misconception that all injuries should heal after six weeks; however, clinical experience and follow-up studies (Mendelson 1982; Radanov et al 1994) clearly demonstrate that not all patients necessarily get better and that there is a significant subset who continue to suffer from chronic symptoms (Teasell 1997).

With respect to imaging, if the clinician does not have access to sophisticated imaging facilities, plain X-ray imaging can be used. Photons of X-ray radiation are absorbed in varying degrees within body tissues, which allows differentiation between different parts of the body; for example, *low absorption* implies that many photons reach the photographic plate behind the body, so that region becomes black, whereas *intermediate absorption* gives shades of grey (as in body fat and muscles), and with high absorption few photons reach the photographic plate that remains white (Dijkstra 2007). However, this type of imaging can only be used to great advantage in cases of mechanical spinal pain if images are taken in the *weight-bearing posture*, with or without the inclusion of flexion and extension views in the sagittal plane or left and right lateral bending views. However, X-radiation exposure should always be considered and minimized where possible.

Historically, diagnostic imaging procedures have evolved over the years beginning with the use of recumbent i.e. *non weight-bearing* plain film radiography (first introduced in approximately 1895), myelography (first introduced in 1920), discography (first introduced in 1948), recumbent computerized tomography (CT; first introduced in 1971), technetium-99 m bone scans (bone scintigraphy; first introduced in 1971), positron emission tomography (PET) scan (first introduced in 1977), recumbent magnetic resonance imaging (MRI; first introduced in 1977 and later modified to be used for whole-body magnetic resonance neurography (MRN; first introduced in 1991)) to selectively visualize the peripheral nervous system (PNS) over long trajectories in a single examination (Yamashita et al 2009). Excellent delineation of small calibre structures such as nerve roots, denticulate ligaments, adhesion bands, and thin walls of intraspinal cysts is now possible using MRI CISS/FIESTA-C (Li et al 2019). Various diagnostic chemical agents used in some forms of imaging can be helpful in cases of mechanically induced disc injury; however, they can be harmful, for example when such chemicals injected into IVDs extravasate into the epidural space (Weitz 1984; Adams et al 1986; MacMillan et al 1991) between the spinal dura mater and other soft tissue structures within the vertebral canal, causing complications due to contact between them and neural structures (Dyck 1985; Merz 1986; Watts et al 1986). The anatomical complexity of the spine often makes roentgenographic interpretation difficult (Le-Breton et al 1993), and sometimes there are multifactorial causes of pain at a given level of the spine (Haldeman 1977; Gross 1979), for example injury to the IVD, the zygapophysial facet joints, and the associated segmental soft tissue structures. In 2007 the first commercially available EOS standing X-ray imaging system was used (Illés et al 2012)—a Slot-scanning 3D X-ray imaging system (Hasegawa et al 2018) that uses 50–80% less radiation than conventional X-rays, while being most useful in relation to scoliosis and sagittal balance and having the advantage of allowing measurement of torsional deformity, which classically requires a CT scan (Melhem et al 2016); EOS allows simultaneous acquisition of A-P and lateral images of the entire body in a natural, erect position (Haouimi et al 2021).

Having mentioned the previous imaging techniques and the limitations of some diagnostic imaging procedures, it is important to note the very advanced progress that has been made with the advent of *erect posture functional/kinetic MRI* (first introduced in 1996 by Stand-Up MRI, Fonar Corp, Melville, NY)—the great value of this advanced diagnostic MR imaging technique will be discussed later in this chapter.

With respect to symptoms, there may be several types of spinal pain that closely mimic each other (Haldeman 1977). A further important point is that a central disc herniation may cause spinal pain alone without radiculopathy (Postacchini et al 1999(a)), whereas a posterolateral or far lateral disc herniation will, in all likelihood, also cause radicular pain (Keim et al 1987).

The nerve root compression that occurs in lumbar disc herniation—and lumbar canal stenosis—often results in a range of symptoms, including low back pain, sciatic pain, sensory disturbances, and muscle weakness in the legs

(Kobayashi et al 2005). Summers et al (2005) point out that the degree of back or leg pain caused by an acute disc prolapse depends, in part, on the position, size, and level of the disc prolapse.

There often is disagreement on which imaging procedures have diagnostic validity for non-specific spinal pain of mechanical origin, although it is generally agreed that, for plain film X-ray examinations, two views of the same anatomical region at right angles is the minimum requirement (Henderson et al 1994); erect posture radiography (Giles et al 1981) and functional views (Weitz 1981) are far more useful than recumbent views. Furthermore, Buirski et al (1993) correctly noted that MRI can only be used as an assessment of nuclear anatomy and not for symptomatology. In addition, Osti et al (1992) concluded that lumbar discography is more accurate than MRI for the detection of annular pathology. However, according to Shalen (1989), lumbar discography is a controversial examination that is regarded by some radiologists and spine surgeons as barbaric and non-efficacious (Wiley et al 1968; Clifford 1986; Shapiro 1986) and may cause serious side effects. For lumbar spine CT and MR imaging, Willen et al (1997) showed that the diagnostic specificity of spinal stenosis will increase considerably when the patient is subjected to an axial load, and Danielson et al (1998) concluded that, for an adequate evaluation of the cross-sectional spinal area, CT or MR imaging studies should be performed with *axial loading* in patients who have symptoms of lumbar spinal stenosis. Now that *erect posture* MRI is available, it has been shown that in scanning of symptomatic patients, 761 in the *recumbent* position, and 725 in an *upright* sitting position, stenosis rates ranged between 38.5% (recumbent) and 56.7% (weight bearing) (Gilbert et al 2011), illustrating the important role of weight bearing MRI.

In summary, it is only rarely possible to validate a diagnosis in cases where pain arises from the spine (White et al 1982) in cases of mechanical spinal pain and, because it is not possible to establish the pathological basis of spinal pain in 80–90% of cases (Chila et al 1990; Spratt et al 1990; Pope et al 1993), this leads to diagnostic uncertainty and suspicion that some patients have a 'compensation neurosis' or other psychological problem, as previously mentioned. It is also appropriate at this time

to recognize the role of *psychosocial* factors in spinal pain. Although the complex interaction of psyche and soma in the aetiology of spinal pain is not well understood, a *psychogenic component* may be *primary* (conversion disorder), *secondary* (depression caused by chronic pain), *contributory* (myofascial dysfunction), or *absent* (Keim et al 1987). Nonetheless, clinicians must have a good understanding of the possible causes of a patient's symptoms and of the possible underlying mechanical spinal pathology, for example patients presenting with symptoms of *tethered cord syndrome* (Yamada 1996; Giles 2003(a); Yamada et al 2004).

Common sources of spinal pain that are identified through medical history or physical examination include vertebrae, muscles, fascia, and ligaments, and some may be confirmed as such by radiography, computed tomography (CT), MRI, or electromyography (EMG)/nerve conduction velocity (NCV) testing (Kim et al 2011). When nerve root dysfunction is suspected, electromyography and nerve root conduction studies can be helpful (Hoppenfeld 1977).

It is reasonable to broadly classify *acute spinal pain* as being of 7–28 days or less duration, which may be followed by a *sub-acute* stage of up to 12 weeks; after this time interval the pain can be considered *chronic* (Skouen et al 2002).

Patient History of Spinal Pain

As previously mentioned, the importance of a *thorough case history* cannot be overemphasized, and it should take into account facts such as the patient's age, occupation, onset of pain, previous injuries, medication, recreational activities, pain aggravation and characteristics, location, distribution, and any related neurological symptoms (numbness, paraesthesiae, muscle weakness) and whether compensation is involved regarding an injury. Some conditions provide reasonably characteristic patterns, while others do not. For example, spinal pain that occurs at night and that is relieved by aspirin may be associated with an osteoid osteoma, i.e. a benign tumour of bone (Keim et al 1987). Night pain per se should be considered as being of probable serious pathological change. Likewise, spinal pain patients with night sweats may suggest a serious underlying pathology, so appropriate laboratory or imaging tests may be necessary to rule out organic disease.

If a thorough history is not taken, there is a great risk of the clinician making the wrong diagnosis, as Dahm et al (2021) found that interactions between patient and clinician where there is a diagnostic error had a

shorter history-taking period as one component of the interaction.

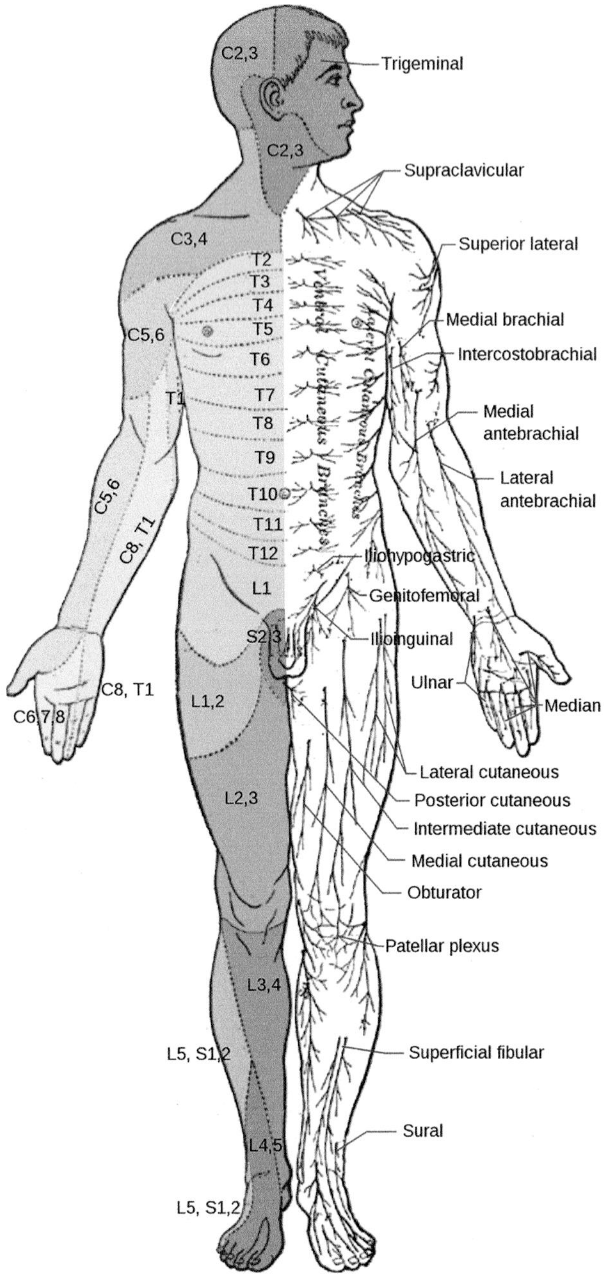

Neurological Concepts

Bearing in mind the previously mentioned findings of Slipman et al (1998) and others, a couple of important neurological concepts that need to be considered during the examination relate to (i) *dermatomes* and (ii) *myotomes* of the human body.

Dermatomes of the human body i.e. the distribution of *cutaneous* areas supplied with afferent nerve fibres by single *posterior* (sensory) spinal nerve roots

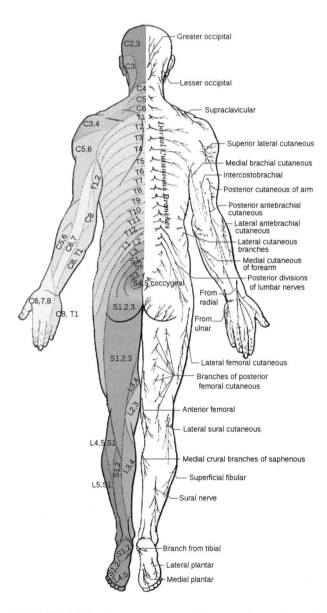

FIGURE 1.1A Dermatomes on the anterior surface of the body. A dermatome is an area of skin that is primarily supplied by a single nerve root communicating sensation from this skin region to the brain.

Source: Reproduced with permission from Mikael Häggström https://commons.wikimedia.org/wiki/File: Dermatomes_and_cutaneous_nerves_-_anterior.svg https://creativecommons.org/licenses/by/4.0/.

FIGURE 1.1B Dermatomes on the posterior surface of the body.

Source: Reproduced with permission from Mikael Häggström https://commons.wikimedia.org/wiki/File: Dermatomes_and_cutaneous_nerves_-_posterior.svg https://creativecommons.org/licenses/by/4.0/.

(Dorland's *Illustrated Medical Dictionary* 1974; Barr et al 1983), have been fairly well established (Figures 1.1A and B) and enable deficits of a specific nerve root to be accurately localized during sensory examination (Keim et al 1987).

Myotomes are the segmental innervation of *skeletal muscle* by the *anterior* (motor) root(s) of spinal nerves i.e.

a group of muscles innervated from a single spinal segment (Dorland's *Illustrated Medical Dictionary* 1974). Like dermatomes, myotomes have been fairly well established (Figure 1.2), and muscle weakness may be present due to mechanical nerve compromise.

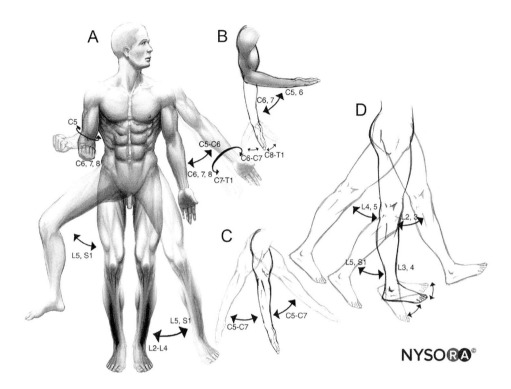

FIGURE 1.2 Functional innervation of the muscles (myotomes). **(A)** Medial and lateral rotation of shoulder and hip, pronation and supination of wrist and forearm. Abduction and adduction of shoulder and hip. **(B)** Flexion and extension of elbow and wrist. **(C)** Flexion and extension of shoulder. **(D)** Flexion and extension of hip and knee, dorsiflexion and plantar flexion of ankle.

Source: Reproduced with permission from Carrera A, Lopez A.M., Sala-Blanch X et al 2020 Functional Regional Anesthesia Anatomy, New York School of Regional Anesthesia (NYSORA) www.nysora.com/foundations-of-regional-anesthesia/anatomy/functional-regional-anesthesia-anatomy/.

Intervertebral Foramen

Before discussing areas of the lumbosacral spine that may cause spinal pain, with or without radiculopathy, it is important to define the region commonly referred to as the '*intervertebral foramen*' (*canalis intervertebralis*) that lies between the pedicle above and the pedicle below. The word '*foramen*' does not convey the significance of the *length* of this root canal—or tunnel— that extends from the vertebral foramen medially to the lateral opening—or outer boundary—of the root canal i.e. the *exit zone* of this canal (Schmorl et al 1971; Dommisse 1975; Porter 1998). The *true foramen* is the *foraminal region* of the canal (Newell 2008) through which pass the nerve root, the segmental mixed spinal nerve and its sheaths, posterior root ganglion (PRG), radicular artery, veins, and lymphatics that may be

stabilized by transforaminal ligaments (Choi 2019). In addition, also located in the foramen are from two to four recurrent meningeal nerves, variable numbers of spinal arteries, and plexiform venous connections between the internal and external vertebral venous plexuses (Newell 2008).

The length of the intervertebral foramen [canal] in the lumbar spine from L1–2 to L5-S1 levels in 20–35-year-old males and females, respectively, ranges from 9.1 (± 2.0) to 22.5 (± 4.3) mm for males and from 8.1 (± 1.8) to 18.8 (± 4.1) for females (Twomey et al 1988). Therefore, it can be seen that the nerve root canal is a tubular canal of variable length arising from the lateral aspect of the dural tube (Crock 1981).

The same principle applies to the length of the root canal between the sacral *anterior* and *posterior* foramina at each level of the sacrum, with the upper root canal levels being longer than those at the lower levels because of the greater anterior to posterior depth of the sacrum superiorly.

Among various structures that may be involved in a patient's symptoms are ligamentous structures that are found within the intervertebral foramen i.e. from the entrance zone to its exit zone. The *internal transforaminal ligaments* (TFLs) may be involved in a patient's symptoms (Amonoo-Kuofi et al 1988; Giles 1992(a); Cramer et al 2002; Akdemir 2010; Zhao et al 2016) as they reduce the space available for the spinal nerve root within the intervertebral foramen (Min et al 2005) and thus may play a role in giving rise to severe pain and paraesthesiae along the distribution of a nerve, due to direct mechanical pressure on the neural complex (Amonoo-Kuofi et al 1997). The *extra-foraminal ligaments* i.e. just outside the intervertebral foramen, are believed to protect against traction and compression of the nerves by positioning the nerve in the intervertebral foramen (Kraan et al 2009). Lumbar *extra*-foraminal ligaments have been described by Zhong et al (2017).

TFLs can successfully be imaged with low-field-strength MRI; if a radiologist identifies a TFL, there is an 87% chance that one is present, and, if a radiologist does not identify a TFL in an intervertebral foramen, there remains a 51% chance that one is present (Cramer et al 2002). Furthermore, *high-resolution far-lateral* MR images through the spinal neural foramen yield relevant information concerning the neural foramina, alterations in the posterior spinal facet joint, pedicle, IVD, and its margins—such images may be complemented by information gained from high-resolution far-lateral thin-section stacked axial CT images (Jinkins 2004(a)).

From the previous evidence, it is clear that clinicians need to be familiar with both normal and abnormal spinal anatomy in order for them to think laterally when confronted with challenging mechanical spinal pain syndromes, and this text aims to achieve this.

Imaging for Spinal Mechanical Dysfunction

Imaging of the degenerative spine is a frequent challenge in radiology (Kushchayev et al 2018). Nonetheless, routine radiographs of the lumbar spine and pelvis and, when indicated by the history and symptoms, the chest, should be taken to establish a baseline and to rule out metabolic, inflammatory, and malignant conditions (Keim et al 1987), bearing in mind the limitations of plain X-ray examinations and recumbent spinal images. As long as proper coning of the X-ray beam is used in conjunction with up-to-date imaging equipment, minimal radiation should be received by the patient. As previously stated, lumbosacral spine and pelvis radiographs should be taken in the *weight-bearing erect posture*, whenever possible, using carefully standardized procedures specifically to look for *mechanical dysfunction*; for example, to accurately determine whether possibly significant leg length inequality (LLI) is present with corresponding pelvic obliquity causing scoliosis in the spine (Giles et al 1981; Giles 1984(a)). Furthermore, a *lateral lumbosacral X-ray view* may show thinning of a disc space height that usually produces a degree of subluxation of the zygapophysial joint's facet articular surfaces, with narrowing of the intervertebral foramen (Hadley 1936). Disc narrowing with *retrolisthesis* of the vertebra above the disc is most likely a sign of posterior or posterolateral disc bulging or protrusion (Giles et al 2006); an example of a normal lumbosacral (L5-S1) joint level, followed by an example of disc thinning is shown in Figures 1.3A and B.

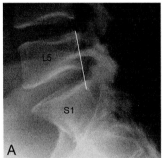 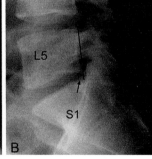 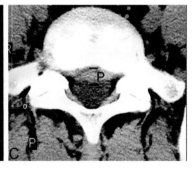

FIGURE 1.3 **(A)** Lateral lumbosacral plain X-ray view with normal disc height and *without retrolisthesis*. A line drawn along the posterior margin of the L5 vertebral body to the sacrum does not fall behind the sacral base (S1). **(B)** A line drawn along the posterior margin of the L5 vertebral body to the sacrum in this case falls *behind* the posterior margin of the sacral base (arrow), indicating *retrolisthesis* of L5 on S1 due to disc narrowing, suggesting a disc bulge or protrusion is present. As a matter of interest, the X-ray report stated *"minor narrowing at L5-S1 disc space is probably developmental rather than pathological"*. **(C)** An axial CT (Computerized Tomography) scan of the patient shown in Figure **B** shows a broad-based posterior central disc protrusion (P) that encroaches upon the pain sensitive anterior aspect of the thecal sac indenting it and the associated nerve roots.

If, following a history and a physical examination, the clinician suspects that the patient may have a lumbar disc herniation but there is no access to sophisticated imaging, a mechanical evaluation of the lumbar spine can be made using plain X-ray *dynamic* lateral flexion images (Weitz 1981), with the patient in the erect posture (Figure 1.4).

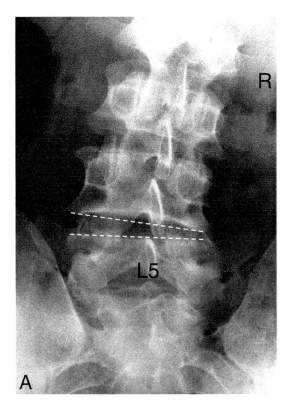 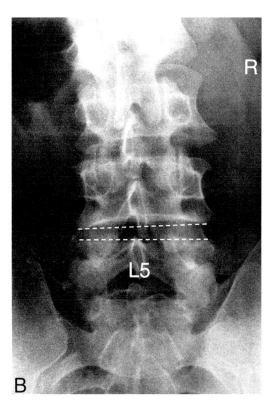

FIGURE 1.4 Erect posture right and left lateral flexion X-ray images of a 34-year-old male who presented with recent onset acute low back pain and mild left sided radiculopathy, made worse on coughing. **(A)** Right lateral flexion shows that the L4–5 disc space functions normally i.e. it is wider on the left side than on the right side; also the overall lateral flexion contour of the spine is normal with disc spaces narrower on the right. **(B)** Left lateral flexion shows that the L4–5 disc space does not function normally i.e. there is minimal wedging of the L4–5 disc space on the left side; also the lateral flexion contour of the spine is limited. Follow-up at a sophisticated imaging facility showed a left sided posterolateral disc herniation of the L4–5 intervertebral disc.

With reference to low back pain, guidelines recommend that imaging should not routinely be used as part of early management (Foster et al 2018; Oliveira et al 2018). This recommendation—and Bogduk's (1999) "modified criteria for the use of plain films in low back pain"—that are based on the work of Deyo et al (1986), are of concern, as I believe they overlook the importance of possible *mechanical abnormality and function*. Bogduk (1999) states "plain films may be used as a screening test for 'red flag' conditions if a patient presents with any of the following features: history of cancer, significant trauma, weight loss, temperature > 37.6 degrees C, risk factors for infection, neurological deficit, minor trauma in patients (over 50 years of age, known to be osteoporotic or taking corticosteroids), and no improvement over a 1-month period". Jarvik et al (2002) state that for adults younger than 50 years of age, with no signs or symptoms of systemic disease, symptomatic therapy without imaging is

appropriate, and Kasch et al (2021) who conducted a lumbar MRI study support current guidelines that recommend restrictive imaging for low back pain. Again, in my opinion, unless there is a contraindication such as pregnancy, it is important for *appropriate* plain X-ray imaging to be used i.e. *weight-bearing and functional imaging views* that can be *much more useful* from a diagnostic perspective, as the *frequently used* non-weight-bearing and static imaging may miss many spinal *mechanical* and early functional *degenerative conditions*. Such imaging at the *onset* of symptoms, rather than risking possible misdiagnosis and mismanagement, both of which would be disadvantageous to patients, is important. This is particularly relevant when treatment by spinal manipulation is considered, as the application of mechanical forces to a spine that may have degenerative changes, let alone overt pathological changes, potentially could be harmful. In my opinion, not looking at the spine and pelvis in all cases prior to using *mechanical treatment* may well explain the occurrence of occasional adverse events, even though most authors have reported a very low rate of adverse events associated with spinal manipulation.

In addition, more sophisticated imaging procedures may be necessary. These include (i) *MRI*, which can provide very good detail of soft tissue structures in and about the spinal column, importantly without the need of radiation, and frequently without the need for contrast; (ii) *computerized tomography scans*, which are particularly good at showing bony structures but use X-radiation; (iii) *bone scans* when tumour, infection, or small fracture(s) are suspected; and (iv) *discography*, when indicated, to show tears in the IVD with internal disc disruption. The usefulness of a *PET* scan, used heavily in clinical oncology, should not be underestimated. When *invasive* imaging is being contemplated, the possible complications of such a procedure should always be considered.

Unfortunately, all the preceding procedures have some limitations, for example plain film radiographs will not show an osseous erosion until approximately 40% decrease in bone density has occurred (Michel et al 1990; Perry 1995), and Schellhas et al (1996) and Osti et al (1992) found that discography is more accurate than MRI for the detection of annular pathology in the lumbar and cervical spines, respectively. The limitations of present diagnostic imaging procedures in not being able to show all soft tissues are an unfortunate but obvious fact (Finch 2006).

The following comments are of interest regarding some limitations of imaging procedures. With respect to the lumbar spine, Vernon-Roberts (1980) wrote: *"It may be a minor consolation to clinicians and others who have to deal with the problem of low back pain to know that even clinically and radiologically 'normal' spines can have pathological changes which, until proved otherwise, could be a cause of much stress to both doctor and patient".*

Furthermore, the imaging report often states 'degenerative disc disease' or 'normal examination', in spite of a patient's considerable symptoms. Therefore, in this book some possible reasons for this are presented.

In spite of the advantage of MRI, which is considered to be the major medical imaging development of the century (Wong et al 2007), in that it is a *non-invasive* procedure, without any recognized biological hazard, that combines a strong magnetic field and radiofrequency energy to study the distribution and behaviour of hydrogen protons in fat and water (Weir et al 2003), a normal MRI *does not exclude* significant changes in the peripheral structure of the IVD that can produce spinal pain (Osti et al 1992).

A limitation of MR imaging is the resolving power (i.e. ability to distinguish small or closely adjacent structures) of the MRI machine; this has to be taken into account when considering what cannot be seen. As an example, for brain tissue a 3-T MRI machine can resolve details as small as 1 mm (1,000 microns) while the resolution of a 7-T machine can be as fine as 0.5 mm (500 microns)

(Nowogrodzki 2018); any lesion smaller than this would not be seen. For this reason, with regard to small injuries, imaging reports may fail to indicate the cause of mechanical spinal pain.

Several routine (recumbent) MRI studies have shown that 20–76% of asymptomatic adults exhibit abnormalities of lumbar discs (Boden et al 1990; Buirski et al 1993; Jensen et al 1994; Deyo 1994; Boos et al 1995; Jarvik et al 2001), but Kleinstück et al's (2006) lumbar spine MRI study showed that symptomatic adults with *chronic, non-specific low back pain* appear to have an overall higher prevalence of structural abnormalities than previously reported for asymptomatic individuals. In addition, *many times, but not always, MR imaging findings do correlate with the clinical presentation* (Bartynski et al 2007), and Haldeman et al (2002) concur, stating that even the most severe degenerative changes can occur in the absence of symptomatology but that back pain is more common in individuals who do demonstrate these degenerative changes. The specific difficulties encountered with MRI studies to date may relate to the fact that *recumbent* MRI technology was used; new technology, allowing for comparisons between *upright, weight-bearing, dynamic, positional MRI* and traditional recumbent MRI has shown that there often is a very significant difference between the pathology visualized between the two MRI procedures; therefore, the diagnostic information that can be derived from routine recumbent MRI studies is limited (Jinkins JR, personal communication, 2007).

In a study to review the general clinical utility of the first dedicated MRI unit enabling *upright, weight-bearing positional evaluation* of the spinal column (pMRI) during various *dynamic-kinetic manoeuvres* (kMRI) (Fonar 0.6 T unit with images acquired with a lumbar solenoidal radiofrequency receiver coil) in patients with degenerative conditions of the spine, Jinkins et al (2003(a)) concluded that: the *potential relative beneficial aspects of using upright, weight-bearing (pMRI), dynamic-kinetic (kMRI) spinal imaging* include (i) the revelation of occult disease dependent on true axial loading, (ii) the unmasking of kinetic-dependent disease, and (iii) the ability to scan the patient in the position of clinically relevant signs and symptoms, while this imaging unit also demonstrated low claustrophobic potential and yielded relatively high-resolution images with little motion/chemical shift artifact.

Thus, Professor Jinkins and colleagues' considerable pioneering work in comparing recumbent and upright, dynamic-kinetic MRI has clearly added valuable insight for diagnosing mechanical and degenerative spinal pain syndromes.

'Functional' MRI and its ability to detect load-dependent and motion-dependent disc herniations, stenosis, instabilities, and combinations of these pathologies not seen during recumbent imaging (Jinkins et al 2003(b); Elsig et al 2006) is a great advance in diagnostic MR imaging. In addition, 3 Teslar (T) MRI units are becoming available that can provide even higher-quality images than those obtained at 1.5 T (Tanenbaum 2006).

In an evaluation of IVD *herniation* and *hypermobile intersegmental instability* in symptomatic adult patients undergoing recumbent and upright MRI of the cervical and lumbosacral spines, Perez et al (2007) concluded that overall, upright-seated MRI was superior to recumbent MRI of the spine, where, in 89 patients recumbent imaging missed pathology (n:10) and recumbent imaging underestimated pathology (n:42) i.e. 52/89 total patients

(58%), validating the importance of weight-bearing imaging of the spine.

In order to demonstrate the concept of using appropriate *upright dynamic-kinetic MR imaging* for *mechanical* spinal pain syndromes, the following images (courtesy the Late Professor R Jinkins 2007 from his collection of images) clearly show the important diagnostic difference between *recumbent* and *weight-bearing kinetic MR images* of the lumbar spine (Figure 1.5). A brief clinical comment on different mechanical changes in the diagnosis between the various postures is provided by Professor Jinkins.

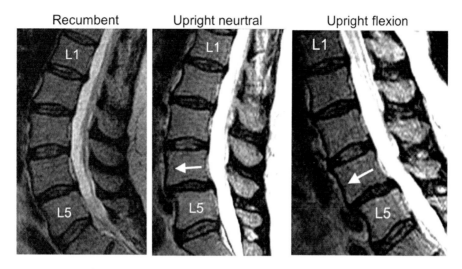

FIGURE 1.5 Salient History: A patient with chronic progressive low back pain when upright. The MRI initial diagnosis, based on the *recumbent MRI*, was *L4–5 Degenerative Disc Disease*. In the upright neutral and flexion postures, the MRI final diagnosis was *L4–5 Hypermobile Intersegmental Instability with anterolisthesis of L4 on L5*, therefore providing an indication for intersegmental fusion at this spinal level. This provides an example of increased imaging *sensitivity* and *specificity*.

From Figure 1.5, it is clear that an *appropriate* type of imaging for the patient's presenting condition is imperative if the imaging is to be contributory to the *diagnosis* and *treatment* and that imaging of the spine in the erect standing (and seated) position adds *significantly* to the diagnostic ability of MRI (Smith et al 2004), especially in situations where symptomatic radiculopathy is present without any abnormalities demonstrated on conventional MRI (Zou et al 2008).

As Professor Jinkins has indicated (Personal Communication 2007), with appropriate weight-bearing kinetic MR images (p/kMRI) that show increased *sensitivity* and *specificity*, the radiologist can show the physician the entire *radiological problem*; the physician is then in a position to treat the patient's clinical condition, with the possibility that he will remedy the patient's clinical symptoms. Furthermore, the clinical-radiological relevance of p/kMRI relates to: (i) patient care considerations due to improvement of imaging sensitivity over that of recumbent examinations, (ii) medicolegal aspects regarding revelation of diagnoses missed or underestimated on recumbent examinations, (iii) workers' compensation

regarding revelation of occult pathology not found on recumbent examinations, and (iv) economic factors due to nations' burgeoning spinal pain syndrome costs when using only recumbent MRI investigations for diagnosis (Jinkins et al 2003(b)). In addition, one has to consider what are the possible implications for patients' *pain* and *psychological management*.

In various lumbar spine studies, it has been shown that a significant association exists between some structural abnormalities and the *presence* (Parkkola et al 1993; van Tulder et al 1997; Paajanen et al 1997; Luoma et al 2000), *frequency* (Videman et al 2003; Videman et al 2004), or *severity* (Videman et al 2003; Peterson et al 2000) of *low back pain*.

Using flexible fibrescopes (external diameter of 0.6–1.5 mm), Tobita et al (2003) stated, with respect to the entire spine: "*Although the diagnosis of spinal disease has been greatly improved by CT and MRI, there are still many conditions that are difficult to diagnose by these means as pathological changes were seen by fibrescopic examinations in patients in whom no abnormal changes were found by MRI or CT*".

The aforementioned findings raise questions about the morphology-based understanding of pain pathogenesis in patients with disc abnormalities (Boos et al 2000). Furthermore, Karppinen et al (2001) found that recumbent MRI scans from 160 patients with unilateral sciatic pain suggested that a *discogenic pain mechanism* other than nerve root entrapment generates the subjective symptoms among sciatic patients.

A further difficulty is that the nomenclature and classification of lumbar *disc* pathology is not standardized (Fardon et al 2001), although Pfirrmann et al (2001) and Kushchayev et al (2018) have suggested a method for grading disc degeneration on T2-weighted MRI (See Figure 2.42). Changes in *vertebral body* bone marrow with MR imaging have been well documented by Modic et al (1988(a and b)) who described three types: (i) *marrow oedema*, (ii) *fatty degeneration*, and (iii) *bony sclerosis* (Figure 1.6).

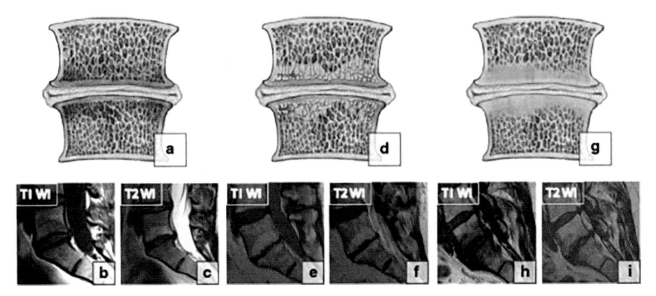

FIGURE 1.6   Degenerative bone marrow (Modic) changes: (a-c) Type 1 changes; (d-f) Type 2 changes; (g-i) Type 3 changes.

Source: **Reproduced with permission from Kushchayev et al 2018 ABCs of degenerative spine. Insights into Imaging 9: 253–274; Creative Commons Attribution 4.0 International License. http://creativecommons.org/licenses/by/4.0/.**

Signal intensity changes seem to reflect a spectrum of vertebral body marrow changes associated with degenerative disc disease (Modic 1988(a)), and a lumbar disc herniation is a strong risk factor for developing Modic changes (especially Type I) during the following year (Albert et al 2007). Modic changes are the MRI-image representation of inflammatory vertebral endplate damage that are often related to general disc degeneration; however, in a subgroup of patients, *disc infection* may be the causal factor, so it is relevant to consider 'disc infection'—most commonly involving Propionibacterium acnes, in which case long-term antibiotics may be effective (Manniche 2014).

It is important to note the following comments regarding imaging shown in this text:

- Most plain film anteroposterior radiographic images of the spine and or pelvis are printed as if the clinician were looking at the patient's back; i.e. a marker showing 'R' indicates the patient's right side.
- Spinal axial CT and MRI scans are viewed, as usual, from 'below'; i.e. remember that the clinician 'looks up' the patient's spinal canal with the patient recumbent, so the patient's right side is marked 'R' on the left side of the axial scan images.

- MRI T1-weighted images produce essentially a fat image in which structures containing fat (bone marrow, subcutaneous fat) appear bright, while structures containing water (oedema, neoplasm, inflammation, cerebrospinal fluid (CSF), sclerosis, large amounts of iron) appear dark (Yochum et al 1996).
- MRI T2-weighted images produce essentially a water image in which structures containing predominantly free or loosely bound water molecules (CSF, healthy nucleus pulposus, oedema, inflammation, neoplasm) appear bright, while substances with tightly bound water (ligaments, menisci, tendons, calcification, sclerosis, or large amounts of iron) appear dark (hypointense) (Yochum et al 1996).
- In all cases, patient identification details have been deleted to maintain patient confidentiality.

When imaging has been performed, look at the images to *determine their diagnostic quality*. For example, with plain film radiographs, to determine whether they are of diagnostic value, specifically consider whether there is: (i) correct *exposure* of the X-ray film and (ii) correct *positioning* of the patient.

Neurocentral Joints of Immature Spines

To conclude this General Introduction, although this text refers to the lumbosacral spine anatomy of *adults*, it is worth noting that, at birth, each typical vertebra consists of *three* bony parts i.e. the centrum (body) and two halves of the neural arch posteriorly (Grant 1962). The neural arch and the body are united by hyaline cartilage and fusion of the paired (i.e. left and right) *neurocentral* junction *cartilaginous growth plate* (Rajwani et al 2002; Schlösser et al 2013), or *neurocentral* synchondrosis (NCS) (Zhang et al 2010; Blakemore et al 2018) in the vertebra remains 100% open in all three regions of the spine in the one-to-three-year age group. The *lumbar NCS* is nearly fully closed by 11–12 years of age, the *thoracic NCS* remains open up to 14–17 years of age, and the *cervical NCS* is the first to close, with completion about 5–6 years of age (Rajwani et al 2002; Blakemore 2018). It is interesting to note that overall the NCS appears to close sooner in males than in females, even though females mature faster and reach skeletal maturity sooner than males (Blakemore et al 2018).

The issue of non-fusion of the lumbar spine neurocentral joints is shown in Figure 1.7, using the upper lumbar spine of an eight-year-old male.

In summary, Blakemore et al (2018) performed a gross anatomical study of cadaveric osteological specimens from the spines of 32 children aged 1 to 18 years, whereas Rajwani et al (2002) and Zhang et al (2010) used MRI. In a retrospective study of 43 non-scoliotic children who had previously required CT scans of the thorax and abdomen for unrelated medical conditions, Schlösser et al (2013) showed that the age of closure of the neurocentral junction in the lumbar and thoracic spines depends on (i) the spinal level and (ii) the left-right asymmetry that depends on age and gender, and that this asymmetry may be associated with idiopathic scoliosis, but they confirmed that their study cannot answer this question, as a specific longitudinal study would be required to do so.

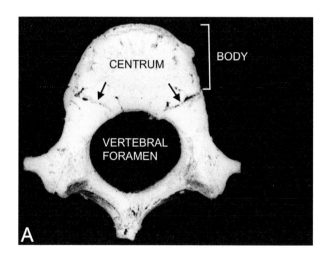 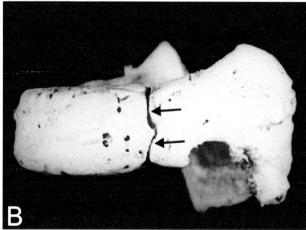

FIGURE 1.7 **(A)** Superior view of an upper lumbar spine vertebra from an eight-year-old male showing incomplete fusion of the paired hyaline cartilaginous neurocentral synchondroses (arrows). **(B)** Lateral partly oblique view of the same vertebra. Note the cartilaginous neurocentral joint (arrows), which is seen to be largely unfused in this projection.

Source: **Photographed by the author at the R A Dart collection of Modern Human Skeletons, University of the Witwatersrand, Johannesburg, South Africa.**

Chapter 2
NEUROANATOMY SUMMARY OF THE LUMBOSACRAL SPINE

Abstract: This chapter presents a brief anatomical overview of the spinal cord, spinal nerves, and cauda equina with supporting diagrams and histological sections, including one axial view of the spinal cord with its membranes, grey matter, and white matter. An axial view schematic diagram of the spinal cord and its descending and ascending pathways is shown. Diagrams of the ensheathment of peripheral myelinated nerve fibres, the recurrent meningeal nerve (sinuvertebral nerve), and the neuroanatomy across a lumbar vertebral level as well as the sympathetic and parasympathetic divisions of the peripheral nervous system are shown. Arteries and veins of the spinal cord, nerve roots, and cauda equina are illustrated. The anatomical and physiological basis of pain sensation, mechanisms, sensory nerve receptors, fibre types, and pathways to the central nervous system, as well as blood vessels and their histological anatomy and innervation are discussed. Lumbosacral spine innervation in general and the relationship of the nerve roots to the cerebrospinal fluid and the arachnoid villi in the spinal root sleeves, and their contact with the epidural venous plexus, are illustrated. Lumbosacral mechanical spinal pain syndromes due to structures such as the cluneal nerves, furcal nerves, and the sacroiliac joint are presented. A sequence of radiological axial CT scans from the lumbosacral level to the lowest part of the sacroiliac joint are presented as is a brief summary of the muscles of the back with their basic function and innervation.

Key words: neuroanatomy, recurrent meningeal nerve, sinuvertebral nerve, pain, vascular pain, root sleeves, cerebrospinal fluid, spinal membranes, spinal arachnoid villi, sacroiliac joint, spinal neuroanatomy

Contents

DOI: 10.1201/9781003315964-2

Introductory Overview

The following is a brief summary of human spinal neuroanatomy in order to present an understanding of basic neuroanatomy for the reader. The terms (i) anterior or ventral and (ii) posterior or dorsal are used interchangeably.

The nervous system consists of all the nerve tissue in the body and is comprised of two parts i.e. the brain and spinal cord that form the *central nervous system* (CNS) and the *PNS* with its sympathetic and parasympathetic divisions consisting of nerves, ganglia, and receptors (Ross et al 1985). Spinal nerves are part of the PNS (Moore et al 2018).

The overall divisions of the nervous system can be classified as shown in Figure 2.1.

In this text, the emphasis is on the human nervous system with regard to the lumbosacral spine and its involvement in low back pain syndromes.

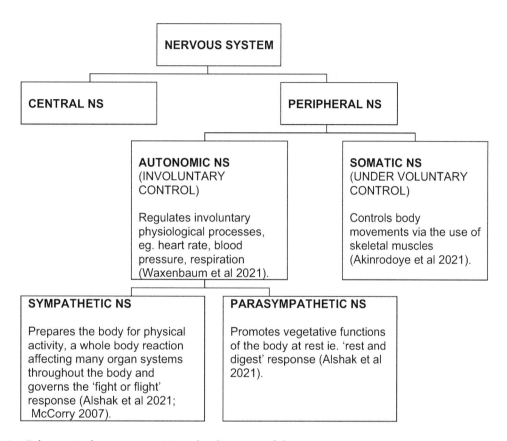

FIGURE 2.1 Schematic chart summarizing the divisions of the nervous system.

Anatomy of the Spinal Cord, Spinal Nerves, and Cauda Equina

Spinal Cord

The spinal cord is an extension of the CNS from the brain (AANS 2020), and it begins at the superior border of the first cervical vertebra and extends to the upper border of the second lumbar vertebra as an elongated cylindrical mass of nerve tissue that occupies the upper two-thirds of the vertebral canal and is usually 42–45 cm in length in adults (Chusid 1985).

The spinal cord divides into 31 segments: cervical 8, thoracic 12, lumbar 5, sacral 5, and coccygeal 1—these segments consist of 31 pairs of *spinal nerves*, with their respective *spinal root ganglia* located on the posterior root of each spinal nerve, composed of the unipolar nerve cell bodies of the sensory neurons—also called sensory ganglion (Dorland's Illustrated Medical Dictionary 1994). Neurons are the structural and functional units of the nervous system specialized for rapid communication and are composed of a cell body with long processes (extensions) called dendrites and an axon, which carry impulses to and away from the cell body, respectively, with some axons being myelinated (Moore et al 2018). (See Definitions for neuron figures).

The cord has two significant *enlargements* i.e. at the cervical and lumbar regions for the *brachial* and *lumbosacral* plexuses, to innervate the upper and lower limbs, respectively; the cervical one is present between C3 and T1, and the lumbar one is present between L1 and S2 (Dafny 2020). The cord is a structure of nervous tissue composed of *white* matter consisting of various ascending and descending tracts of myelinated axon fibres and *grey* matter composed of cell bodies (Dawodu 2018). This *grey matter* is made up of two symmetric halves joined across the midline by a transverse connection i.e. the anterior and posterior grey *commissures*, through which runs the minute *central canal* (Chusid 1985) (Figure 2.2) that is continuous with the fourth ventricle in the brain and contains Original proof correctly showed the wording 'cerebrospinal fluid (CSF)' CSF (Ganapathy et al 2020), an ultrafiltrate of plasma providing a constant source of nutrients for the regulation of neuronal functioning and removal of waste products of neuronal metabolism (May et al 2019).

A schematic diagram (Figure 2.2) shows the *posterior median sulcus*, and the *posterolateral sulcus* on either side of it, to which the posterior nerve *rootlets* are attached; the anterior nerve *rootlets* exit bilaterally at the *anterolateral sulcus.*

As this diagram does not show the *three* membranes surrounding the spinal cord, a histological section from a cadaveric thoracic spine, photographed using darkfield microscopy to illustrate these membranes, as well as the white and grey regions, including the 'H'-shaped internal mass of grey substance between *T1 and L2* (Ganapathy et al 2020), is shown in Figure 2.3.

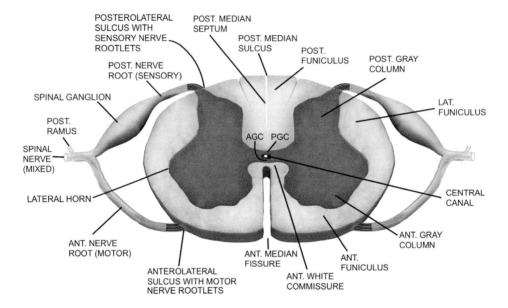

FIGURE 2.2 Diagram of an upper lumbar spinal cord segment showing mode of formation of a typical spinal nerve and the gross relationships of the grey and white matter. Note the posterior nerve rootlets that exit at the posterolateral sulcus, while the anterior nerve rootlets exit at the anterolateral sulcus. The anterior and posterior nerve roots join to form the *mixed* spinal nerve.

Source: **Modified from Blaus B, https://commons.wikimedia.org/wiki/File:Spinal_Cord_Sectional_Anatomy.png.**

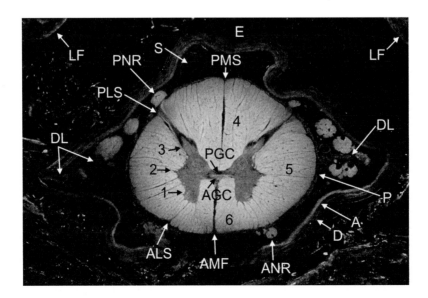

FIGURE 2.3 A 200-μm-thick axial view histological darkfield photomicrograph through the thoracic spinal cord of a 40-year-old male. AGC and PGC = anterior and posterior grey commissures; ALS = anterolateral sulcus to which anterior nerve rootlets (ANR) are attached; AMF = anterior median fissure that is usually about 3 mm deep and

FIGURE 2.3 (Continued)
contains a double fold of pia mater and a groove for the anterior spinal artery; D = dura mater of the dural tube with associated arachnoid mater (A); P = pia mater that closely covers the spinal cord; DL = denticulate ligament; E = epidural fat space that surrounds the spinal cord; LF = ligamentum flavum posterolaterally; PLS = posterolateral sulcus, a vertical furrow to which posterior nerve rootlets (PNR) are attached; PMS = posterior median sulcus (usually 4 to 6 mm deep); S = subarachnoid space that contains the CSF, which surrounds the pia mater of the spinal cord; 1 = anterior column (horn) of grey matter; 2 = lateral column of grey matter (lateral horn) that consists of the *cell bodies* of the presynaptic neurons of the *sympathetic nervous system* and is found in the thoracic and upper lumbar regions (T1-L2 or L3) (Moore et al 2018) and is the central element of the sympathetic division of the autonomic nervous system; 3 = posterior column of grey matter. The funiculi: 4 = posterior funiculus, 5 = lateral funiculus, 6 = anterior funiculus—the funiculi are mostly made up of glial cells and myelinated axons.

The CSF is found in the ventricles of the brain, in the cisterns around the outside of the brain, and in the subarachnoid space around both the brain and the *spinal cord* (Hall et al 2020). The, spinal cord serves as a conduit for the ascending and descending fibre tracts that relay information from the spinal and peripheral nerves to the brain, and it is immersed in CSF (Dawodu 2018).

A diagrammatic axial view of the spinal cord to illustrate the overall approximate location of the motor and descending (*efferent*) pathways and the sensory and ascending (*afferent*) pathways of the spinal cord is shown in Figure 2.4. (*Efferent* nerve fibres convey *motor* impulses *away* from the CNS toward the periphery, classified according to function as *somatic* efferent and *visceral* efferent neurofibres) (Dorland's 1994). *Afferent* nerve fibres convey *sensory* impulses from the periphery *to the CNS*, classified according to function as *somatic* afferent and *visceral* afferent neurofibres (Dorland's 1994).

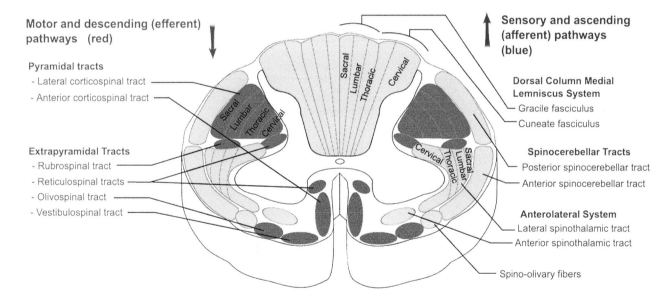

FIGURE 2.4 Schematic axial overall view of the spinal cord illustrating the *descending* and *ascending* pathways.

Source: Reproduced with permission from Polarlys and Mikael Häggström, CC BY-SA 3.0 https://commons.wikimedia.org/wiki/File:Spinal_cord_tracts_-_English.svg <https://creativecommons.org/licenses/by-sa/3.0>, via Wikimedia Commons.

Typically, there are two routes for signal transmissions to be conducted i.e. (i) *ascending* pathway (carrying sensory information from the body via the spinal cord to the brain) and (ii) *descending* pathway (where nerves go downward from the brain to the reflex organs via the spinal cord) (Yam et al 2018).

Ascending pathways that are involved with, for example (i) the posterior column medial-lemniscal pathway that carries the sensory modalities of *fine touch, proprioception*, and *vibration*, and (ii) the spinothalamic tract that is responsible for relaying signals concerning the perception of pain, temperature, crude touch, and pressure from the skin to the somatosensory area of the thalamus (Al-Chalabi et al 2021) are shown in Figure 2.5.

The sensation of pain is associated with the activation of the receptors in the primary afferent fibres, which is inclusive of the unmyelinated C-fibre and myelinated A-delta fibre; both nociceptors remain silent during homeostasis in the absence of pain and are activated when there is a potential of noxious stimuli (Yam et al 2018).

Thus, the spinal cord (i) carries *sensory* information (sensations) from the body, and some from the head, to the CNS via *afferent* fibres (i.e. toward the brain), and it performs the initial processing of this information, (ii) has *motor* neurons in the anterior column that project their axons into the periphery to innervate skeletal and smooth muscles that mediate voluntary and involuntary reflexes, and (iii) contains neurons whose descending

axons mediate autonomic control for most of the visceral functions (Dafny 2020).

The spinal cord is sheathed in the same three meninges as is the brain: the pia, arachnoid, and dura as shown in Figure 2.3, the latter being the tough outer sheath beneath which the arachnoid lies, while the pia closely adheres to the surface of the cord that is attached to the dura by a series of lateral *denticulate ligaments* emanating from the pial folds and allow the cord to 'float' in the spinal canal (Dafny 2020). The *pia*, which is delicate and highly vascular (Adeeb et al 2013), extends over the exiting spinal nerve roots and blends with their epineurium (Sinnatamby 2011).

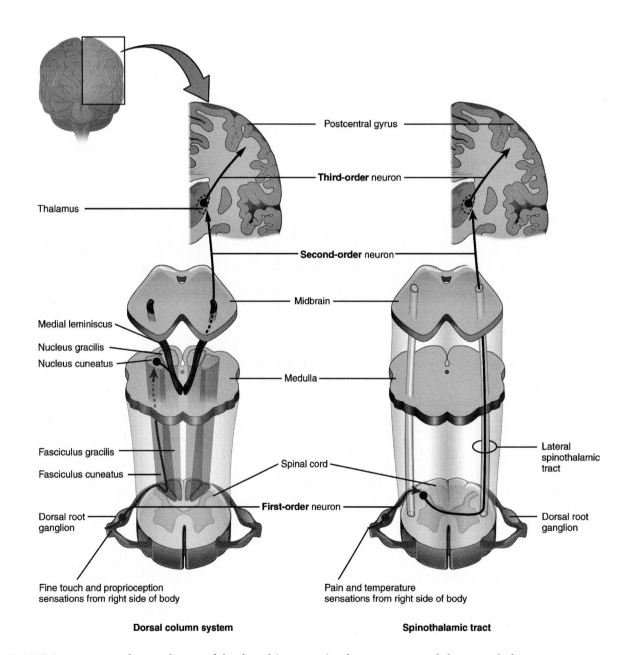

FIGURE 2.5 Ascending pathways of the dorsal (posterior) column system and the spinothalamic tract.

The *dentate ligaments* (Figure 2.3), which are extensions of the pia mater, are flat, fibrous sheets situated on each side of the spinal cord between the anterior and posterior spinal roots (Epstein 1966; Moini et al 2020) and extend laterally through the arachnoid, usually in a series of 21 triangular folds that insert into the dura mater—the first dentate ligament is at the level of the foramen magnum and the first cervical root, and the last merges with the pia mater surrounding the filum terminale (Epstein 1966). It is widely believed that the main function of dentate ligaments is to stabilize and protect the spinal cord in its protective cylinder of CSF within the vertebral canal (Sutton 1973; Ceylan et al 2012), and they are especially concerned with the transmission of biomechanical forces i.e. the uniform distribution of physiological tensile forces over the length and cross-section of the spinal cord (Breig 1960).

Spinal Nerves

Spinal nerves arise from the spinal cord as anterior and posterior *rootlets* that converge to form two nerve roots i.e. the *anterior nerve root*, consisting of motor (efferent) fibres passing from nerve cell bodies in the anterior horn of spinal cord grey matter to effector organs located peripherally, and a *posterior nerve root*, consisting of sensory (afferent) fibres from cell bodies in the *spinal root ganglion* that extend peripherally to sensory endings and centrally to the posterior horn of spinal cord grey matter; the posterior and anterior nerve roots unite, within or just proximal to the intervertebral foramen, to form a mixed (motor and sensory) *spinal nerve*, which immediately divides into two *rami* (branches) i.e. a *posterior ramus* and an *anterior ramus* that carry both motor and sensory fibres, as do all their subsequent branches (Moore et al 2018). The extension of the subarachnoid space is continued along the nerve roots, usually as far as the ganglion, occasionally involving its inner pole but never to envelop it completely; the dural layer is continued along the nerve roots for a short distance before finally blending with the anterior root and the ganglion to form an outer fibrous sheath for these structures, and this connective tissue is continued outwards to become the strong *perineurial sheath* of the single bundle of nerve fibres of the spinal nerve formed by the fusion of the two roots (Sunderland 1975). The somewhat condensed layer of *epidural tissue* on the surface of the dura is continuous with the epineurium of the spinal nerve, and the formation of this perineurial-epineurial sheath adds to the thickness of the spinal nerve (Sunderland 1975).

Figure 2.6 shows the nerve complex and its meningeal coverings that occupy about 1/6 to 1/4 of the foramen and which are surrounded by a generous reserve cushion space containing blood vessels, lymphatics, fat, and areolar tissue in the normal intervertebral foramen (Hadley 1950).

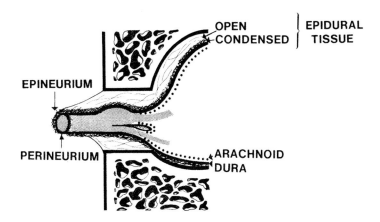

FIGURE 2.6 The nerve complex and its meningeal coverings in the intervertebral foramen, although the arrangement is not to scale and has been drawn to accentuate relative relationships (Sunderland 1975). The pia mater covering the neural structures is not shown. The neural structures are surrounded by epidural fat.

Source: **Reproduced with permission from Sunderland S 1975 Anatomical perivertebral influences on the intervertebral foramen. In: Goldstein M (ed) The research status of spinal manipulative therapy. US Department of Health, Education, and Welfare, Public Health Service, National Institutes of Health, National Institute of Neurological and Communicative Disorders and Stroke, Bethesda, Maryland. NINCDS Monograph No 15, p. 129–140.**

The spinal nerve root ganglion is covered by the *dural sleeve* consisting of pia mater, arachnoid mater, and dura mater that terminate at the beginning of the spinal nerve where the dural sleeve blends with the epineurium of the spinal nerve (Bogduk 1997). The epineurium forming the outermost covering of the nerve includes fatty tissue, *blood vessels*, and *lymphatics* (Moore et al 2018).

The anterior and posterior roots receive innervation from the *nervi nervorum*, and they are sensitive to stretching and pressure on the nerve (Gharries 2018). The *nervi*

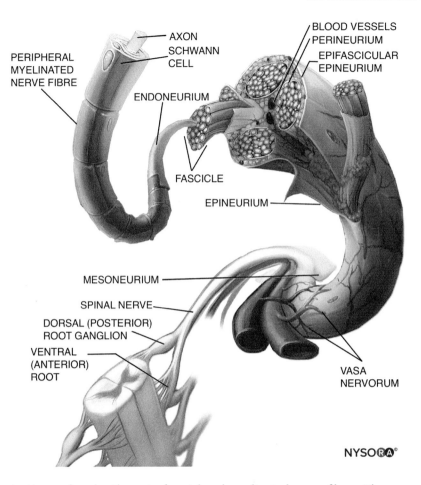

FIGURE 2.7 Organization and ensheathment of peripheral myelinated nerve fibres. The nerves are comprised of bundles of nerve fibres, layers of connective tissue, and blood vessels (*vasa nervorum*).

Source: **Reproduced with permission from Carrera A, Lopez AM, Sala-Blanch X et al 2020 Functional Regional Anesthesia Anatomy, New York School of Regional Anesthesia (NYSORA) www.nysora.com/foundations-of-regional-anesthesia/anatomy/functional-regional-anesthesia-anatomy/. Lettering modified.**

nervorum (small nerve filaments innervating the epineurium (sheath) of a larger nerve) are located on the outside of the epineurium and innervate and regulate the function and discharge of sensory, motor, or mixed-modality nerves (Lam et al 2020). In addition, mild compression of the *vasa nervorum* (small blood vessels that provide the blood supply to peripheral myelinated nerves (Figure 2.7) would first affect venous outflow with potential stasis and accumulation of toxin at the affected part of the nerve (Lam et al 2020).

Figure 2.7 shows the anatomy of a peripheral myelinated nerve fibre.

The *spinal nerve* contains *motor, sensory*, and autonomic nerve fibres (Ganapathy et al 2020) passing to and from all parts of the body, and each spinal cord segment innervates a *dermatome* (Dafny 2020).

Immediately distal to the spinal root ganglion where the anterior and posterior roots unite to form the *spinal nerve* that emerges through intervertebral foramen,

they divide into *anterior* and *posterior* rami (Berry et al 1995), and the anterior ramus gives off recurrent meningeal branches (von Luschka 1850) (Figure 2.8A). Since the German anatomist Hubert von Luschka first described the *sinuvertebral* nerve in 1850 as being a nerve that *originates from the anterior ramus* of the *spinal nerve* that *re-enters* the spinal canal via the intervertebral foramina to innervate multiple meningeal and non-meningeal structures (Shayota et al 2019)—for example, posterior longitudinal ligament, ligamentum flavum, the anterior dura mater, epidural fat tissue, and veins and the walls of blood vessels that supply the vertebral bodies (Haldeman 1980), it has acquired many other names. These include (i) the recurrent nerve of Luschka, (ii) recurrent meningeal nerve, and (iii) meningeal branch of the spinal nerve (Shayota et al 2019). In this text, the term *recurrent meningeal nerve* will be used to describe these nerves that supply both *proprioceptive* fibres (receiving stimuli within the tissues of the body, as within muscles and tendons (Dorland 1994)) and *nociceptive* fibres, and the nerve can be traced as far as the outer three layers of the IVD lamellae in healthy patients, but it can go as far as the nucleus pulposus in degenerative discs and has been implicated in *discogenic pain* (Shayota et al 2019).

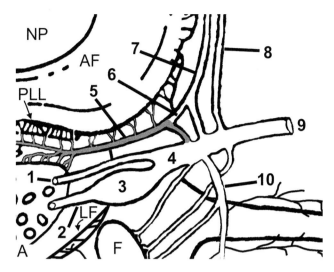

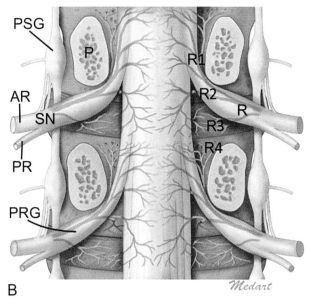

FIGURE 2.8 **(A)** An axial view schematic diagram showing the recurrent meningeal nerve (sinuvertebral nerve), coloured grey, and its associated structures. 1 = anterior nerve root; 2 = posterior nerve root; 3 = posterior root spinal ganglion; 4 = main trunk of spinal nerve; 5 = recurrent meningeal nerve (coloured grey) with branches carrying sympathetic fibres to the dural tube and the posterior longitudinal ligament, respectively; 6 = autonomic (sympathetic) branch to the recurrent meningeal nerve; 7 = *grey ramus communicans* (multilevel irregular lumbosacral distribution); 8 = *white ramus communicans* (myelinated)—not found above T1 or below L2–3–4; 9 = anterior ramus of spinal nerve; 10 = posterior ramus of spinal nerve; AF = annulus fibrosus; F = facet; LF = ligamentum flavum; PLL = posterior longitudinal ligament; NP = nucleus pulposus.

The rami communicans (or communicantes) connect the spinal nerves with the sympathetic trunk (Rickenbacher et al 1985) (Figures 2.8A). Thus, at or distal to its origin, each *anterior spinal ramus* receives a *grey ramus communicans* from the corresponding sympathetic ganglion, while the thoracic and first and second lumbar, (and sometimes third lumbar) anterior spinal rami, each contribute a *white ramus communicans* to the corresponding paravertebral ganglia (Berry et al 1995); *grey rami communicantes*, passing from all ganglia to the lumbar spinal nerves, are long and accompany the lumbar arteries around the sides of the vertebral bodies, medial to the fibrous arches to which the psoas major muscle is attached (Berry et al 1995).

A coronal view mid-pedicle cut across the lumbar spine is shown in Figure 2.8B to illustrate the extensive distribution of the recurrent meningeal nerve and some of its branches.

Cauda Equina

The lumbosacral enlargement extends from T11 through S1 segments of the spinal cord, inferior to

FIGURE 2.8 **(B)** The *recurrent meningeal nerve* (R) gives rise to several branches: R1 = ascending branch, which goes intraosseous and gives rise to the *basivertebral nerve* (R4) near the pedicle. (The basivertebral nerve is a paired nerve believed to play an important role in endplate pain nociceptive transmission). R2 = descending branch supplying the adjacent posterior longitudinal ligament (not seen) and the disc; R3 = direct branches to the IVD. PSG = paraspinal sympathetic ganglion; P = pedicle; PRG = posterior root ganglion. The recurrent meningeal nerve is both somatic and sympathetic.

Source: Reproduced with permission from Kim HS, Wu PH, Jang I-T 2020 Lumbar degenerative disease Part 1: Anatomy and pathophysiology of intervertebral discogenic pain and radiofrequency ablation of basivertebral and sinuvertebral nerve treatment for chronic discogenic back pain: A prospective case series and review of literature. Int. J. Mol. Sci 21(4): 1483. License granted http://creativecommons.org/licenses/by/4.0/; Medart. Lettering modified.

which the cord continues to diminish as the *conus medullaris* (Moore et al 2018) (Figure 2.9). Nerve roots descend within the spinal canal as individual rootlets, collectively termed the *cauda equina* (Jones et al 2021(a)) (Figure 2.9). Inferior to the conus medullaris, a strand of fibrous tissue called the filum terminale extends to the coccyx (Jones et al 2021(a)) (Figure 2.10) initially as the filum terminale *internum* while it is within the dural tube (sac), beyond which it becomes the filum terminale *externum* (Newell 2008).

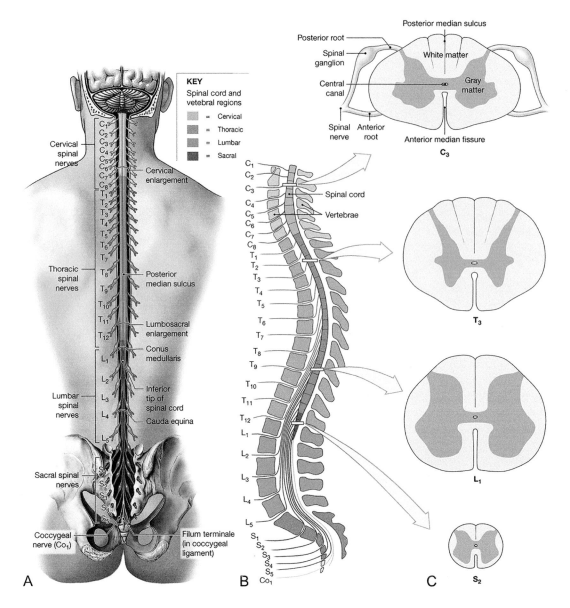

FIGURE 2.9 **(A)** The superficial anatomy and orientation of the adult spinal cord. The numbers to the left identify the spinal nerves and indicate where the nerve roots leave the vertebral canal. The spinal cord extends from the brain only to the level of vertebrae L1–2; **(B)** Lateral view of vertebrae and spinal cord. Note that the sacral spinal cord segments are [approximately] level with the T12-L1 vertebrae. **(C)** The spinal segments found at representative locations are indicated in the transverse sections and show the arrangement of grey matter and white matter.

Source: Reproduced with permission from www.seekpng.com/ipng/u2w7w7i1e6u2q8r5_nerves-of-the-spine-png-spinal-cord/.

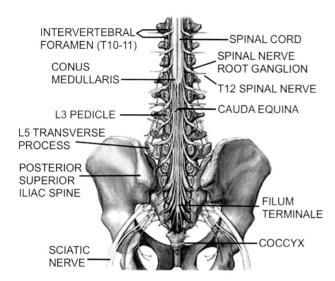

FIGURE 2.10 Schematic diagram showing exposed spinal and sacral canals with the nerve roots of the cauda equina in the subarachnoid space. On the posterior and anterior surfaces of the sacrum are four pairs of sacral foramina for the exit of anterior and posterior rami of the spinal nerves.

Source: **Reproduced with permission from Mr Arifnajafov, https://commons.wikimedia.org/wiki/File: Onur%C4%9Fa_beyni_at_quyru%C4%9Fu.jpg;https:// creativecommons.org/licenses/by-sa/4.0/. Lettering modified.**

In a large study of adults who had no spinal deformity and who underwent MR imaging in the supine position, it was found that the *conus medullaris* can extend to the lower third of the L2–3 disc space both in women and men (Karabulut et al 2016).

The cauda equina nerve roots are immersed in CSF, as is part of the filum i.e. the filum terminale *internum* that extends to the termination of the dural tube/thecal sac that usually ends at the S2 level but can range from the L5-S1 IVD level to the upper third of the S3 vertebra (Binokay et al 2006). The filum terminale continues as the filum terminal *externum* outside the dural tube to anchor to the coccyx posteriorly (DeSai et al 2020) to give longitudinal support to the cord (Jones et al 2021(a)).

The collection of cauda equina nerves in the lumbosacral vertebral column that extends from the spinal cord provides *sensory* innervation to the perineal or saddle area (S2-S3), *motor* innervation to the anal and urethral sphincters, and *parasympathetic* innervation to the bladder and lower bowel (Dawodu 2018; Goodman 2018).

See colour plate Figure 2.11 that illustrates the extensive neurovascular anatomy of the lumbar and sacral regions of the spinal cord.

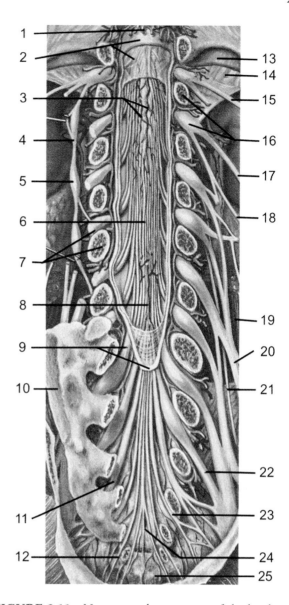

FIGURE 2.11 Neurovascular anatomy of the lumbosacral region of the spinal cord. 1 = posterior internal vertebral venous plexus; 2 = spinal dura mater and arachnoid mater; 3 = posterior spinal artery and vein; 4 = sympathetic trunk; 5 = lumbar sympathetic ganglion; 6 = cauda equina; 7 = third lumbar spinal ganglion and pedicle of L4 vertebra; 8 = posterior median longitudinal spinal vein; 9 = first sacral nerve and dural sac termination; 10 = sacral auricular surface for articulating with the ilium; 11 = third sacral nerve; 12 = fifth sacral nerve; 13 = pleura; 14 = lumbar part of diaphragm; 15 = twelfth thoracic nerve; 16 = pedicle of L1 vertebra and first lumbar ganglion; 17 = iliohypogastric nerve; 18 = ilioinguinal nerve; 19 = psoas major muscle; 20 = femoral nerve; 21 = obturator nerve; 22 = second sacral nerve; 23 = fourth sacral nerve; 24 = filum terminale externum; 25 = coccyx.

Source: **Part of a colour plate by Professor Paul Peck. Modified and reproduced from Atlas of Normal Anatomy, Medical Student Edition, Lumbar and Sacral Regions of the Spinal Cord, Plate 48, 1956. Lederle Laboratories, American Cyanamid International, Pearl River, N.Y. © 1974.**

Arteries and Veins of the Spinal Cord and Cauda Equina

The arteries supplying the spinal cord are branches of the vertebral, ascending cervical, deep cervical, intercostal, lumbar, and lateral sacral arteries (Moore et al 2018), depending on the region of the spine.

Spinal Cord

Basically, the main *blood supply* to the spinal cord is via the *anterior single spinal artery* and the *two posterior spinal arteries* (Gofur et al 2020) providing the spinal cord with an adequate blood supply and anastomoses, and the *lumbar* and *cervical enlargements* have additional blood flow; the anterior spinal artery supplies the anterior area of the spinal cord, while the pair of posterior spinal arteries supply the posterior one-third of the cord (Ganapathy et al 2020). A schematic diagram providing an outline of the arterial blood supply to—and venous drainage from—the spinal cord is shown in Figure 2.12 followed by a more detailed figure (Figure 2.13).

The spinal cord drains via the *anterior* and *posterior spinal veins*, one each in the anterior and posterior median fissures and four others, often incomplete, one pair being posterior, the other anterior to the anterior and posterior nerve roots (Berry et al 1995). The veins, in turn, drain into the *internal venous plexus* located in the *epidural space*, and these veins eventually empty into the *external vertebral venous plexus* via the *basivertebral* veins (Gofur et al 2020).

The extensive vascular plexuses surrounding the spinal cord protect it from circulatory insufficiency, and it is important to note (i) the segmental arteries supplying the cord and the high compensatory capacity of the pial vascular plexus covering the surface of the spinal cord, (ii) the importance of CSF in supplying nutrients to the spinal cord, and (iii) that the intradural nerve tissues, spinal cord, and nerve roots are devoid of lymphatic vessels but are immersed in the CSF (Yoshizawa 2002).

The important association between the arterial supply and venous drainage of the spinal cord and spinal nerve roots is shown schematically in Figure 2.13.

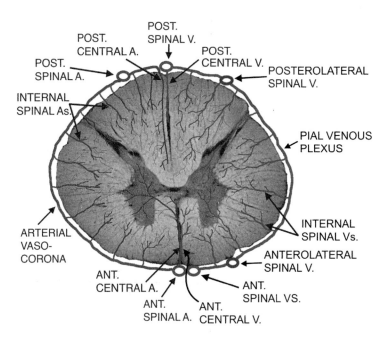

FIGURE 2.12   A schematic diagram of the arterial blood supply to—and venous drainage from—the spinal cord showing half the arterial and venous circulation for each side of the spinal cord, using a thoracic spine section as an example.

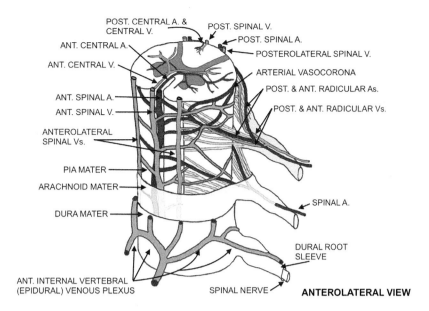

FIGURE 2.13 Arterial supply and venous drainage of spinal cord and spinal nerve roots: (A) The basic pattern of the arterial supply of the spinal cord is from three longitudinal arteries: one anterior lying in the anteromedian fissure and the other two lying posterolaterally, and these vessels are reinforced by medullary branches derived from the segmental arteries. Most proximal spinal nerves and roots are accompanied by radicular arteries. (B) The veins that drain the spinal cord, as well as *internal* vertebral venous plexuses, drain into the intervertebral veins, which in turn drain into segmental veins.

Source: **Modified and reproduced from Hasan S, Arain A. 2021 Neuroanatomy, Spinal Cord Arteries. [Updated 2021 Aug 22]. In: StatPearls [Internet]. Treasure Island (FL): StatPearls Publishing; Available from: www.ncbi. nlm.nih.gov/books/NBK539889/ (http://creativecommons.org/licenses/by/4.0).**

Cauda Equina

The cauda equina spinal nerve roots have a corresponding medullary artery (Berg et al 2020). Rydevik (1993) describes the nerve roots as having a vascular supply that comes from both peripheral and central sources and references the work of Crock et al (1976), Parke et al (1985), and Olmarker (1991) in this regard. Essentially, each nerve root is supplied by the radicular artery arising from the corresponding lumbar, medial and lateral sacral, or iliolumbar artery (Namba 2016). The filum terminale is supplied by the artery of the filum that is a direct extension of the anterior spinal artery (Namba 2016).

The right and left *posterolateral longitudinal arterial trunks* of the spinal cord converge at the inferior point of the conus medullaris, and the *posterior median longitudinal venous channel* of the spinal cord is a large, long vein that courses downward in company with radicles (rootlets) of the cauda equina (Crock et al 1977).

Apart from their arterial supply, all nerve roots derive some of their nutritional supply via diffusion from the surrounding CSF (Rydevik et al 1990).

Peripheral Nervous System and Its Sympathetic and Para-Sympathetic Divisions

The PNS is a complex system of nerves that branch off from the spinal cord as nerve roots and travel outside the spinal canal to the upper extremities, the muscles of the trunk, to the lower extremities, and to the organs of the body; it is by way of the PNS that nerve impulses travel to and from the CNS, facilitating nerve signals between specific locations in the body and the CNS (AANS 2020).

The *autonomic* nervous system (ANS), a division of the PNS that is distributed to the smooth muscle and glands throughout the body, is entirely a motor (efferent) system; it is highly integrated in structure and function with the rest of the nervous system, and it helps maintain the constancy of the internal environment of the body via its *sympathetic* and *parasympathetic* divisions (Chusid 1985).

The *sympathetic* and *parasympathetic* divisions, respectively, are concerned with maintaining a stable internal environment below the level of consciousness; the *sympathetic* nervous system predominates during emergency 'fight-or-flight' reactions and exercise, whereas the *parasympathetic* system predominates during quiet resting conditions (McCorry 2007).

The cell bodies of the *presynaptic* neurons of the *sympathetic* division of the ANS are found in *only one location* i.e. in the *lateral horn intermediolateral cell columns*

(IMLs) or *nuclei* of the spinal cord; the paired right and left IMLs are a part of the grey matter of the thoracic (T1-T12) and the upper lumbar (L1-L2 or L3) segments of the spinal cord (Moore et al 2018). Figure 2.14 illustrates the location of paravertebral ganglia and the left and right sympathetic trunks.

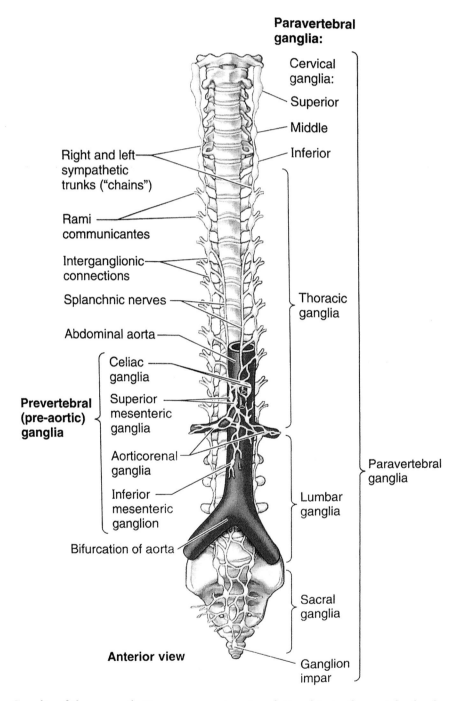

FIGURE 2.14 Ganglia of the sympathetic nervous system in relationship to the vertebral column. In the sympathetic nervous system, cell bodies of *postsynaptic* neurons occur either in the *paravertebral ganglia* of the sympathetic trunks or in the *prevertebral ganglia* that occur mainly in relationship to the origins of the main branches of the abdominal aorta. Prevertebral ganglia are specifically involved in the innervation of abdominopelvic viscera. The cell bodies of postsynaptic neurons distributed to the remainder of the body occur in the *paravertebral* ganglia.

Source: **Reproduced with permission from Moore KL, et al, Clinically Oriented Anatomy, 8th Edn, © Wolters Kluwer, 2018.**

Motor axons of presynaptic neurons leave the spinal cord through anterior roots and enter the anterior rami of spinal nerves T1-L2 or L3 and, almost immediately after entering, all the presynaptic sympathetic fibres leave the anterior rami of these spinal nerves and pass to the sympathetic trunks through *white rami communicates* (communicating branches) (Moore et al 2018).

The cell bodies of *postsynaptic* neurons of the sympathetic nervous system occur in two locations, the *paravertebral* and *prevertebral* ganglia (Figure 2.14) that are linked to form the right and left sympathetic trunks (chains) on each side of the vertebral column and extend essentially the length of this column from the superior paravertebral ganglion (the *superior cervical ganglion* of each sympathetic trunk) that lies at the base of the cranium and continues inferiorly to where the two trunks

unite as the *ganglion impar* at the level of the coccyx (Moore et al 2018).

It should be noted that the thoracic sympathetic chain ganglia can be identified on precontrast 3D-CISS MR imaging (Chaudhry et al 2018).

Figure 2.15 illustrates part of the spinal cord and its relationship to the paravertebral and prevertebral ganglia.

The sympathetic efferents leave via anterior roots from levels T1 to L2, enter the spinal nerves, then form *white rami communicantes* (myelinated) to the paravertebral ganglia of the sympathetic trunks (Figure 2.15) (Wilkinson 1986). Having synapsed, some re-join the spinal nerves by *grey rami communicantes* (non-myelinated) as vasomotor, sudomotor, and pilomotor fibres (Wilkinson 1986).

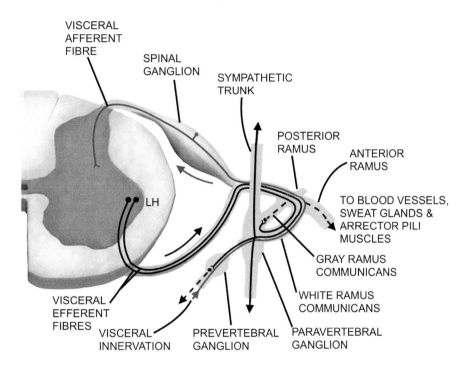

FIGURE 2.15 A schematic diagram showing sympathetic afferent and efferent fibres; postganglionic efferents are represented by dashed lines. LH = lateral horn.

Figure 2.16A illustrates how the *sympathetic division* of the ANS arises from preganglionic cell bodies located in the IML of the 12 thoracic and upper lumbar segments of the spinal cord (Chusid 1985).

The axons of these cells (*preganglionic fibres*) are mostly myelinated fibres that form the *white communicating rami* of the thoracic and upper lumbar nerves, through which they reach the trunk ganglia of the sympathetic chain, lying on the lateral sides of the bodies of the thoracic and lumbar vertebrae, where they may synapse with ganglion cells, or pass up or down the sympathetic trunk to synapse with ganglion cells at a higher or lower level, or pass through the trunk ganglia and out to one of the collateral, or intermediary, sympathetic ganglia (e.g. the

celiac ganglion)—the *grey communicating rami* join all of the spinal nerves (Chusid 1985).

The *parasympathetic division* of the ANS (Figure 2.16B) arises from *preganglionic cell bodies* in the grey matter of the brain stem via *cranial nerves* III, VII, IX, and X (Chusid 1985; Wilkinson 1986) and via the second to fourth *sacral nerves* (Wilkinson 1986) (pelvic splanchnic nerves) (Moore et al 2018). Its distribution, in contrast to that of the sympathetics, is confined entirely to *visceral structures*, and most of its preganglionic neurons run without interruption from their central origin to the wall of the viscus they supply or to where they synapse with *terminal ganglion cells* associated with the plexuses of Meissner and Auerbach in the intestinal tract (Chusid 1985).

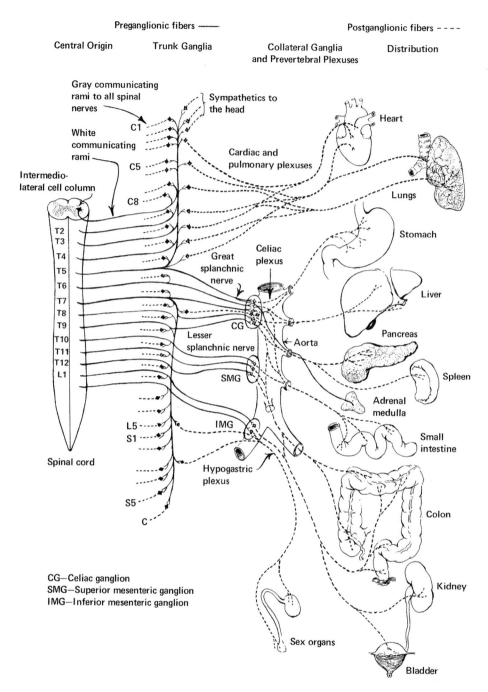

FIGURE 2.16A   The sympathetic (or thoracolumbar) division.

Source: Reproduced with permission from Chusid JG 1985 Correlative neuroanatomy and functional neurology, 19th edition, © McGraw Hill.

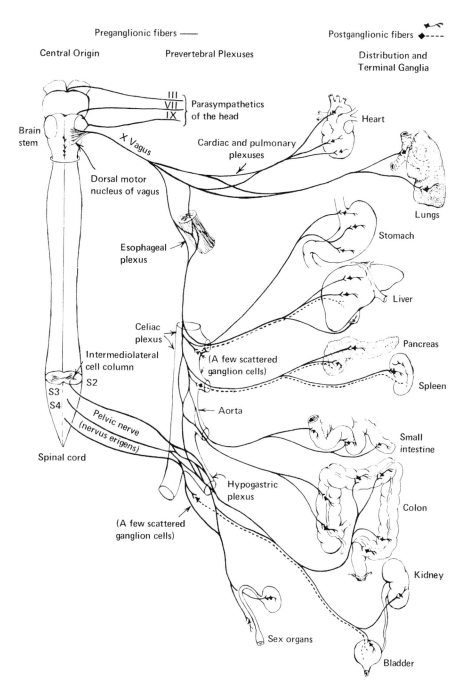

FIGURE 2.16B The parasympathetic (or craniosacral) division.

Source: Reproduced with permission from Chusid JG 1985 Correlative neuroanatomy and functional neurology, 19th edition, © McGraw Hill.

As a brief summary of this section, the *autonomic—or visceral*—reflex arcs with central connections in the CNS differ anatomically from the *somatic* reflex arcs in that the *preganglionic efferent components* of the former make synaptic connections with ganglion cells in the autonomic ganglia, whereas the efferent components of the latter terminate in direct relation to effector organs (Kuntz 1953) (Figure 2.17). The efferent limb of the *autonomic* reflex arc consequently comprises *two neurons*, whereas that of the *somatic* reflex arc are comprised of *one neuron*—the portion of either the autonomic or the somatic reflex arc that is located within the CNS may be confined to a single segment, or it may involve two or more segments; the *preganglionic* component of the *autonomic* reflex arc likewise may make synaptic connections in one or more autonomic ganglia (Kuntz 1953).

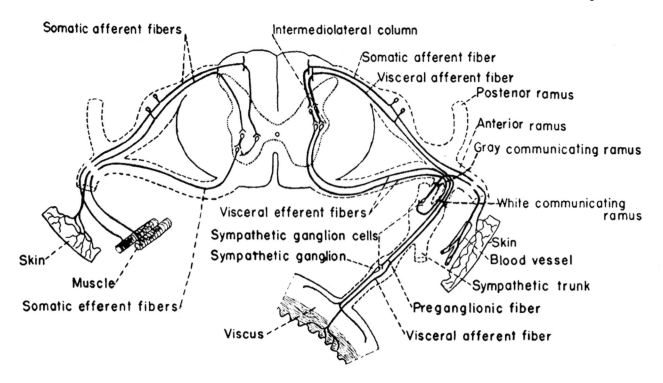

FIGURE 2.17   Diagrammatic illustration of somatic (left) and visceral (right) reflex arcs.

Source: Reproduced with permission from Kuntz A, The Autonomic Nervous System, 4th Edn. Lea and Febiger, Philadelphia, © Wolters Kluwer, 1953.

Pain: Its Anatomical and Physiological Basis with Reference to the Low Back

General Introduction

This text is primarily concerned with the anatomical basis of pain generation in structures in the lumbosacral spine, so the general topic of the pathophysiology of pain will now be briefly considered. It is not within the scope of this text to consider the phenomenon of 'behavioural pain' that has been discussed at length in the literature (Fordyce 1976; Crown 1980; Wood 1980; Keefe et al 2007). The following is an historical overview of knowledge in the area of pain sensation over the years.

Pain Sensation

The perception of pain is an unpleasant sensory and emotional experience associated with actual—or potential—tissue damage (Raja et al 2020); it is a complex experience (Willis 1985; Wang et al 1987; Editorial 2020) that normally occurs when tissue is damaged (Wall 1974). Pain serves the purpose of preventing tissue damage and protecting the body while it is healing, but, under certain conditions, pain can become maladaptive and persist as *chronic pain* (Schug et al 2011).

While all pain is perceived 'centrally' in the cortex, it is a sensation that normally results from noxious stimulation of peripheral nociceptive nerve endings by chemical or physical agents (e.g. pressure, tension, heat, and cold) (Sherrington 1906; Keele 1967; Monnier 1975; Dubin et al 2010). The particular nerve terminal that is considered to act as the pain receptor is the *free nerve ending*

(Haldeman 1980; Daube et al 1986); these endings are by far the most common of all the general sensory end organs (Arey 1965), with some of the free nerve endings arising from small myelinated fibres (Lipton 1978). Painful stimuli are detected by nociceptors located in tissues and organs (Schug et al 2011) that respond to abnormal conditions by setting up impulse discharges that travel over specific or alternative afferent pathways to the sensory cortex, where the activity evoked is interpreted as pain (Sunderland 1968).

There are two distinct types of nociceptors (Schug et al 2011):

- High threshold *mechanoreceptors* that stimulate small diameter *myelinated* A-delta -fibres and transmit a well-localized sharp or pricking sensation that lasts as long as the stimulus. (This is known as *fast pain* (Daube et al 1986)).
- *Polymodal* nociceptors that stimulate small *unmyelinated* slowly conducting C-fibres. (This *slow pain* may outlast the actual stimulus (Daube et al 1986)). As well as responding to mechanical stimuli, these receptors are activated by thermal and chemical stimuli e.g. hydrogen ions, potassium ions, bradykinin, serotonin, adenosine triphosphate, and prostaglandins (Shug et al 2011).

Noxious stimuli to the body, whether external or internal to the body, create physical change that induces afferent input in the nervous system, with or without sensory experience or behavioural response; a noxious stimulus is actually—or potentially—damaging to tissue and liable to cause pain (Cervero et al 1996). Information regarding the damaging impact of these stimuli on bodily tissues is transduced to neural pathways and transmitted through the PNS to the CNS and to the ANS, respectively—this form of information processing is known as nociception (Garland 2012). Somatic pain is pain that results from noxious stimulation of one of the musculoskeletal components of the body (Bogduk 1997), for example the vertebral column and peripheral nociceptive afferent fibres (less than 5 micron in diameter) transmit the sensation centripetally (Wyke 1979).

The small diameter of pain fibres presents practical difficulties in physiological research (Iggo 1974) during microneurography, a technique involving the insertion of a microelectrode into a peripheral nerve to register axonal electrical activity from individual neurons in awake, relaxed humans (Ackerley et al 2018). The latter authors concluded that microneurography presents a technically demanding, yet insightful, approach for studying the function of individual C-fibre afferent responses from nociceptors, thermoreceptors, and mechanoreceptors in humans. In addition, unmyelinated C-tactile afferents can be recorded in humans via microneurography; they are highly sensitive mechanoreceptors, with low activation threshold, that show characteristic responses to mechanical, thermal, electrical stimuli (Ackerley 2022). Microneurography fits in well with exploring the human nervous system, although to attain single discrimination is a matter of trial and error, but it is possible to discriminate impulse trains in a single nerve fibre (Vallbo 2018).

Pain Mechanisms

When there is a noxious stimulus, the nociception mechanism undergoes three events—*transduction* (the process by which a sensory receptor converts a stimulus from the environment into an action potential for transmission to the brain (Dorland's 1994), *transmission* (an impulse across a synaptic junction through the medium of a chemical substance (neurotransmitter) (Dorland's (1994), and *modulation* of the nociceptive signals i.e. the process by which the body alters a pain signal as it is transmitted along the pain pathway (Kirkpatrick et al 2015).

Nociceptors are widespread in the superficial layers of the skin as well as in certain internal tissues such as the periosteum, arterial walls, and joints, whereas most other deep tissues are sparsely supplied; nevertheless, any widespread tissue damage can still summate to cause the slow chronic (i.e. not acute) aching type of pain in most of these areas, and pain can be perceived with the activation of nociceptors by multiple stimuli classified as three main types i.e. *mechanical*, *thermal*, and *chemical* stimuli (Guyton et al 2000; Dubin et al 2010). Referred pain is pain that is felt in a part of the body remote from the tissue in which the activated nociceptors are located, for example it may be initiated in one of the visceral organs for it to be referred to an area on the body surface (Hall et al 2020) or to the back (Beers et al 2006).

Axons (nerve fibres) are the main component of a neuron that functions to conduct action potentials in a unilateral direction from the dendrites to the axonal terminals, as well as from one neuron to another—axons can be myelinated or unmyelinated, and the presence of a myelin sheath, with its nodes of Ranvier, increases the propagation speed of impulses as they travel along the myelinated fibre via *saltatory conduction* (generation of action potential at each node of Ranvier) and acts as an insulator to prevent electrical impulses from leaving the axon during transmission; for unmyelinated fibres, the impulses move continuously at a much slower pace (Yam et al 2018).

Sensory Nerve Receptors

The sensory system is the portion of the nervous system responsible for processing input from the environment, and sensory nerves have different types of nerve fibres depending on their associated receptors (Koop et al 2021). The peripheral endings of the different types of sensory fibres are differently located, are differentially sensitive to different forms of energy, and have different properties such as adaptation, threshold, refractoriness, and after-discharge (Bishop 1946). Non-neural elements associated with nerve fibre terminals, such as *encapsulating cells*, are the structures that must be deformed to excite the nerve endings (Burgess et al 1973). There are five basic types of sensory receptors: (i) *nociceptors* (detect damage occurring in the tissues, whether physical or chemical damage), (ii) *chemoreceptors* (detect taste in the mouth, smell in the nose, oxygen level in the arterial blood, and other factors that make up the chemistry of the body), (iii) *thermoreceptors* (detect changes in temperature, some of which detect cold and others warmth), (iv) *mechanoreceptors* (detect mechanical compression or stretching of the receptor or of tissue adjacent to the receptor), and (v) *electromagnetic* receptors (detect light on the retina of the eye) (Hall et al 2020). Receptors may show more than one form of behaviour, for example, both position and velocity detection (Burgess et al 1973).

Nerve Fibre Types and Pain Pathways

Nerve fibres are classified in a number of ways (Gasser et al 1927; Lloyd 1943), but for practical purposes Wang et al (1987) suggest that *primary afferent fibres* be divided into two groups on the basis of *different diameters* and *conduction velocities* i.e.: (i) unmyelinated C-fibres and small myelinated A-delta fibres, which transmit pain when strongly stimulated (Bishop 1946; Lipton 1978; Loeser 1985) and (ii) large myelinated fibres, which give rise to sensations of touch and pressure when stimulated (Lipton 1978). These large myelinated fibres have a lower threshold (Lipton 1978) but conduct rapidly and transmit impulses from elaborate special receptors in the periphery; the small unmyelinated fibres and the small myelinated fibres conduct slowly and transmit impulses from less specialized receptors in the periphery (Schaumburg et al 1975).

Information relating to the nature, quality, and intensity of the sensation is transmitted along individual fibres as a pattern of activity or frequency code (Sunderland 1968). This pattern is dependent, in part, on the velocity of conduction in the particular fibre; it is also determined by the time intervals between successive impulses and the total amplitude of the impulse discharge, which depends on the intensity of the stimulus (Sunderland 1968).

Central Nervous System Connection

Temporal summation is documented for dull, delayed C-fibre pain, which is different in quality and less accurately projected than the fast, sharp pain from high threshold A-delta nociceptors (Torebjork 1985). Most small afferent fibres terminate in the more superficial laminae of the dorsal horn and the nociceptive neurons in lamina I of the cord, which receive exclusively nociceptive inputs from myelinated and unmyelinated afferents, and project, at least in part, to the thalamic and brain stem regions (Iggo et al 1985).

It is suggested that there are two parallel C-fibre primary afferent pathways carrying similar sensory information into different areas of the dorsal horn; the evidence supporting this hypothesis is largely derived from observations of the skin but may equally apply to joints, muscles, and viscera (Hunt et al 1985). The central events and pathology that may underlie chronic pain states must take into account the different contributions made by the peptide- and non-peptide-containing C-fibre sensory pathways in nociception (Hunt et al 1985).

Blood Vessels and Their Innervation

Briefly, blood circulates through the body via the vascular tree that consists of arteries, veins, and capillary beds (Rahman et al 2021). Most commonly, small arteries open into muscular arterioles that branch into terminal arterioles forming the typical capillary bed arrangement of (i) terminal arterioles, (ii) metarterioles (i.e. precapillary sphincter area), (iii) capillaries, and (iv) postcapillary venules (Rhodin 1974; Hall et al 2020). The postcapillary venules are connected by collecting venules to the muscular venules (Rhodin 1974). An overall schematic diagram of this arrangement is shown in Figure 2.18.

Aside from capillaries, blood vessels are made up of three layers (Tucker et al 2021). Arterial vessels have:

- The *tunica externa* [*tunica adventitia*] or outer layer that provides structural support and shape to the vessel. (This is composed of a substantial sheath

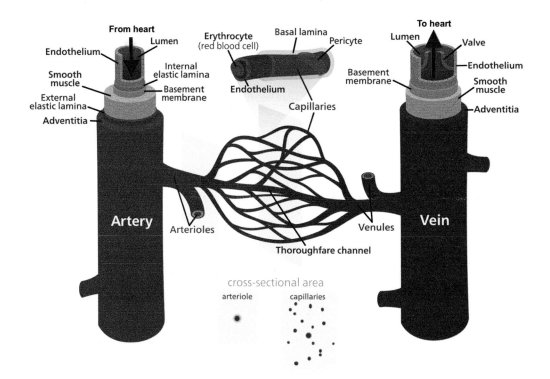

FIGURE 2.18 Schematic diagram of artery, aterioles, capillaries, venules, and veins that also shows cross-sectional area differences. Arterioles providing blood to the organs are chiefly composed of smooth muscle, and the autonomic nervous system influences the diameter and shape of the arterioles; capillaries are thin-walled vessels composed of a single endothelial layer that allows the exchange of nutrients and metabolites to occur by diffusion (Tucker et al 2021). Venules are the smallest veins and they receive blood from the capillaries; they also play a role in the exchange of oxygen and nutrients for water products—there are post-capillary sphincters located between the capillaries and the thin-walled venules that then allow blood to flow into the larger veins, and one-way valves inside veins allow for blood flow toward the heart (Tucker et al 2021).

Source: Reproduced with permission from https://commons.wikimedia.org/wiki/File:Blood_vessels-en.svg, https://creativecommons.org/licenses/by-sa/3.0/deed.en.

of connective tissue, consisting primarily of collag-enous fibres with some bands of elastic fibres (Betts et al 2019); within the connective tissue lie *nerve fibres* and blood vessels i.e. the *vasa vasorum* or 'blood vessels of blood vessels' (DiFiore 1967)).

- The *tunica media* or a middle layer composed of elastic and muscular tissue that regulates the internal diameter of the vessel. (There are fine elastic fibres interspersed within the circular smooth muscle fibres (DiFiore 1967)).
- The *tunica intima* or an inner layer consisting of an endothelial lining that provides a frictionless path-way for the movement of blood. (This is composed of a smooth muscle layer that contains one layer of endothelial cells and the rest is smooth muscle and elastin (Mercadante et al 2021)).

Within each layer, the amount of muscle and collagen fibrils varies, depending on the size and location of the vessel (Tucker et al 2021).

A *medium sized vein* has a large lumen and a relatively thin wall comprised of the following layers (DiFiore 1967):

- The *tunica externa* [*adventitia*] composed of a wide layer of connective tissue.
- The *tunica media* composed of a thin layer of circu-lar smooth muscle fibres.
- The *tunica intima* composed of only the endothe-lium; sometimes the tunica intima of a vein also has a thin layer of fine collagenous and elastic fibres.

Cross-sectional schematic and histological views to illustrate the anatomy of the arteries and veins are shown in Figure 2.19.

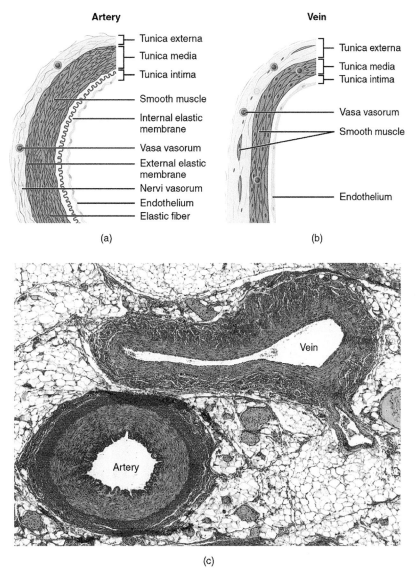

FIGURE 2.19   Cross sectional schematic and microscopic views of arteries and veins.

Source: **Reproduced with permission from OpenStax College, Anatomy and Physiology, Connexions Website. http://cnx.org/content/col11496/1.6 https://commons.wikimedia.org/wiki/File:2102_Comparison_of_Artery_and_Vein.jpg https://creativecommons.org/licenses/by/3.0/deed.en including the micrograph provided by the Regents of the University of Michigan Medical School © 2012.**

Vascular Pain

Naturally occurring biological substances have been implicated by Sicuteri et al (1974) as producing pain in vascular disorders; these include bradykinin, 5-hydroxy-tryptamine, potassium and adenosine triphosphate and are grouped under the term 'vasoneuroactive substances'.

Postganglionic sympathetic nerve fibres are localized to the adventitial-medial border of most arteries, arterioles, and veins throughout the body; venules and capillaries, which lack smooth muscle, are not directly innervated by sympathetic nerves (Thomas 2011). Nonetheless, Rahman et al (2021) state that sympathetic fibres are also extensively distributed in the capillary sphincter, and Rhodin (1974) found, near to the smooth muscle cells of the metarteriole (precapillary sphincter area), unmyelinated nerve fibres and denuded terminal axons with granular and agranular vesicles present.

Thus, sympathetic nerve fibres carried in the recurrent meningeal nerve (Figure 2.8) are thought to innervate blood vessels (Shayota et al 2019).

Neurotransmission in Sensory Nerves

It is worth noting that immunohistochemical studies indicate that *substance P* is not confined to primary sensory neurons (McGeer et al 1979); it is concentrated in certain neurons of the posterior root ganglia, basal ganglia, hypothalamus, and cerebral cortex (Schwartz 1981). It is present in 10–20% of spinal sensory neurons and is found within synaptic vesicles in the central terminals of sensory neurons located in laminae I and II of the posterior horn of the grey matter in the spinal cord (Jessell 1982).

It is considered that the presence of substance P in nerve fibres indicates a probable nociceptive function in these fibres (Henry 1982; Liesi et al 1983). Substance P may be involved in the mediation of mechanical nociception (Salt et al 1982), and the probable involvement of substance P containing fibres in conveying nociceptive information is reinforced by immunohistochemical observations following the application of the chemical desensitizing agent capsaicin (8-methyl-N-vanillyl-6-noneamide) (Cuello 1984). Further direct evidence of the role of substance P in nociception has been presented by Rossell (1982) who administered a substance P antagonist (D-Pro/2,D-Trp/7,9)-SP intrathecally to conscious rats, which caused hypoalgesia in the hot-plate test. According to Korkala et al (1985), substance P is known to participate in the sensory, especially nociceptive, transmission of neural impulses. Furthermore, in monkey spinal cords, substance P is present only in laminae of the dorsal horn which receive peripheral pain fibres (Carpenter 1985).

Although it is not possible to associate substance P with certainty with any specific sensory modality (McGeer et al 1979), it is suggested that it is associated with input for pain (Henry 1976; Jessell et al 1977), and Liesi et al (1983) suggest that it is involved in the primary pain transmission of low back pain.

This brief review of the role of substance P in spinal pain mechanisms has relevance to the innervation of synovial folds in the zygapophysial joints of the lumbar spine as discussed in Chapter 4.

Finally, radiating nerve root pain is likely to be based on structural changes in nerve fibres such as demyelination, including ischaemic factors (Rydevik 1993).

Lumbosacral Spine Innervation

General Overview

The overall basic pattern of innervation of the lumbosacral spine is briefly outlined in the schematic diagram shown in Figure 2.20.

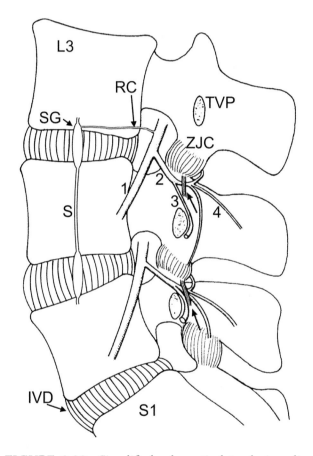

FIGURE 2.20 Simplified schematic lateral view diagram showing part of the lower lumbar (L3 to S1) spinal innervation. 1 = anterior ramus of the spinal nerve, suppling the psoas major muscles (via anterior rami of L1 to L4 (Siccardi et al 2021)) and quadratus lumborum muscles (via anterior branches of T12 and L1-L4 nerves (Moore et al 2018)); 2 = posterior ramus and its branches, supplying the deep layers of the intrinsic back muscles, although a few are also innervated by anterior rami (for example the intertransversarii and the quadratus lumborum muscles (Moore et al 2018)), and the zygapophysial joint capsule (ZJC); 3 = lateral branch of the posterior ramus suppling the iliocostalis lumborum muscles (via posterior rami) (Nomizo et al 2005); 4 = medial branch of the posterior ramus supplying the upper (adjacent) and

FIGURE 2.20 (Continued)

lower 'facet' joints before providing branches to the multifidus muscles (Saito et al 2013); RC = ramus communicans (grey) at the L3 spinal nerve level between the spinal nerve and the sympathetic chain (S); IVD = intervertebral disc; SG = sympathetic ganglion as part of the sympathetic chain that extends from C1 to the ganglion impar (Moore et al 2018); TVP = transverse process remains; arrows = mamillo-accessory ligaments that form an osseofibrous tunnel for the medial branch of the posterior ramus.

Source: Modified and reproduced with permission from Giles LGF, Anatomical basis of low back pain. Baltimore, Williams and Wilkins, © Wolters Kluwer, 1989). See Saito et al (2013) for detailed anatomy of the posterior ramus of the lumbar spinal nerve.

In order to provide a different perspective of the site of branching of a lumbar posterior ramus and its branches in the axial plane, see Figure 2.21.

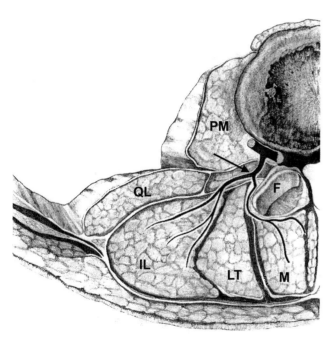

FIGURE 2.21 Diagram illustrating the site of branching (arrow) of a lumbar *posterior ramus* at the bottom of a tissue plane between the multifidus muscle (M) medially, and the longissimus thoracis muscle (LT) laterally. The course of the medial branch (> 1 mm diameter) is also shown in relation to the zygapophysial joint. F = facet of zygapophysial joint; IL = iliocostalis lumborum muscle; PM = psoas major muscle; QL = quadratus lumborum muscle. The lateral branch (~1.5 mm diameter) terminal fibres are not shown.

Source: Modified and reproduced with permission from Sunderland S 1975 Anatomical perivertebral influences on the intervertebral foramen. M Goldstein, Ed. *The research status of spinal manipulative therapy.* US Department of Health, Education, and Welfare,

FIGURE 2.21 (Continued)

Public Health Service, National Institutes of Health, National Institute of Neurological and Communicative Disorders and Stroke: Bethesda, Maryland 129–140. NINCDS Monograph No 15. Public Domain.

Usually, *white* and *grey* communicating rami are found between the levels of C8 and L2, while only grey rami are present above and below that area (Groen et al 2000). However, there is some ambiguity in the literature regarding the lowest level of white rami communicantes as Wilkinson (1986) suggests L2, Barr et al (1983) and Berry et al (1995) suggest sometimes to L3, Moore et al (2018) suggest L2 to L3, and Chusid (1985) suggests sometimes to L4. Below the L2 level, each anterior ramus receives a grey ramus communicans from the corresponding sympathetic ganglion (Kayalioglu 2008). Branches from the anterior rami of the S2-S4 spinal nerves join the pelvic plexus of the ANS (Kayalioglu 2008).

Figure 2.22A shows that each zygapophysial joint receives innervation from at least two adjacent spinal levels, in agreement with Sunderland (1975) who found that fine branches from the rami of at least two spinal nerves supply each joint. The posterior ramus nerve is responsible for transmitting pain generated in the facet joints, the periosteum of the posterior vertebral arch, the following ligaments: flaval, *posterior* longitudinal, interspinous, supraspinous, intertransverse (Figures 2.22B–D), as well as the superficial fascia and the deep muscles of the back (Gharries 2018).

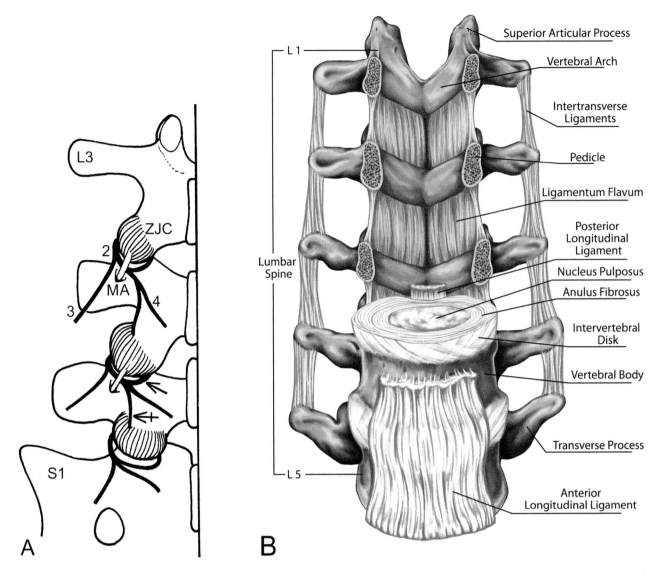

FIGURE 2.22 **(A)** Schematic posterior view diagram showing part of the lower lumbar spine innervation. Spinal nerves: 2 = posterior ramus and its branches supplying the posterior spinal muscles and zygapophysial joints; 3 = lateral branch of the posterior ramus; 4 = medial branch of the posterior ramus with an adjacent zygapophysial joint capsule (ZJC) articular branch (arrow), and a descending articular branch to the ZJC one joint lower (tailed arrow); MA = mamillo-accessory ligament. **(B)** Anterior to posterior view showing some spinal ligaments, while further detail for the ligaments is illustrated in the lateral view **(C)**, and in the posterior to anterior view **(D)**. (Also see Figure 2.33 that shows the ligamentous attachment of the lumbar spine to the sacrum.)

Source: **(A) Reproduced with permission from Giles LGF 1989 Anatomical basis of low back pain. Baltimore, Williams and Wilkins; (B, C, and D) Reproduced with permission from Shutterstock.com.**

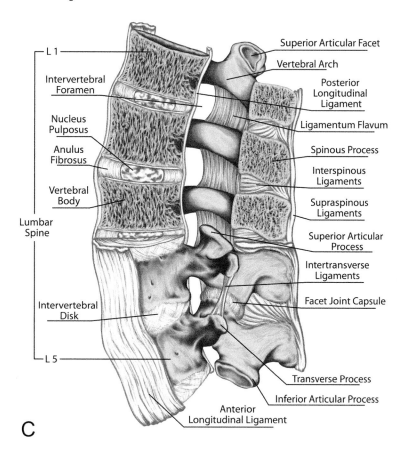

C

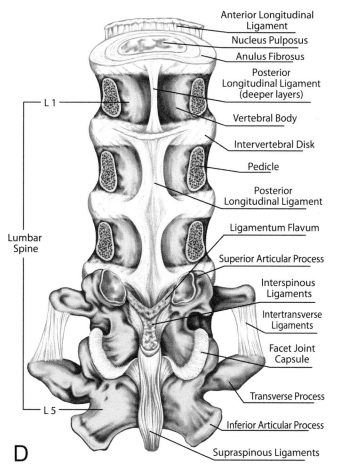

D

FIGURE 2.22   (Continued)

Briefly, ligaments are fibrous bands or sheets of connective tissue linking two or more bones, cartilages, or structures together, to provide joint stability and movement (Bridwell 2021). Three of the more important ligaments in the spine are the anterior and posterior longitudinal ligaments and the ligamenta flava (Bridwell 2021). The *anterior longitudinal ligament* is attached to the basilar occipital bone rostrally, extends to the anterior tubercle of the atlas (C1) as well as the front of the body of the axis (C2), then runs caudally to the anterior of the sacrum (Bannister et al 1996; Jones et al 2021(b)). The *posterior longitudinal ligament* rostrally is continuous with the tectorial membrane (Jones et al 2021(b)) and runs inside the spinal canal to extend from the C2 body to the sacrum (Bridwell 2021). As it attaches to the vertebral bodies from C2 to the sacrum, it often bridges the [epidural] fat and blood vessels between the ligament and bony surfaces (Moore et al 2018). In the lumbar region, part of it takes a horizontal path and extends out to the intervertebral foramen (Figure 2.22D), covering the lower half of the annulus fibrosus, and attaching to the lateral opening of the intervertebral foramen (Lang 1993; Jones et al 2021(b)). The *ligamenta flava* connect the lamina of the adjacent vertebrae (Jones et al 2021(b)) and form a cover over the dura mater to protect the spinal cord (Bridwell 2021). Inferiorly, the lateral portion of each ligamentum flavum extends to the midpoint between two pedicles and forms the anterior capsule of the zygapophysial joint (Jones et al 2021(b)). The *supraspinous ligament* connects the tips of the spinous processes from C7 to the sacrum (Moore et al 2018). The *interspinous ligament* connects adjoining spinous processes, attaching from the root to the apex of each process (Moore et al 2018) and extending between the supraspinous ligament posteriorly and the ligamenta flava anteriorly. The *intertransverse ligament* extends from the inferior border of one transverse process to the superior border of the adjacent transverse process (Bannister et al 1996). The *iliolumbar ligament* bilaterally extends from the tip of the anteroinferior aspect of the L5 transverse process, as well as the L4 transverse process in some cases, and it radiates laterally to attach to the pelvis (Bannister et al 1996; Jones et al 2021(b)). The lumbar *facet capsular ligament* fully encases the facet joint (Jones et al 2021(b)) by covering it in a rostral to caudal direction with a non-uniform thickness, which may vary from approximately 2.0 mm thick posteriorly, while being as much as 3.2 mm thick anteriorly (Jaumard et al 2011).

The innervation of the *anterior* longitudinal ligament is by the sympathetic trunk and grey rami communicantes nerves that are responsible for transmitting pain generated in this ligament, while the *posterior* longitudinal ligament is innervated by the recurrent meningeal nerve, which is responsible for transmitting pain generated in this ligament (Gharries 2018).

Free nerve endings are also present in the *posterior ligamentous structures* of the human lumbar spine i.e.

supraspinous ligament, interspinous ligaments, and ligamenta flava (Yahia et al 1989). In addition, the posterior ligamentous structures contain Paciniform and Ruffini corpuscles, suggesting that these posterior ligamentous structures could be involved in the spinal control system (Yahia et al 1989). In a scanning electron microscopy and immunohistochemical study of the *interspinous* and *longitudinal* ligaments, Yahia et al (1993) confirmed that nerve fibres are localised in the superficial layers of the ligaments as well as in the deeper ligamentous substance, and the immunohistochemical staining for neurofilament protein (NFP) clearly confirmed the presence of sensory nerve endings, most of which terminated as simple free endings thought to be nociceptors.

The sympathetic fibres carried in the recurrent meningeal nerve are thought to innervate much of the surrounding vasculature, including the vessels that supply blood to the outer annulus, endplates, vertebral bodies, and bone marrow (Shayota et al 2019). Furthermore, Nencini et al (2016) found that both the periosteum and the marrow cavity of bones must be innervated by primary afferent neurons capable of transducing and transmitting nociceptive information—these bone afferent neurons provide the CNS with information that elicits primary pain arising from bone.

The recurrent meningeal nerves, at every level of the vertebral column, are made up of plexiform branches of *rami communicantes* (Groen et al 1990). The column of vertebral bodies and IVD s is surrounded in its entire length by a continuous network of interlacing nerve fibres, and *anteriorly* this network is made up of the nerve plexus of the *anterior longitudinal ligament*, present at the lumbar, thoracic, and cervical levels, while *posteriorly* it consists of the nerve plexus of the *posterior longitudinal ligament* continuing from the cervical to the lumbosacral regions; contributions to both nerve plexuses are derived from the sympathetic trunks, rami communicantes, and perivascular nerve plexuses of segmental arteries (Groen et al 1990).

Furthermore, the *recurrent meningeal nerve* is responsible for transmitting pain generated in the posterior longitudinal ligament, the anterior surface of the spinal dura mater, the periosteum of the posterior aspect of a vertebral body, the posterior aspect of the IVD, and the epidural adipose tissue and veins (Gharries 2018). The *sympathetic trunk* and *grey rami communicantes* nerves are responsible for transmitting pain generated in the periosteum of the lateral and anterior aspects of the vertebral bodies, the anterior aspect of the IVD, and the anterior longitudinal ligament (Gharries 2018).

The segmental innervation of the lumbar spine is extensive as is shown in an axial view diagram illustrating parts of the IVD and the vertebral body (Figure 2.23). Note the extensive plexuses of nerves that accompany the anterior and posterior longitudinal ligaments (Groen et al 1990) and how the posterior longitudinal ligament plexus also innervates the dura mater and the associated root sleeves (not illustrated in Figure 2.23)

(Groen et al 2000). It should be recalled that the discs are innervated only in the *outer annulus fibrosus* by sensory and sympathetic perivascular nerve fibres, branches from the *recurrent meningeal nerve*, the anterior rami of spinal nerves, or from the *grey rami communicantes* (Tomaszewski et al 2015) and that the sensory fibres of the spinal nerve are intimately related to the zygapophysial joint (Sunderland 1978).

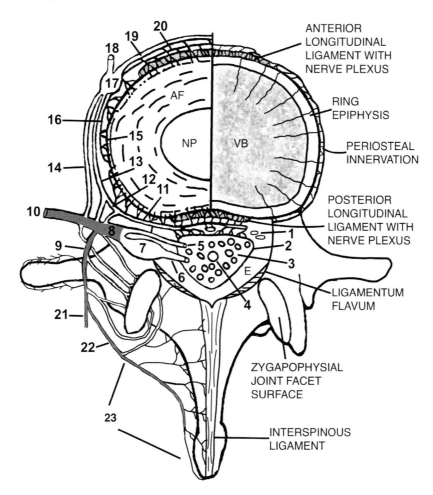

FIGURE 2.23 A schematic and not to scale axial view showing an upper lumbar vertebra (at approximately L3 level) with part of its intervertebral disc on the left and part of the top of the vertebral epiphysial ring and bone plate on the right. Detailed and extensive neuroanatomy is shown on the left side of this figure, and only a simplified neuroanatomical outline to the bone and periosteum from the grey ramus communicans is shown on the right side: 1 = epidural vasculature in the epidural fat space (E); 2 = dural tube; 3 = intrathecal nerve roots of cauda equina; 4 = filum terminale internum; 5 = anterior nerve root; 6 = posterior nerve root; 7 = posterior root spinal ganglion; 8 = main trunk of spinal nerve (coloured grey) formed by the junction of the anterior and posterior nerve roots just beyond the spinal ganglion where it is enclosed in the dural sheath surrounded by epineurium; 9 = posterior ramus of spinal nerve (coloured grey) that provides *sensory innervation of the zygapophysial joints* (Epstein 1976); 10 = anterior ramus of spinal nerve (coloured grey); 11 = recurrent meningeal nerve with branches carrying sympathetic fibres through the epidural space to supply the dural tube; 12 = autonomic (sympathetic) branch to the recurrent meningeal nerve; 13 = *grey ramus communicans* (*multilevel* irregular lumbosacral distribution); 14 = *white ramus communicans* (myelinated; not found above T1 or below L2–3–4 *); 15 = lateral sympathetic efferent branches projecting from grey ramus communicans; 16 = lateral paraspinal afferent sympathetic ramus projecting to paraspinal sympathetic ganglion (PSG—17); 18 = paraspinal sympathetic chain; 19 = anterior paraspinal afferent sympathetic ramus projecting to PSG; 20 = anterior sympathetic efferent branches projecting from PSG; (Note: afferent and efferent sympathetic paraspinous branches/rami may be partially combined in vivo); 21 = lateral branch of posterior ramus (coloured grey) to posterior peri-spinal tissues; 22 = medial branch of posterior ramus (coloured grey); 23 = neural fibres associated with zygapophysial joints, lamina, spinous process, interspinous and supraspinous ligaments.

Source: Reproduced with permission from Jinkins JR, The anatomic and physiologic basis of local, referred and radiating lumbosacral pain syndromes related to disease of the spine, Journal of Neuroradiology; 31(3): 163–80. © 2004 Elsevier Masson SAS. All rights reserved. Modified *There appears to be some ambiguity in the literature regarding the lowest level of the *white ramus communicans*, as previously mentioned.

Essentially, the IVDs and related ligaments, psoas major and quadratus lumborum muscles are innervated by various branches of the *anterior* rami and sympathetic nervous system, while the *posterior* elements of the vertebral column, including the zygapophysial joints and back muscles, are innervated by branches of the posterior rami of the spinal nerves (Bogduk 1997). In a study of the human foetus vertebral column, Groen et al (1990) showed that the *anterior nerve plexus* consists of the nerve plexus associated with the anterior longitudinal ligament; this longitudinally orientated nerve plexus has a bilateral supply for many small branches of the sympathetic trunk, rami communicantes, and perivascular nerve plexuses of segmental arteries. The *posterior nerve plexus* is made up of the nerve plexus associated with the posterior longitudinal ligament and is more irregular and receives contributions only from the recurrent meningeal nerves that originate from the rami communicantes (Groen et al 1990).

A lateral view diagram in which the spinal dura is represented as a cylinder with dural sleeves to emphasize the dural tube's highly innervated *anterior surface* is shown in Figure 2.24. Although the *anterior* dura is heavily innervated (Groen et al 1988), the *posterior* dura is sparsely innervated (Richardson et al 2005).

Figure 2.24 provides insight into how a *posterior or posterolateral* IVD herniation could press upon the anterolateral side of the spinal dura—or the spinal nerve—and the associated spinal branches of the radicular arteries and recurrent meningeal nerves and, therefore, likely result in a sensation perceived as pain when they are activated.

The basic neuroanatomical structures for the lumbar spine intervertebral foramen contents are the anterior and posterior branches and the recurrent meningeal nerve branch (Pallure 2017). Some intervertebral foramen contents are shown schematically in the parasagittal section in Figure 2.25, which does not include any transforaminal ligaments.

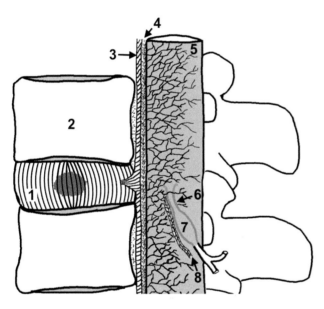

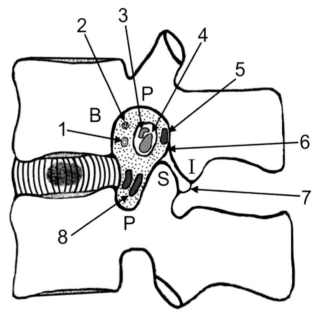

FIGURE 2.24 Schematic lateral view of the *dural tube* with its related structures viewed from the left side, following resection of some bony structures. Note the extensive *recurrent meningeal nerve plexus* on the anterolateral surface of the dura. It is partly supplied by branches from the perivascular nerve plexus of the radicular arteries, and it gives off some branches to lateral parts of the dura, while the middle two quarters of the posterior dura are devoid of nerve fibres (Groen et al 2000). 1 = intervertebral disc with its nucleus pulposus and lamellae; 2 = vertebral body; 3 = posterior longitudinal ligament; 4 = epidural fat space; 5 = dura mater; 6 = nerve root sleeve; 7 = spinal ganglion; 8 = perivascular nerve plexus of radicular arteries.

FIGURE 2.25 Schematic diagram showing a parasagittal section of the intervertebral foramen contents and its boundaries. B = body of upper vertebra; P = pedicles above and below the foramen; I = inferior articular process of upper vertebra; S = superior articular process of lower vertebra. The intervertebral foramen contents within the epidural fat (dotted area) are: 1 = radicular artery; 2 = recurrent meningeal nerve; 3 = anterior root of spinal nerve; 4 = posterior root ganglion of spinal nerve; 5 = radicular vein; 6 = ligamentum flavum; 7 = fibrous joint capsule of the zyapophysial joint; 8 = foraminal veins; no lymphatics are shown, although they are present (Hadley 1950).

The vascular and neural structures, including the dural tube, are surrounded by the epidural fat space (Figure 2.26)—this space extends from the foramen magnum of the skull to the sacral hiatus (Ellis 2006). The epidural fat does not usually adhere to these structures, allowing mobility of the dura within the vertebral canal (Reina et al 2009).

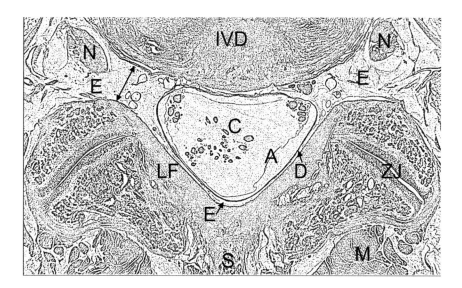

FIGURE 2.26 Schematic diagram showing an axial (horizontal) view of some of the contents of the spinal canal and the intervertebral foramina in order to illustrate their epidural fat (E) distribution and some of its adjacent structures, such as the dural tube (D), ligamentum flavum (LF), neural complex (N), and intervertebral disc (IVD). In addition, the following structures are shown: A = arachnoid mater; C = cauda equina; M = muscle; S = remains of spinous process; ZJ = zygapophysial synovial joint; arrow shows the dimension of the intervertebral foramen.

In summary, other than the zygapophysial joints being innervated by *articular branches* of the *medial branches* of the *posterior rami*, the vertebral column is innervated by *recurrent meningeal nerve branches* of the spinal nerves (Figure 2.27) that are distributed to (i) the anterolateral aspect of the vertebral bodies and IVDs, the periosteum and anterior longitudinal ligament and (ii) the contents of the spinal canal including blood vessels, posterior longitudinal ligament, posterior and posterolateral aspect of the IVDs, ligamenta flava, periosteum covering the posterior vertebral bodies, pedicles and laminae, and the spinal dura mater (Moore et al 2018). The function of these afferent and sympathetic fibres is unclear, although it is known that the afferent fibres supply *nociceptors* that could be involved in the referred pain characteristic of spinal disorders and become activated when there is inflammation of the meninges (Moore et al 2018).

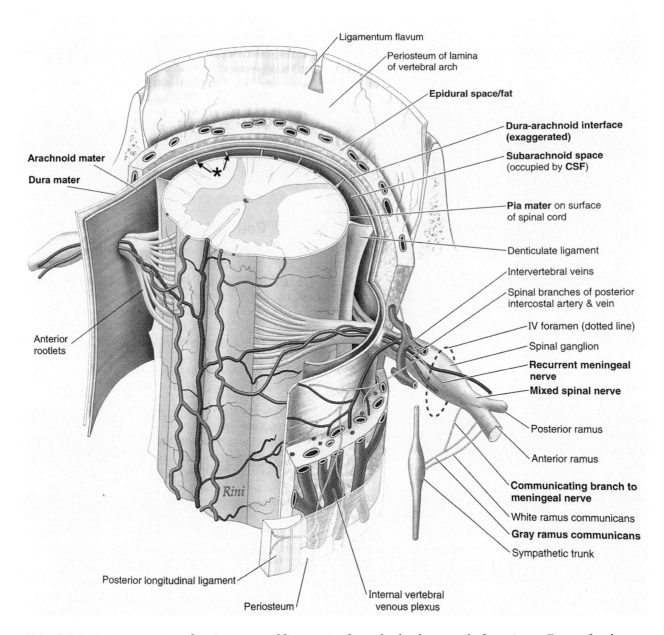

Ligamentum flavum

Periosteum of lamina
of vertebral arch

Epidural space/fat

**Dura-arachnoid interface
(exaggerated)**

Subarachnoid space
(occupied by **CSF**)

Pia mater on surface
of spinal cord

Denticulate ligament

Intervertebral veins

Spinal branches of posterior
intercostal artery & vein

IV foramen (dotted line)

Spinal ganglion

**Recurrent meningeal
nerve**

Mixed spinal nerve

Posterior ramus

Anterior ramus

**Communicating branch to
meningeal nerve**

White ramus communicans

Gray ramus communicans

Sympathetic trunk

Arachnoid mater

Dura mater

Anterior
rootlets

Rini

Posterior longitudinal ligament

Periosteum

Internal vertebral
venous plexus

FIGURE 2.27 Innervation of periosteum and ligaments of vertebral column and of meninges. Except for the zyg-apophysial joints and external elements of the vertebral arch, the fibroskeletal structures of the vertebral column (and the meninges) are supplied by the *(recurrent) meningeal* nerves. Although usually omitted from diagrams and illustrations of spinal nerves, these fine nerves are the first branches to arise from all 31 pairs of spinal nerves and are the nerves that initially convey localized pain sensation from the back produced by acute herniation of the IV disc or from sprains, contusions, or fractures of the vertebral column itself. [Note the arachnoid trabeculae (*) spanning the subarachnoid space.]

Source: **Based on Frick H, Kummer B, Putz R. Wolf-Heidegger's Atlas of Human Anatomy, 4th ed. Basal, Switzerland: Karger AG, 1990:476. Modified and reproduced with permission from Moore KL, et al, Clinically Oriented Anatomy, 8th Edn, © Wolters Kluwer, 2018, and Frick HF, et al., Wolf-Heidegger's Atlas of Human Anatomy, 4th edn, © S Karger AG, Basel, 1990.**

Central Nervous System and Its Relationship to Cerebrospinal Fluid

As previously mentioned, the spinal cord is enclosed in the *dura, arachnoid*, and *pia maters*—these structures are separated from each other by the *subdural* and *arachnoid* spaces, the former being merely *potential* and the latter containing the CSF (Berry et al 1995). Delicate strands of connective tissue, the *arachnoid trabeculae* (Figure 2.27), span the subarachnoid space connecting the spinal arachnoid and pia maters (Moore et al 2018). These three membranes surround, support, and protect the spinal cord and spinal nerve roots, including those of the cauda equina, in conjunction with the CSF in which these structures are suspended (Moore et al 2018).

The spinal cord and nerve roots are devoid of lymphatic vessels, as previously mentioned, and their vascular supply is via radicular arteries and veins, while physiochemical homeostasis is maintained by the diffusion barrier in the deep arachnoid layer and by the blood-nerve barrier in the intraneural vascular endothelial cells; also CSF 'flow' must play an important role in replacing the lymphatic vessels that the spinal cord and nerve roots lack (Yoshizawa 2002). CSF 'movement' (rather than 'circulation') (Oreskovic et al 2014) is affected by the downward pull of gravity, the continual process of secretion and absorption, blood pulsations in contingent tissues, respiration, and body movements (Encyl Brit 2018). Such movement plays vital functions including providing nourishment and elimination of wastes (Spector et al 2015) as the considerable metabolic activity of the CNS requires an efficient system of tissue drainage and detoxification (Thomas et al 2019).

Ultimately, the lymphatic system does play an important role in CSF absorption (Sokolowski et al 2018) by removing foreign material (Richardson et al 2005) such as solutes, lipids, immune cells, and cellular debris (Dupont et al 2019). In the spinal subarachnoid space, the part of the CSF absorbed by the epidural venous plexus and spinal nerve sheaths enters the lymphatic system, while the remaining CSF 'flows' rostrally towards the cranial subarachnoid space (Sakka et al 2011). It is important to understand the anatomical and physiological relationships between CSF and its drainage into the lymphatic system as arachnoid villi function like 'valves' that allow CSF and its contents to flow readily into venous blood, while not allowing blood to flow backward in the opposite direction (Hall et al 2020).

Patients with disc herniation and sciatica have increased concentrations of neurofilament and S-100 proteins in CSF, which indicates damage of axons and Schwann cells in the affected nerve root (Brisby et al 1999) and which is assumed to be due to leakage of plasma proteins into CSF from the nerve root (Skouen et al 1997), probably through the blood-nerve root barrier (Skouen et al 1993; Skouen et al 1994).

The CSF also dynamically conveys signals modulating the development and the activity of the nervous system, an observation that implies that cues from the CSF could act on neurons in the spinal cord and brain via bordering receptor cells; candidate neurons to enable such modulation are the cerebrospinal fluid-contacting neurons (CSF—cNs) that are located precisely at the interface between the CSF and neuronal circuits (Djenoune et al 2017). The atypical apical extension of CSF-cNs bears a cluster of microvilli bathing in the CSF, indicating putative sensory or secretory roles in relationship with the CSF (Djenoune et al 2017). Altogether, neurons contacting the CSF appear as a novel sensory modality enabling the detection of mechanical and chemical stimuli from the CSF and modulating the excitability of spinal circuits underlying locomotion and posture (Djenoune et al 2017).

The spinal arachnoid villi were first described in humans by Hassin (1930) and Tubbs et al (2007) quantified their numbers regionally in the spinal dural nerve sleeve region (excised 1 cm lateral and medial to the intervertebral foramina), describing them in detail to aid in understanding the physiological characteristics of CSF absorption. Their study found that the arachnoid villi/arachnoid granulations in the human spinal dural nerve sleeves are 50 to 170 microns long (mean 110 microns) and noted that the majority of villi protruded into—or were juxtaposed with—an adjacent radicular vein (Figure 2.28).

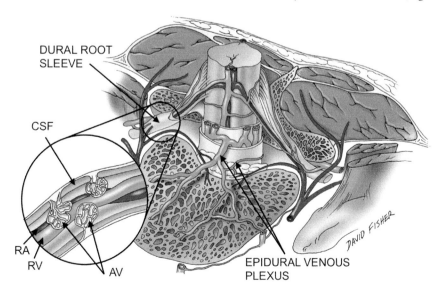

FIGURE 2.28 A drawing showing the arachnoid villi (AV) as found in the spinal *dural root sleeves*. CSF = cerebrospinal fluid; RA = radicular artery; RV = radicular vein. Note the epidural venous plexus.

Source: Reproduced with permission from Tubbs RS, et al., Human spinal arachnoid villi revisited: immunohistological study and review of the literature. J Neurosurg Spine 7:328–31, 2007; American Association of Neurological Surgeons; lettering modified.

As a clear coupling of these structures was demonstrated, it seems reasonable that these structures may have the ability to convey CSF to regional veins and thus recirculate this fluid and that such a vast surface area, as is afforded by the spine, would certainly rival the ratio of arachnoid villi to dural venous sinuses as seen intracranially and ostensibly make this region at least as important in CSF absorption (Tubbs et al 2007). A lumbar region photomicrograph illustrates a dense collection of arachnoid cells (Figure 2.29).

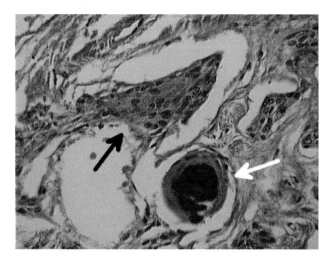

FIGURE 2.29 Photomicrograph illustrating a dense collection of arachnoid cells (black arrow) from the lumbar region, with psammoma-like calcification (white arrow) forming a small arachnoid villus. (H and E stain. Original magnification x132).

Source: **Reproduced with permission from Tubbs RS, et al., Human spinal arachnoid villi revisited: immunohistological study and review of the literature. J Neurosurg Spine 7:328–31, 2007; American Association of Neurological Surgeons.**

This study demonstrated that *spinal arachnoid villi* exist in the lumbar, thoracic, and cervical regions and have an *intimate relationship with adjacent radicular veins* (Tubbs et al 2007).

Furthermore, Kido et al (1976) found that *human spinal arachnoid villi and granulations* were either (i) located entirely internal to the dura, (ii) extended into the dura, or (iii) penetrated the dura completely; most venous sinuses were closely related to arachnoid proliferations.

At the entrance point of posterior *rootlets* in the spinal cord, *arachnoid cisterns* were described by Dauleac et al (2019), and *lymphatics* are present around the region of the nerve root even though they are absent in the nerve root itself (Richardson et al 2005), as mentioned previously. *Lymphatics of the epidural space* are concentrated in the region of the *dural roots* where they remove foreign materials including microorganisms from the subarachnoid and epidural spaces (Niharika et al 2017).

Absorption of CSF from the dural tube and nerve roots is shown schematically in Figure 2.30.

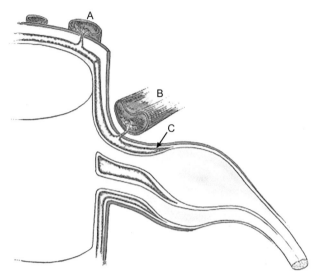

FIGURE 2.30 Cerebrospinal fluid absorption by spinal arachnoid villi and meningeal sheaths of spinal nerves. Spinal arachnoid villi in contact with the epidural venous plexus (A) and adjacent to spinal nerve roots (B). Absorption surfaces in the meningeal recess of spinal nerve roots (C).

Source: **Reproduced with permission from Sakka et al. Anatomy and physiology of cerebrospinal fluid. European Annals of Otorhinolaryngology, head and neck diseases 2011; 128: 309–316. Copyright © 2021 Elsevier Masson SAS. All rights reserved.**

The constant secretion of CSF contributes to complete CSF renewal four to five times per 24-hour period in the average young adult (Telano et al 2020), and the fine balance between the secretion, composition, volume, and turnover of CSF is strictly regulated (Bothwell et al 2019). Thus, the CSF has the function of *hydromechanical protection* of the neuraxis (Sakka et al 2011), while also playing an essential role in maintaining the *homeostasis* of the CNS and *draining into both the venous and lymphatic systems* (Matsumae et al 2016).

The vascularity of the spinal cord and spinal nerve roots (Figure 2.27) is important as pressure on these structures may cause pain of ischaemic origin (Sunderland 1975; Rydevik et al 1984) due to accumulation of lactic acid in the tissues, formed as a consequence of anaerobic metabolism that occurs during ischaemia; it is also probable that other chemical agents, such as bradykinin and proteolytic enzymes, are formed in the tissues because of cell damage and that these, rather than lactic acid, stimulate the pain nerve endings (Hall et al 2020). Spinal nerve root compression, including the PRG, alters nerve root conduction and compromises the nutritional support of spinal nerve roots (through intrinsic and extrinsic vascularity and CSF percolation) (Garfin et al 1995).

In view of the foregoing, it could be *hypothesized* that, if decreased spinal movement occurs, this may lead to sluggish CSF movement and its drainage of metabolic waste products into the vertebral veins due to the intimate relationship between the spinal CSF and the venous system. This possible build-up of metabolic waste products around the anterior and posterior nerve roots within the intervertebral foramen may affect basic physiological functions that are required for normal nerve function. For example, it may cause impaired nerve action potentials due to a possible breakdown of the sodium pump mechanism, in turn leading to an abnormal flow of impulses along the associated nerve fibres, with related breakdown of the cell's Krebs citric acid cycle. Therefore, it seems sensible to encourage people to *keep active*, just as activity is encouraged for other good health lifestyle outcomes. This is an area requiring animal laboratory research.

Additional Anatomical Structures That May Give Rise to Lumbosacral Pain Syndromes

It is important to consider the following brief summary of some anatomical structures that may give rise to lumbar, sacroiliac, hip, and groin pains, with or without radicular symptoms, as low back pain is now the number one cause of disability globally (Hartvigsen et al 2018).

Cluneal Nerves

The pivot of the rotation of the trunk is at the T12 level i.e. at the thoraco-lumbar junction, where most of the rotation of the trunk takes place in everyday activities; this may result in a lesion or dysfunction of the corresponding facet joint that has a close relationship with the posterior ramus of a spinal nerve at the thoraco-lumbar junction (Maigne 1974), resulting in irritation of the nerve.

The lateral branches of the posterior ramus of the thoraco-lumbar junction (Maigne et al 1989) at the T12, L1 or L2 levels innervate the cutaneous area of the iliac crest as their branches become superficial as *cluneal* nerves i.e. sensory nerves that innervate the skin (Maigne 1980; Maigne et al 1991; Maigne 1996; Quon et al 1999). As a schematic example of a T12 posterior ramus and its emerging superficial cutaneous branches as superior cluneal nerves at the iliac crest, see Figure 2.31.

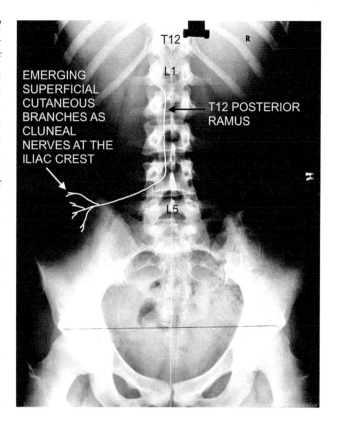

FIGURE 2.31 Schematic diagram of the approximate path of the T12 posterior ramus with the cluneal nerves at the iliac crest.

Apart from *cluneal nerves* being associated with low back pain in the region of the posterior iliac crest (Maigne 1980, 2000), they can also be associated with pain projecting into the buttock (Maigne et al 1997) (Figure 2.32).

The origin of Maigne's thoraco-lumbar syndrome due to a segmental dysfunction of the facet joints is highly treatable with spinal manipulation, injections and percutaneous rhysotomy (Maigne 1997; Maatman et al 2019). In fact, when Maigne's syndrome is suspected, the diagnosis is confirmed by alleviation of pain following manipulation or injection into the involved zygapophysial joints (Bernard et al 1999).

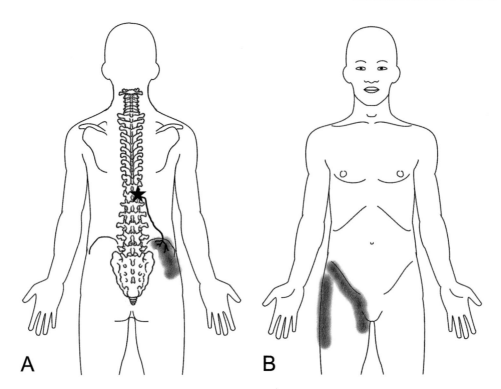

FIGURE 2.32   Maigne's Syndrome. **(A)** Unilateral low back pain referred via the *cluneal* nerves supplying the skin near the iliac crest from the T11-L1 region. Tenderness to deep palpation over the area of pain is approximately 7 cm from the midline of the spine. **(B)** Pain may be felt on the lateral aspect of the hip region and groin area via the lateral cutaneous branch of the subcostal and iliohypogastric nerves.

Furcal Nerves

The *furcal* nerve is a common cause of atypical presentation of sciatica/radicular symptoms—it is an independent nerve that is present most commonly at L4 level (Izci et al 2005) and the majority of furcal nerves bifurcate extra-foraminally (Harshavardhana et al 2014). The furcal nerve is an accessory spinal nerve originating from the cord independently of other lumbar nerve roots that includes an anterior and a posterior component; the furcal nerve can be found in all subjects, is generally single, and, in most cases, its roots emerge from the spinal cord and run within the thecal sac beside the L4 root (Kikuchi et al 1986; Postacchini et al 1999(b)). Occasionally, two furcal nerves may be present, i.e. L3 and L4 or L4 and L5; sometimes only one L5 furcal nerve is present. The posterior root of the furcal nerve has a ganglion situated, as for the normal posterior roots, at the level of the intervertebral foramen; once the nerve has left the intervertebral foramen with the roots proper of that level, with which it constitutes a single radicular nerve, it gives off three branches, contributing to form, respectively, the femoral nerve, the obturator nerve, and the lumbosacral trunk (Postacchini et al 1999(b)). The clinical relevance of the furcal nerve is that disc herniation, or other pathological

conditions, may impinge upon both the radicular nerve proper of that level and on the furcal nerve, thus causing atypical bi-radicular syndromes (Kikuchi et al 1986; Postacchini et al 1999(b)). According to Haijiao et al (2001), MRI provides accurate information on lumbosacral nerve root anomalies.

Sacroiliac Joint

The understanding of low back pain would be seriously hampered by neglecting the sacroiliac (SI) joints (Vleeming et al 1996) as they are known to be a source of low back pain (Aprill 1992; Quon et al 1999; Barros et al 2019), which is widely overlooked (Barros et al 2019), often with referral to the buttock, the posterior thigh, and sometimes the calf (Quon et al 1999). In view of this, it is necessary to consider the anatomy of some of the pelvic bony and associated ligamentous soft tissue structures (Figure 2.33).

Stability of the *SI joints* that consist of a cartilaginous and a fibrous or ligamentous compartment (Kampen et al 1998) is provided by a strong articular capsule and the powerful posterior sacroiliac and interosseous sacroiliac ligaments (IOSILs) (Figures 2.33) that tightly knit and strengthen the joint, while allowing minimal movement (Rickenbacher et al 1985; Weisel 1955; Sturesson et al 1989).

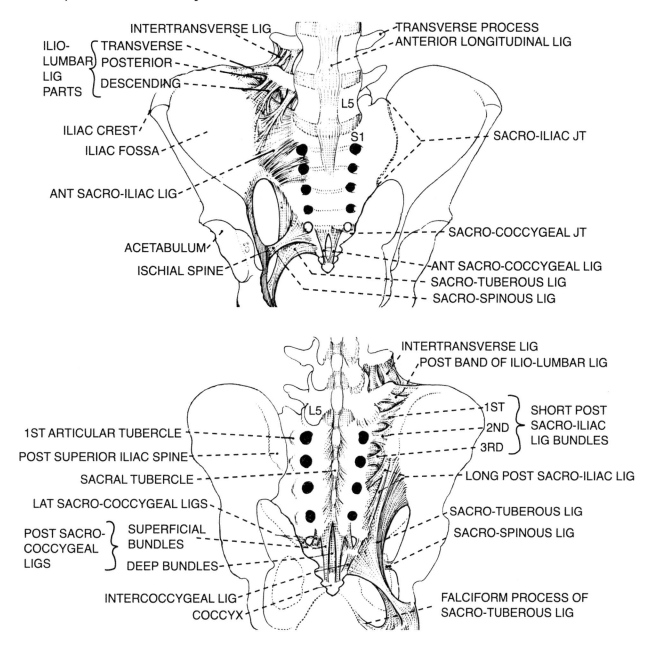

FIGURE 2.33 The anterior and posterior ligaments are shown. The three ligaments that stabilize the pelvis, sacrum, and the fifth lumbar vertebra are the iliolumbar, sacrotuberous, sacrospinous ligaments, respectively (Hanson et al 1994).

Source: Modified from Pauchet B, Dupret S, Pocket Atlas of Anatomy, 3rd edn, London, Oxford University Press, 1965. Reproduced with permission of the Licensor through PLSclear.

The positions of the sacral *auricular surface* and the adjacent sacral *tuberosity* that is rough and deeply pitted by attachment of ligaments (Soames 1995) are shown in a slightly oblique posterior view of the sacrum (Figure 2.34A). The internal aspect of the left hip bone with its auricular surface and iliac tuberosity is shown in Figure 2.34B.

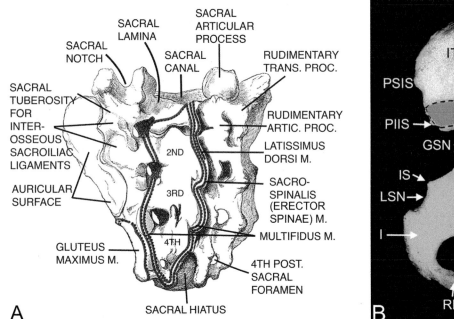

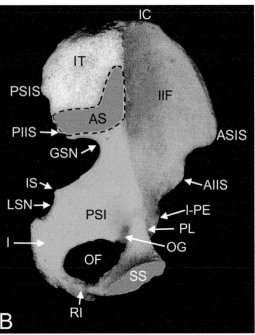

FIGURE 2.34 **(A)** This slightly oblique view particularly illustrates the auricular surface—which is covered by articular cartilage—and the *tuberosity* of the sacrum. The positions of the sites of origin for the muscles named on the posterior of the sacrum are illustrated as shown by the dotted lines. **(B)** Internal aspect of the left hip bone showing its auricular surface (AS)—which is covered by articular cartilage—and the iliac tuberosity (IT) to which the interosseous and posterior sacroiliac ligaments are attached, spanning the gap between the iliac and sacral tuberosities. AIIS = anterior inferior iliac spine; ASIS = anterior superior iliac spine; GSN = greater sciatic notch; I = ischium; IIF = internal iliac fossa; I-PE = ilio-pubic eminence; IS = ischial spine; LSN = lesser sciatic notch; OF = obturator foramen; OG = obturator groove; PIIS = posterior inferior iliac spine; PL = pectineal line; PSI = pelvic surface of ischium; PSIS = posterior superior iliac spine; RI = ramus of ischium; SS = symphysial surface. To this is firmly attached a thin lamina of hyaline cartilage, which in turn blends with the surface of a thick, strong, but deformable pad (or disc) of fibrocartilage (Soames 1995) that is sandwiched between the articular surfaces of paired pubic bones to form the pubic symphysis (Becker et al 2010).

Source: (A) Modified and reproduced with permission from Gray H 1858 Anatomy of the Human Body. Philadelphia, Lea and Febiger. Public Domain. https://commons.wikimedia.org/wiki/File:Gray96.png), (B) Reproduced with permission from Giles LGF, Crawford CM, Sacroiliac Joint. In: Giles LGF, Singer KP The Clinical Anatomy and Management of Low Back Pain, Edinburgh, Butterworth-Heinemann, © Elsevier, 1997(b), p. 173–182.

An anteroposterior X-ray view showing the upper region of the pelvis with its S-I joints (Figure 2.34C) and an axial CT myelogram scan across the sacroiliac joints (Figure 2.34D) are shown.

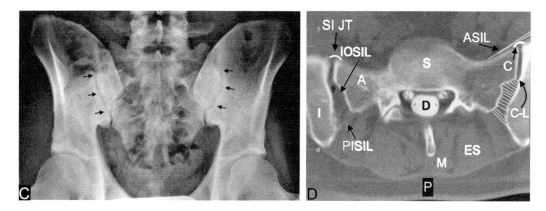

FIGURE 2.34 **(C)** Plain X-ray view showing SI joints bilaterally (arrows). **(D)** CT myelogram axial image through the S1–2 level showing the corresponding SI joints at this level (SI JT). The synovial part of the joint is located *anteriorly*; the *posterior* ligamentous part contains the *interosseous sacroiliac ligament* (IOSIL) and the adjacent *posterior interosseous sacroiliac ligament* (PISIL)—both of these ligaments are shown schematically for the interosseous part of the joint on the right side of the image. A = ala of sacrum; C= thin joint capsule anteriorly covered by the *anterior sacroiliac ligament* (ASIL); C-L = the change from the *anteriorly* situated cartilage of the synovial joint to the *posterior* ligamentous compartment. D = dural tube; ES = erector spinae muscle; I = ilium; M = multifidus muscle; S = sacrum.

The sacroiliac joint is a diarthrodial synovial joint—it is surrounded by a fibrous capsule containing a joint space filled with synovial fluid between its articular surfaces (Wong et al 2020). The histological structure of the sacroiliac joints is shown in Figures 2.34E and F.

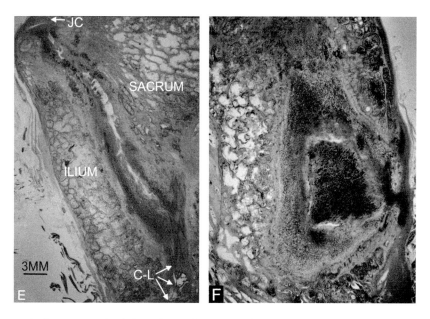

FIGURE 2.34 **(E and F)** 200 μm thick histological sections from the synovial joint regions of the SI joints of a 59-year-old female showing some osteoarthritic changes. **(E)** Was cut in a slightly oblique axial plane and shows the length of the cartilaginous part (at this level for this cadaver) between its iliac and sacral cartilages and their adjacent bone marrow. JC = thin *joint capsule* anteriorly that lies beneath the anterior sacroiliac ligament; the change from the synovial joint's cartilaginous region to the posterior ligamentous compartment is shown (C-L); there is no capsule posteriorly because the interosseous sacroiliac ligaments form the posterior margin of the joint space. **(F)** A section cut through the plane of the auricular surface of the SI joint's cartilaginous area to illustrate its ridges and depressions, albeit in a one plane section.

There is no true joint capsule superiorly where the IOSILs are located but, inferiorly, the joint does have an *innervated synovial lined joint capsule* and cartilaginous surfaces that probably contain a mixture of hyaline and fibrocartilage (Bernard et al 1997).

The anteroposterior rotatory movement appears to range from 2 degrees (Egund et al 1978) to 12 degrees (Lavignolle et al 1983). The anteroposterior rotation occurs around the transverse axis about 5–10 cm vertically below the sacral promontory (Weisel 1955).

The *articular part* of the sacral side usually involves the first, second, and third sacral levels (Solonen 1957; Rosse et al 1997; Forst et al 2006, Butler et al 2012). It is a complex joint with two parts, as mentioned earlier, i.e. an anterior *synovial* part and a posterior *ligamentous* part (Herregods et al 2016). The synovial joint area is located in the *anterior* and *lower third* of the joint with cartilage on the joint surfaces (Figure 2.34E) surrounded with synovium, while the ligamentous part is located in the *posterior* and *upper two-thirds* of the joint, where the sacrum and the ilium are connected with restraining ligaments (anterior and posterior sacroiliac, interosseous, sacrotuberous, and sacrospinous ligaments) (Puhakka et al 2004; Herregods et al 2016). In addition, thin section light microscopy has shown that the cartilage on the *iliac side* consists of a mixture of hyaline and fibrous cartilage, whereas there is pure hyaline cartilage on the *sacral side* (Hermann et al 2014).

The depth of the cartilage on the sacral surface ranges from 0.2 to 2.4 mm, while on the iliac surface the range is 0.1–1.8 mm, indicating that the sacral cartilage is, on average, 1.7 times thicker than that of the iliac surface (Walker 1986). In addition, Vleeming et al (1990) showed the presence of cartilage covered ridges and depressions that are complimentary on the opposing auricular surfaces of the sacroiliac joints.

A series of CT axial images (Figure 2.35A-L) beginning at the lumbosacral level superiorly, then progressing inferiorly through the sacrum to show the anatomy of the bilateral SI joints of a 55-year-old male (involved in a minor pelvic injury), illustrates the *anterior* location of the joint's synovial and cartilaginous part, as well as its *posterior* ligamentous part. The left sided L5-S1 posterior IVD bulge was reported as were some minor degenerative changes in the SI joints—all muscles of the pelvic girdle were reported as being normal.

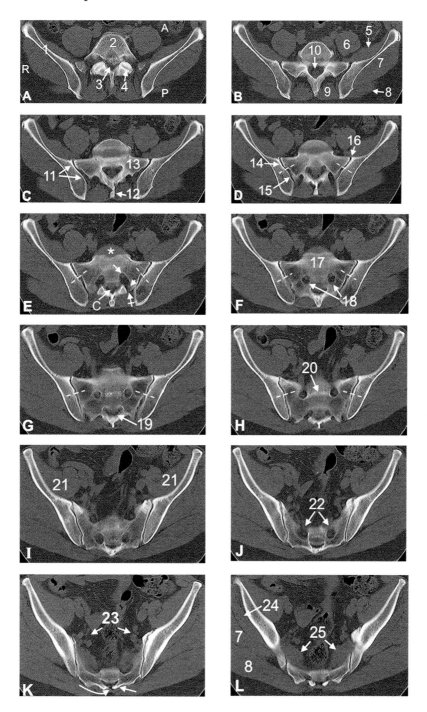

FIGURE 2.35 A series of CT axial images beginning at the lumbosacral level are illustrated in this figure. **(A)** A = anterior; P = posterior; R = right side of scans; 1= ilium; 2 = upper part of sacrum; 3 = lumbosacral canal with significant left sided posterior intervertebral disc bulge causing spinal stenosis with encroachment on the left L5-S1 neural foramen; 4 = left L5-S1 zygapophysial 'facet' joint; **(B)** 5 = iliacus muscle (m); 6 = psoas m; 7 = gluteus medius m; 8 = gluteus maximus; 9 = multifidus/erector spinae ms; 10 = dural tube/thecal sac within the central sacral canal and two bilateral S1 nerve roots; **(C)** 11 = right S-I joint; 12 = sacral tubercle; 13 = sacral ala. This section indicates that the sacral canal now has a triangular configuration. **(D)** 14 and 15 = the synovial cartilaginous part of the S-I joint anteriorly and the ligamentous part posteriorly. The dashed lines across the S-I joint in some of the images illustrate where the anterior cartilaginous synovial joint transitions to the ligamentous part posteriorly; 16 = S-I joint; **(E)** (*) = sacral promontory; arrow = the larger S1 anterior nerve root leaving the anterior sacral foramen; tailed arrow = posterior sacral foramen through which the smaller posterior S1 nerve root leaves (arrow head); C = cauda equina within the central sacral canal; **(F)** 17 = sacrum; 18 = bilateral posterior sacral foramina containing S2 nerve roots; **(G)** 19 = central sacral canal; **(H)** 20 = site of fusion between sacral bodies; **(I)** 21 = iliopsoas m; **(J)** 22 = bilateral anterior sacral foramina; **(K)** 23 = external and internal iliac arteries and veins; the sacral hiatus (curved arrow) with adjacent left and right sacral cornua (arrow); **(L)** 24 = gluteus minimus m; 25 = piriformis muscle.

As early as 1905, Goldthwait and Osgood emphasized mobility of the sacroiliac joint and suggested that an *acute or chronic slip*, or *subluxation*, of the joint could cause pain and suggested that the variability of symptoms may be attributable to differing degrees of mobility. Furthermore, as the cartilage-covered ridges and depressions are normally complementary on opposing auricular surfaces (Vleeming et al 2012), when the joints are subjected to abnormal [mechanical] loading conditions, they may be forced into a new position where the ridges and depressions are *no longer complementary*, theoretically causing a *blocked joint* (Vleeming et al 1990), resulting in low back pain due to the innervation of the SI joints.

The superior surface of a block of osteoligamentous tissues, cut in the axial plane through the sacrum and parts of its adjacent ilia, at the level of the first left and right sacral foramina, is shown in Figure 2.36.

Part of a histological section, cut in the axial plane from the anatomical block in Figure 2.36, is shown in Figure 2.37. This figure shows part of the IOSIL in the retroarticular space of the SI joint cavity, which is the main determinant of sacral movement (Vukicevic et al 1991). It is a powerful and very strong ligament uniting the ilium and sacrum, which fills the irregular space immediately above and behind the SI joint and is covered by the posterior sacroiliac ligament (Williams et al 1980). The IOSIL is the largest of the sacroiliac joint ligaments (Steinke et al 2010).

Using oblique transaxial thin histological sections through a normal SI joint, Madsen et al (2010) confirmed that the transition between the *anterior cartilaginous* and *posterior ligamentous* parts of the joint space are clearly demarcated. The posteriorly located joint ligaments insert directly into the cartilage anteriorly; there is no synovium and the entire ligamentous joint space is rich in vessels (Madsen et al 2010) (Figure 2.37).

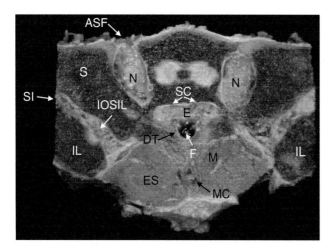

FIGURE 2.36   The superior surface of a block of osteoligamentous tissues showing the sacrum (S), adjacent ilia (IL), first anterior sacral foramen (ASF) containing the anterior root of the first sacral spinal nerve (N) and accompanying vascular structures and epidural fat within the length of the first anterior spinal foramen that is approximately 10–15 mm long (Whelan et al 1982); same orientation for Figure 2.37. The posterior ligamentous parts of the left and right SI joints (SI) are shown at this level. The sacral canal (SC) is seen centrally and contains epidural fat (E), vascular structures, and the lower portion of the dural tube (DT) and the filum terminale (F). ES = erector spinae muscle; IOSIL = interosseous sacroiliac ligament in the posterior region of the SI joint cavity (Vleeming et al 1992(a)) that contains blood vessels and adipose tissue; M = multifidus muscle; MC = median sacral crest.

Source:**Reproduced with permission from Giles LGF, Crawford CM, Sacroiliac Joint. In: Giles LGF, Singer KP The Clinical Anatomy and Management of Low Back Pain, Edinburgh, Butterworth-Heinemann, © Elsevier, 1997(b), p. 173–182.**

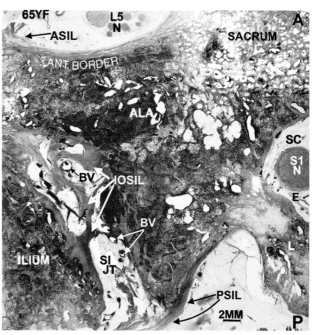

FIGURE 2.37   A 200-µm-thick histological section cut in the axial plane from a 65-year-old female showing parts of the left side of the sacrum and adjacent ilium at the level of the first sacral segment. A = anterior; P = posterior. The anterior border of the sacral ala is shown, with part of the adjacent anterior sacroiliac ligament (ASIL) and neural structures forming part of the fifth lumbar nerve (L5 N). The sacral canal (SC) contains neural structures forming part of the first sacral nerve (S1 N) and epidural (E) adipose tissue containing vascular structures. Part of the posterior interosseous sacroiliac ligament (PSIL) behind the upper recess is seen bridging between the sacrum and the ilium i.e. across the ligamentous part of the SI joint cavity (SI JT); BV = blood vessels, some

FIGURE 2.37 (Continued)
of which are seen coursing through the adipose tissue within the joint's upper recess; IOSIL = parts of the interosseous sacroiliac ligament in the retro-articular space.

Source: **Reproduced with permission from Giles LGF, Crawford CM, Sacroiliac Joint. In: Giles LGF, Singer KP The Clinical Anatomy and Management of Low Back Pain, Edinburgh, Butterworth-Heinemann, © Elsevier, 1997(b) p. 173–182.**

The adult SI joint will accept a volume of 1–2 cc of injectate but the addition of more fluid distends the joint (Aprill 1992) that most often remains patent throughout life (Cassidy 1992) as there is still a demonstrable joint space well into the eighth and ninth decades (Greenman 1992). However, during old age, the SI joint can become partially ossified, especially in men, and calcification in the anterior sacroiliac ligaments makes the joint cavities

less visible on radiographs, even though they are still present (Moore 1992). The adipose tissue with blood vessels seen within the joint's posterior upper recess (Figure 2.37) may serve as a shock-absorbing function for the incongruent surfaces, vessels, and ligaments (Poilliot et al 2019).

The *innervation* of the lower lumbar and sacral region is summarized in Figures 2.38A and B where the fifth lumbar nerve (N5) descends in a groove on the ala of the sacrum, immediately lateral to the articular facet, and it can be traced downwards as the lateral division before it joins the lateral division of the first sacral nerve (S1) (Bradley 1974). The medial division of the L5 nerve curves under the lumbosacral zygapophysial joint, sending tiny branches to it; the lateral division of the L5 nerve, supplies the posterior sacroiliac ligament and joint (Bradley 1974). The nerve plexus on the posterior aspect of the sacrum has also been described by various authors such as Bernard et al (1997) and Murakami (2019).

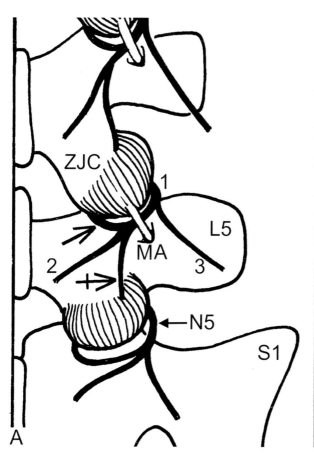
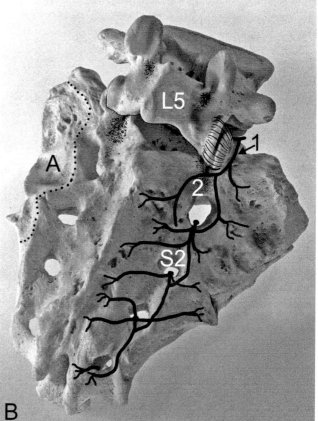

FIGURE 2.38   **(A)** A schematic diagram showing part of the lower lumbar spinal innervation (posterior view). 1 = posterior ramus of the L4 spinal nerve; 2 = medial branch of the posterior ramus with an adjacent ZJC (articular) branch (arrow) and a descending articular branch to the ZJC one joint lower (tailed arrow); 3 = lateral branch of the posterior ramus; MA = mamillo-accessory ligament that forms an osseofibrous tunnel for the medial branch; ZJC = zygapophysial joint capsule. The L5 posterior ramus (N5) is shown providing branches to the posterior first sacral (S1) level. **(B)** A schematic diagram showing only the nerve plexus formed on the right posterior aspect of the sacrum by the posterior rami of the lower lumbar and sacral nerves that also innervate the sacroiliac joint and its overlying ligaments. 1 = posterior ramus of the L5 spinal nerve;

FIGURE 2.38   (Continued)

2 = medial branch of the posterior ramus with an adjacent ZJC (articular) branch; S2 = second sacral foramen branches. A = auricular surface of the sacrum for articulating with the auricular surface of the ilium. As the branches of the posterior rami of the sacral nerves emerge through the posterior sacral foramina they are accompanied by branches of the sacral arterial and venous vessels (Rickenbacher et al 1985).

Source: **(A) Reproduced with permission from Giles LGF, Anatomical basis of low back pain. Baltimore, Williams and Wilkins, © Wolters Kluwer, 1989.**

Thus, sacroiliac joint innervation *posteriorly* is via the sacral nerve plexus' posterior rami (Bradley 1974) and is considered to be from the posterior rami of L5 to S2 (Rickenbacher et al 1985; Wong et al 2020) and the plexiform arrangement of small nerve branches from the posterior rami from L5, and the sacral foramina, lies on the posterior surface of the sacrum in contact with the IOSIL and the sacrotuberous ligament—it is deeply situated on bone and ligamentous tissue beneath the multifidus and sacrospinalis muscles, with extension to the deep and superficial parts of the posterior sacroiliac ligament (Figure 2.38B) (Bradley 1974; Sunderland 1975). Furthermore, immediately upon emerging from the sacral foramina, the posterior rami of the sacral nerves divide into medial and lateral branches, anastomosing with those of adjacent segments—*lateral branches* run to the skin and the *medial branches* ramify in the muscles, seldom reaching the skin (Rickenbacher et al 1985).

The *anterior* sacroiliac ligament is innervated by anterior branches from the sacral plexus (S1–4) (Rickenbacher et al 1985) and possibly small filaments of the obturator nerve (L2–4) (Sunderland 1968).

Overall, the SI joint is well innervated, with variation among individuals, and innervation may be mainly derived from the sacral posterior rami, which might account for the variable patterns of referred pain from the SI joint (Wong et al 2020). Furthermore, Vilensky et al (2002) demonstrated in a histological study of neural elements in the human sacroiliac joint, the presence of nerve fibres and mechanoreceptors in the sacroiliac ligament indicating that the CNS receives information—certainly proprioceptive—and possibly pain from the sacroiliac joint as immunohistochemical staining for substance P, the neurotransmitter known to signal pain from the periphery, showed reactive elements that may have been nerves.

The anterior *blood supply* to the sacroiliac joint occurs by an anastomosis between the median sacral artery and the lateral branches from the internal iliac artery (Figure 3.12); they enter the anterior sacral foramina and anastomose with the posterior sacroiliac blood supply from the gluteal arteries and venous drainage is from the tributaries from the median and lateral sacral veins (Bernard et al 1997).

Clinical Implications of Sacroiliac Joint Mechanical Dysfunction

Sacroiliac joint dysfunction can be exacerbated by various physical manoeuvres that are thought to stress the joint (Mooney 1992). The syndrome is a common condition likely resulting from a *mechanical derangement* of the joint (Kirkaldy-Willis 1988) and may be associated with a small degree of subluxation, based on the apparent success of manipulation directed at the SI joint (Allan et al 1989; Bowen et al 1991).

The importance of sacroiliac syndromes in the causation of low back pain has gained increasing recognition, partly due to the clinical and radiological studies by Schmid (1980), which showed a larger range of movement in the SI joints than was previously supposed. Shaw (1992) states that SI joint dysfunction is a very common cause of low back pain and, according to Schmid (1980), the main feature of the sacroiliac syndrome is the paroxysmal character of the pain which may fluctuate widely during rest and movement and may not be confined to the vicinity of the SI joint, radiating into the groin, trochanteric area, or distal parts of the posterior thigh, and occasionally, pain may be referred down the lateral or posterior areas of the calf to the ankle, foot, and toes (Quon et al 1999).

Aprill (1992) developed a technique for consistent opacification of the joint space. Schwarzer et al (1995), using SI joint diagnostic blocks under image intensifier protocols, concluded that the SI joint is a significant source of pain in patients with chronic low back pain; in some cases the sacroiliac joint arthrogram showed an anterior capsule tear with leakage of radiographic contrast, although such tears are not pathognomonic of SI joint pain but indicate some form of traumatic disruption of the joint as the injections into the joint were not sufficiently forcible to disrupt a normal joint capsule.

The effect of significant (> 9 mm) LLI on the SI joints is unknown but it is reasonable to assume that it may result in excessive unilateral stress on the SI joint capsule, its ligaments, and its articular cartilage (Dihlmann 1980) (Figure 2.39).

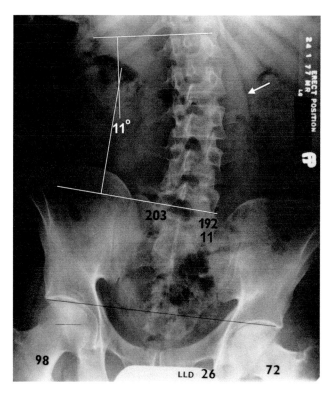

FIGURE 2.39 Radiograph of a 37-year-old male with a right leg length deficiency of 26 mm and a postural scoliosis of 11 degrees using the Cobb (1948) method of measurement. Note the more prominently displayed lateral border of the psoas major muscle (arrow) on the convex side. There is some wedging of the intervertebral discs—particularly at L4–5 with the discs being narrower on the left side.

FIGURE 2.39 (Continued)
Source: Modified and reproduced with permission from Giles LGF, Anatomical basis of low back pain. Baltimore, Williams and Wilkins, © Wolters Kluwer, 1989.

It is generally accepted that the relationship of SI joint dysfunction, osteoarthrosis, and sacroiliac syndrome to LLI is unknown (Bernard et al 1987; Cassidy et al 1992; Dreyfuss et al 1994).

In young individuals, bony structures are sometimes seen within the SI joint but are considered normal (Funke et al 1992). In addition, it should be noted that asymmetry in form and function of the SI joint is normal (Vleeming et al 1992(b)).

Intervertebral Disc Degeneration

Having listed, in Chapter 1 (Table 1.1), numerous possible causes of specific and non-specific lumbosacral spine pain syndromes, many of which would not be seen on imaging, Figures 2.40–2.43 are reproduced from the paper by Kushchayev et al (2018) *"ABCs of the degenerative spine"*, that provides an excellent source of in-depth information on the topic of *overt* degenerative changes, due to mechanical failure or degeneration, that can give rise to pain, for example from IVD and endplate degenerative change.

(A) A Classification of Disc Displacements

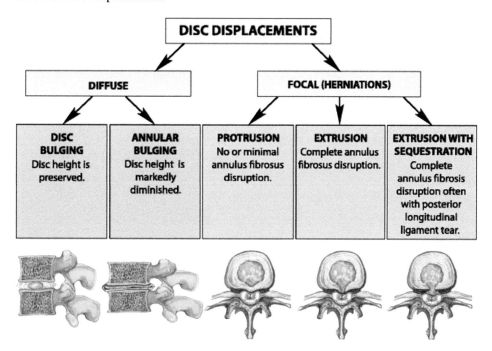

FIGURE 2.40 A schematic diagram illustrating the classification of intervertebral disc displacements.

Source: Reproduced with permission from Kushchayev et al 2018 ABCs of degenerative spine. Insights into Imaging 9: 253–274; Creative Commons Attribution 4.0 International License (http://creativecommons.org/licenses/by/4.0/.

(B) A Classification of Focal Disc Displacements (Herniations)

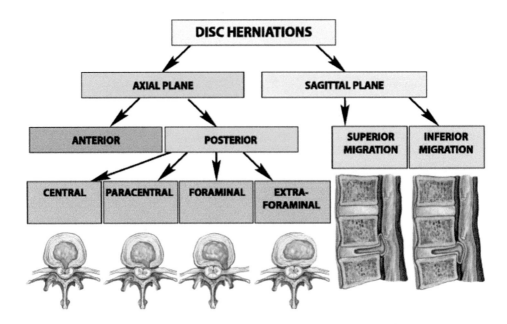

FIGURE 2.41   A schematic diagram illustrating the classification of focal intervertebral disc displacements/herniations.

Source: Reproduced with permission from Kushchayev et al 2018 ABCs of degenerative spine. Insights into Imaging 9: 253–274; Creative Commons Attribution 4.0 International License (http://creativecommons.org/licenses/by/4.0/.

An example of a posterior epidural IVD migration is not shown in Figures 2.40 and 2.41.

(C) A Classification of Endplate Changes

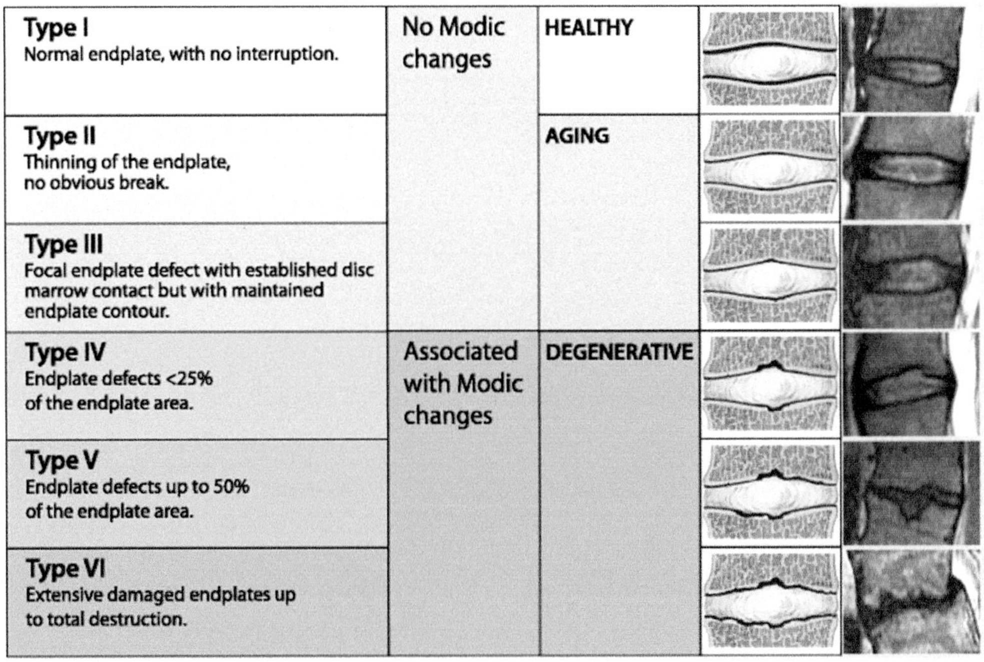

	No Modic changes	HEALTHY		
Type I Normal endplate, with no interruption.	No Modic changes	HEALTHY		
Type II Thinning of the endplate, no obvious break.		AGING		
Type III Focal endplate defect with established disc marrow contact but with maintained endplate contour.				
Type IV Endplate defects <25% of the endplate area.	Associated with Modic changes	DEGENERATIVE		
Type V Endplate defects up to 50% of the endplate area.				
Type VI Extensive damaged endplates up to total destruction.				

FIGURE 2.42   A schematic diagram and MRI illustrations in the sagittal plane to show differences between healthy, aging, and degenerative endplate changes.

Source: Reproduced with permission from Kushchayev et al 2018 ABCs of degenerative spine. Insights into Imaging 9: 253–274; Creative Commons Attribution 4.0 International License (http://creativecommons.org/licenses/by/4.0/.

(D) **A Grading System of Intervertebral Disc Degeneration**

Grade I	Disc has a uniform high signal in the nucleus on T2.	
Grade II	Central horizontal line of low signal intensity.	
Grade III	High intensity in the central part of the nucleus with lower intensity in the peripheral regions of the nucleus.	
Grade IV	Low signal intensity centrally and blurring of the distinction between nucleus and annulus.	
Grade V	Homogeneous low signal with no distinction between nucleus and annulus.	

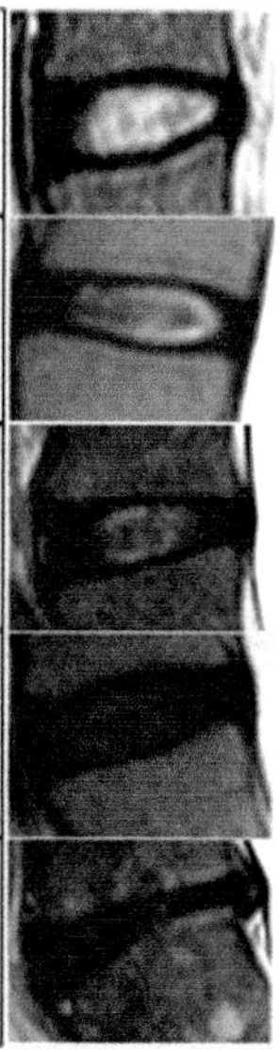

FIGURE 2.43 A series of sagittal plane MR images illustrating the grading system of intervertebral disc degeneration.

Source: Reproduced with permission from Kushchayev et al 2018 ABCs of degenerative spine. Insights into Imaging 9: 253–274; Creative Commons Attribution 4.0 International License (http://creativecommons.org/licenses/by/4.0/.

In a prospective 30-year follow-up MRI study of disc degeneration in young low back pain patients, Sääksjärvi et al (2020) concluded that, in low back patients, early degeneration in lumbar discs predicts progressive degenerative changes in the respective discs but not pain, disability, or clinical symptoms.

Using a study population comprised of 831 twin volunteers from Twins UK (mean age 54 +/− 8 years; 95.8% female), T2-weight magnetic resonance images showed endplate defect is strongly and independently associated with degenerative disc disease at every lumbar disc level (Rade et al 2018).

Brief Summary of the Muscles of the Back: Their Basic Function and Innervation

The function of most muscles in the back is concerned with maintenance of posture and movements of the vertebral column (spine) (Moore 1997). This function is supported by the systems of strong fibrous bands of ligaments that hold the vertebrae and discs together and stabilize the spine by helping to prevent excessive movements; the three major spinal ligaments are the (i) anterior longitudinal ligament, (ii) posterior longitudinal ligament, and (iii) ligamentum flavum Figure 2.22B–D (Eidelson 2021).

There are two major groups of muscles in the back and they are divided into *extrinsic* and *intrinsic* groups (De Sai et al 2020; Henson et al 2021).

The *extrinsic* back muscles include *superficial* and *intermediate* muscles that produce and control limb and respiratory movements, respectively; the *superficial extrinsic* back muscles (trapezius, latissimus, dorsi, levator scapulae, and rhomboids) connect the vertebral column with the pectoral girdle and humerus and produce and control limb movements (Moore et al 2018).

The *intrinsic* (deep) back muscles include muscles that fuse with the vertebral column (Henson et al 2021) and specifically act on the vertebral column, producing its movements and maintaining posture (Rickenbacher et al 1985; Moore et al 2018). They are grouped according to their relationship to the surface i.e. *superficial layer* (splenius capitis, splenius cervicis), *intermediate layer* (erector spinae/sacrospinalis group i.e. iliocostalis, longissimus, spinalis), *deep layer* (transversospinalis group i.e. semispinalis, multifidus and rotatores), and *minor deep layer* (interspinales, intertransversarii, levatores costarum) (Moore et al 2018). The intrinsic deep muscles are enclosed by fascia and are short muscles associated with the spinous and transverse processes (Henson et al 2021).

Some of the intrinsic deep muscles of the back are shown in Figure 2.44, and a partial transverse section of the lumbosacral spine muscles is shown in Figure 2.45, which includes the sacrospinalis muscle i.e. erector spinae group of muscles (Quiring et al 1960).

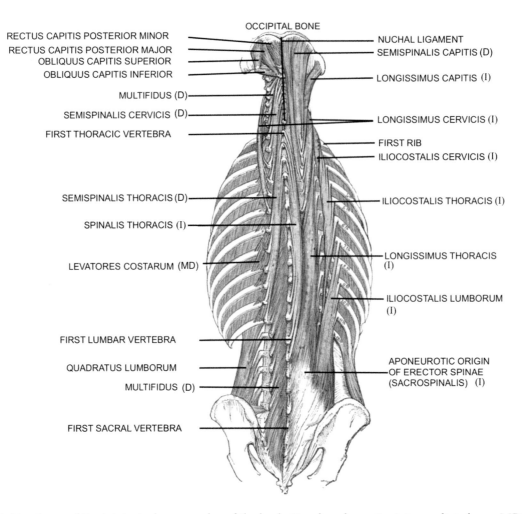

FIGURE 2.44   Some of the intrinsic deep muscles of the back: D = deep layer; I = intermediate layer; MD = minor deep layer.

Source: **Reproduced with permission from Gray H 1858 Anatomy of the Human Body. Philadelphia, Lea and Febiger. Public Domain. https://commons.wikimedia.org/wiki/File:Gray389.png. Lettering modified.**

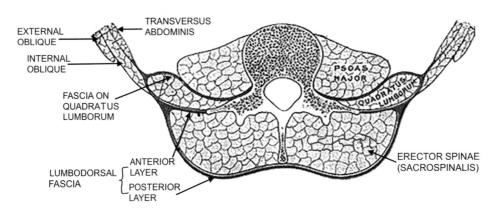

FIGURE 2.45   Partial transverse section of the lumbosacral spine muscles showing the location of the intrinsic back muscles and the layers of fascia associated with them and some of the abdominal wall muscles.

Source: **Reproduced with permission from Gray H 1858 Anatomy of the Human Body. Philadelphia, Lea and Febiger. Public Domain. https://commons.wikimedia.org/wiki/File:Gray388.png. Lettering modified.**

Although the quadratus lumborum muscle is considered to be a deep muscle of the abdomen it resides in the deep, posterior, lateral, and inferior areas of the spine, involving the iliac crest, the transverse processes of the lumbar vertebrae (L1-L4), and the twelfth rib (Bordoni et al 2021).

Although the muscle tracts are listed separately, they form a functional entity (Rickenbacher et al 1985). The clinical significance of back muscles is that their chief pathology is associated with muscle pain, as the muscles develop spasms that may be debilitating—thus, the lower back muscles and the neck muscles are common causes of low back and neck pain, respectively (Henson et al 2021).

The spinal nerve *posterior ramus* is responsible for transmitting pain generated in the superficial fascia and the deep muscles of the back (Gharries 2018), while and the quadratus lumborum muscle innervation is from the spinal nerve *anterior ramus* of T12, L1, L2, L3 (Quiring et al 1960).

Chronic muscle pain remains a significant source of suffering and disability despite the adoption of pharmacologic and physical therapies; it is mediated by free nerve endings distributed through the muscle along arteries (Gregory et al 2014). Mechanical forces, ischaemia, and inflammation are the primary stimuli for muscle pain (Gregory et al 2014).

Chapter 3
GROSS ANATOMY AND HISTOLOGY OF THE LUMBOSACRAL SPINE

Abstract: This chapter illustrates lumbosacral spine anatomy using gross anatomy and histological images to include the spinal canal's epidural space and some of its ligaments. Lumbosacral vertebrae, intervertebral discs, and cartilage endplates are shown in detail with emphasis placed upon the disc-cartilage endplate interface. Cartilage endplates play an irreplaceable role in maintaining the unique physiological environment within the disc with its interface allowing essential diffusion into the disc and removal of waste products of metabolism. Solute transport into the disc is discussed. The basivertebral canal nerve bundle with recurrent meningeal nerves, entering the vertebral body posteriorly via the vascular foramen, with its branches extending toward the endplates, is illustrated. The vertebral column blood supply is summarized, as is the importance of the vertebral spongy bone's marrow spaces bounded by bony trabeculae. Arterial and venous systems of the vertebral bodies and their association with cartilage endplates, arterial and venous capillary buds, and adjacent haematopoietic marrow contact channels is illustrated. The "three-joint complex" is shown radiologically, anatomically, and histologically with the associated vertebral foramen and its contents. Issues relating to degeneration of the intervertebral disc and the zygapophysial facet joint hyaline articular cartilage are discussed. A series of 15 sequential 200-micron thick histological sections from the posterior nerve root ganglion in the mid-zone beneath the pedicle, and progressing to the exit zone, show that in a relatively normal foraminal canal the neurovascular structures have an adequate areolar tissue buffer.

Key words: epidural space, cartilage endplates, solute transport, basivertebral canal nerves, recurrent meningeal nerves, vertebra blood supply, spongy bone, capillary buds/tufts, marrow channels, three-joint-complex

Contents

Introduction

The preceding neuroanatomical/neurophysiological background lays the foundation for the consideration of mechanical spinal pain syndromes that may arise from the *motion segment* (Figure 3.1), so named by Junghanns in 1950 (Schmorl et al 1971). The *motion segment* consists of the IVD (with the *nucleus pulposus, annulus fibrosus, and the cartilaginous endplates*), the anterior and posterior longitudinal ligaments, the zygapophysial joints, the ligamenta flava, the contents of the spinal canal, the left and right intervertebral foramina, and the spaces between the adjacent spinous and transverse processes, as well as the numerous ligaments between the various small joints and vertebral arches and the corresponding muscular parts (Schmorl et al 1971). Many disturbances originate from the motion segment and therapy is the *restoration of normal function* (Schmorl et al 1971).

DOI: 10.1201/9781003315964-3

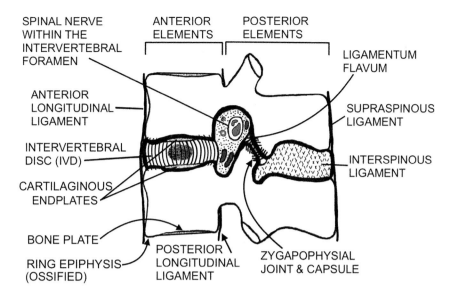

FIGURE 3.1   Schematic and not to scale parasagittal plane diagram of the motion segment surrounded in black. The intervertebral disc is shown with its lamellae, nucleus pulposus, and cartilage endplates. The endplates are within the ring epiphysis. The nucleus pulposus is located slightly posteriorly within the disc, and the inner annular fibres (*lamellae*) attach to the endplates with the outer annular fibres attaching to the ring epiphysis (Cailliet 1995).

The following figures help to set the stage regarding overall orientation for the reader with respect to sectioning planes of gross anatomical specimens and of histological sections, presented in this chapter:

1. Figure 3.2A is a lateral lumbosacral spine plain X-ray image from a 70-year-old female cadaver with its corresponding sagittally bisected anatomical specimen (Figure 3.2B). *Sagittal* and *parasagittal* histology sections are shown in Figures 3.2C and D, respectively.
2. Figure 3.3 is an area of a parasagittally sectioned lumbar spine (L1–2 level) from a 52-year-old female cadaver to show greater anatomical detail of spinal osseous and soft tissue structures, particularly of the *spinal canal contents*, at that level.
3. Figure 3.4 is an axial histological view at the L5-S1 level of a 36-year-old female cadaver, showing the contents of the spinal canal and intervertebral

foramina, with adjacent osseous structures. An *anterior Hofmann's epidural ligament* (Hofmann 1899) is demonstrated. An example of an anterior Hofmann's ligament is also shown on an enlarged MRI axial scan view (Figure 3.5).

All histological sections were stained with *Ehrlich's haematoxylin and light green counterstain*, unless a different staining technique is described in the caption.

In most captions the structures identified have been listed in alphabetical order for the convenience of the reader.

Sharpey's fibres are found at the annular periphery (Kushchayev et al 2018), and they pass from the discs into the bony ridges around the circumference of the adjacent vertebrae and also into the cartilaginous plates on the opposing surfaces of the vertebrae (Rickenbacher et al 1985) (Figure 3.2C).

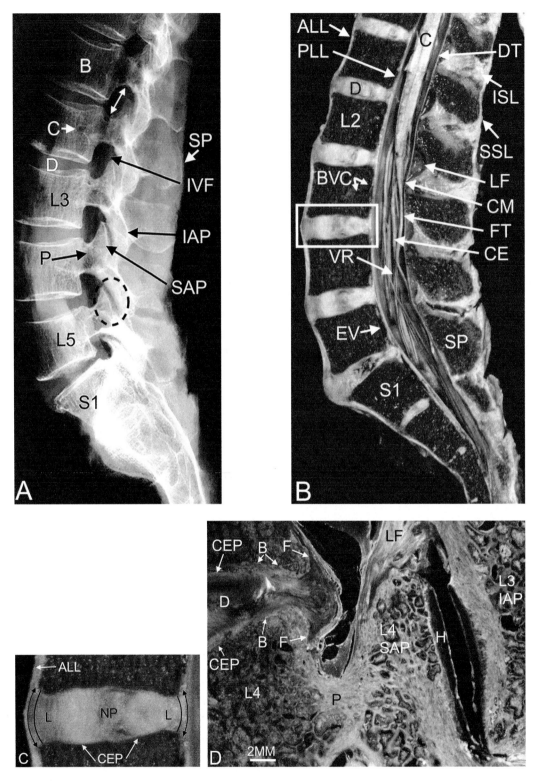

FIGURE 3.2 **(A)** A lateral view X-ray image of the lumbosacral spine of a 70-year-old female showing vertebral bodies (B), with canal for basivertebral nerve and vasculature (C), intervertebral discs (D), intervertebral foramen (IVF), and superior and inferior vertebral notches (double headed arrow); inferior articular processes of the vertebrae e.g. L3 vertebra (IAP) with its facet opposing the facet of the superior articular process (SAP) of the L4 vertebra below—combined they form the synovial *zygapophysial joint* or '*facet joint*' (dashed oval). P = pedicle; SP = spinous process; S1 = first sacral segment. **(B)** Sagittally cut anatomical specimen shown in **(A)**. Vertebral bodies have a posterior canal for the *basivertebral* vasculature (BVC) and the *basivertebral nerve bundle* (not seen at this magnification); EV = *anterior internal vertebral (epidural) venous plexus* in the anterior epidural fat space; D = intervertebral discs; DT = dural tube within the spinal canal containing the lower part of the spinal cord (C) that ends as the conus medullaris (CM) and gives rise to the filum terminale *internum* (FT); CE = cauda equina nerve roots with their blood supply i.e.

FIGURE 3.2 (Continued)

vasa radiculorum (VR); SP = spinous process. Spinal ligaments that can be seen in this plane are the: ALL = anterior longitudinal ligament that is intimately attached to the anterior aspect of the vertebral body, until it reaches the vertebral endplate—at the level of the disc, the ligament is connected to the annulus fibrosus by fairly loose connective tissue (Postacchini et al 1999(b)); ISL = interspinous ligament; LF = ligamentum flavum; PLL = posterior longitudinal ligament, the central portion of which is firmly attached to the vertebral endplates and adjacent *discs* but not to the concavity of the vertebral bodies, thus leaving an epidural fat space occupied by vessels entering—or exiting from—the vertebral body (Postacchini et al 1999(b)). SSL = supraspinous ligament. The rectangle at the L3–4 disc is shown enlarged in (C). **(C)** The nucleus pulposus (NP) is slightly posterior of central; the outermost lamellae (L) of the annulus fibrosus penetrate the vertebral body as Sharpey's fibres (curved arrows) (Johnson et al 1982). ALL = anterior longitudinal ligament; CEP = cartilage endplate (hyaline). **(D)** A 150-μm-thick parasagittal histological darkfield section from a 75-year-old male cadaver showing the following structures. B = *bone plate's* ring epiphysis (see Figure 3.6) with adjacent CEP that covers most of the vertebral body surface (partly shown) of the L3 vertebra; D = intervertebral disc; F = Sharpey's fibres: (MRI is able to distinguish Sharpey's fibres from the remainder of the annulus and nucleus (Yu et al 1989)). L3 IAP = L3 inferior articular process; L4 = L4 vertebral body; LF = ligamentum flavum; P = pedicle. Note the L4 body *marrow spaces* adjacent to both the intervertebral disc's bony ring epiphysis (B) and the *cartilage endplate* (CEP). The L4 superior articular process (L4 SAP) facet's hyaline articular cartilage (H) exhibits (1) adjacent marrow spaces in its normal *upper* half, but its *lower* half has sclerotic changes obliterating the marrow spaces, as is the case with the entire opposing facet subchondral region—this represents *eburnation*, and (2) a dramatically enhanced narrow strip of acellular *lamina splendens* forming its surface (Giles 1992(a)).

Spinal Canal Epidural Space and Some of Its Ligaments

The epidural space lies between the spinal dura mater and the tissues that line the vertebral canal (Figure 3.3); it is closed above by fusion of the spinal dura with the edge of the foramen magnum and below by the posterior sacrococcygeal ligament, which closes the sacral hiatus (Newell 2008). The epidural space contains loosely packed connective tissue, fat, a venous plexus, and small arterial branches, lymphatics, and fine fibrous bands (*meningovertebral ligaments*) that connect the theca with the lining tissue of the vertebral canal and are best developed anteriorly and laterally, while similar bands tether the nerve root sheaths or 'sleeves' within their canals (Newell 2008). Nerve endings are present in the epidural space and the adjacent annulus fibrosus and (diZerega et al 2010).

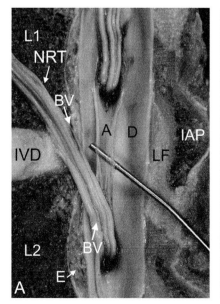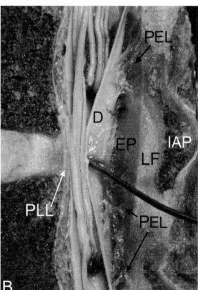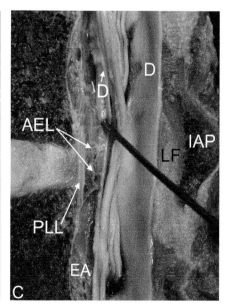

FIGURE 3.3 **(A)** Anatomical specimen cut in the *para-sagittal plane* at the L1 and L2 vertebral levels of a 52-year-old female illustrating the inferior articular process (IAP) of the L1 vertebra. Nerve root trunks (NRT) are invested in pia mater and have vasa radiculorum blood vessels (BV)—the trunks pass to the L1–2 and L2–3 intervertebral foramina, respectively. The lower nerve root trunk has been partially displaced from within the opened dural tube (D) in order to show the arachnoid mater (A) that is elevated by a probe. E = epidural fat space anterolaterally; IVD

FIGURE 3.3 (Continued)
= intervertebral disc; LF = ligamentum flavum that is composed primarily of dense elastic fibres (Johnson et al 1982; Yahia et al 1990). **(B)** Anterior displacement of the *posterolateral* side of the dural tube (D) to display the postero-lateral epidural fat space (EP) with posterolateral epidural ligaments (PEL). PLL = posterior longitudinal ligament. **(C)** Posterior displacement of the *anterolateral* side of the dural tube (D) to display the anterolateral epidural space (EA) with anterolateral epidural ligaments (AEL). As illustrated, the epidural space also contains fat, blood vessels, and connective tissue folds.

Source: Modified from Giles LGF, Introductory graphic anatomy of the lumbosacral spine. In: Giles LGF and Singer KP (eds) Clinical anatomy and management of low back pain, Edinburgh, Butterworth-Heinemann, © Elsevier, 1997(a), p. 35–48.

The parasagittal anatomical dissection (Figure 3.3) shows the general anatomy of the lumbar spinal canal, with associated structures, while demonstrating the relationship between nerve roots and their small diameter blood vessels (*vasa radiculorum*) (Parke et al 1985) as the roots pass into the intervertebral foramina. The human lumbosacral spinal nerve roots in particular are structurally, vascularly, and metabolically unique regions of the nervous system, and the peculiarities of their intrinsic vasculature and supporting connective tissue may account for suspected 'neuroischaemic' responses to pathological *mechanical stresses* and *inflammatory* conditions associated with degenerative disease of the lower spine (Parke et al 1985). This figure also shows the *epidural space*, anteriorly and posteriorly, that contains fat, blood vessels, and connective tissue folds (Richardson et al 2005). Hofmann's (1899) three groups of *anterior epidural* ligaments i.e. *midline, lateral,* and *lateral root* epidural ligaments made of connective tissue bands or ligaments (Dupuis 1999) are distinct from the *posterior epidural* ligaments (PEL) that connect the dural tube to the ligamentum flavum (Connor et al 2013), although no ligaments were identified at the L1-L2 level (Connor et al 2013).

The lumbar (L3-S1) posterior epidural ligaments tether the dural tube to the ligamentum flavum (Connor et al 2013) and may aid in the movement of CSF in the spinal canal (Rimmer et al 2018). The epidural space ligaments tether the spinal dura within the vertebral canal, as well as the spinal roots (Kimmell et al 2011).

With regard to the anterior epidural space, Hofmann (1899) *ligaments* are a normal anatomical finding, present at most levels, that attach to the anterior midline of the dural tube and extend to the posterior longitudinal ligament, providing further support for the dural tube (Wiltse et al 1993; Tardieu et al 2016); specifically they are present at most levels between C7 and L5, with the majority of ligaments limited to a single vertebral segment, although some cross several segments (Wadhwani et al 2004). Hofmann ligaments are anatomically variable fibrous bands (0.5–28.8 mm in length) (Martinez-Santos et al 2021). Part of an anterior Hofmann ligament complex, attached to approximately the anterior midline of the dural tube, is shown histologically in a thinly cut axial section (Figure 3.4).

An example of an anterior Hofmann ligament as seen on MRI is shown in Figure 3.5.

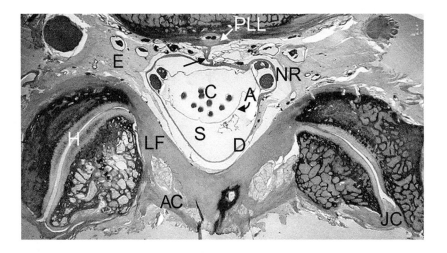

FIGURE 3.4 A 100-μm-thick axial view section from a 36-year-old female at L5-S1 level showing part of a *Hofmann anterior epidural ligament* (arrow) between the anterior midline of the dura mater (D) of the dural tube and the posterior longitudinal ligament (PLL). A = arachnoid mater; AC = ligamentous accessory capsule (Giles 1989); C = cauda equina within the CSF, which is contained within the arachnoid mater; E = epidural fat; H = hyaline articular cartilage on the zygapophysial joint's facet surfaces; JC = joint capsule; LF = ligamentum flavum; NR = nerve root sleeve budding off from the dural tube; S = subdural space.

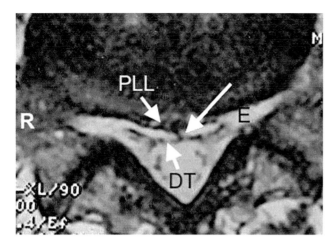

FIGURE 3.5 An axial T2-weighted MRI scan at the L5-S1 level of a 55-year-old male showing part of a Hofmann anterior epidural ligament (long arrow) between the anterior midline of the dural tube (DT) and the posterior longitudinal ligament (PLL). E = epidural fat within the intervertebral foramen; R = right side.

Lumbosacral Vertebrae, Intervertebral Discs and Cartilage Endplates

An axial view from above of a macerated (Todd et al 1928) L4 vertebral body from a mature aged cadaver is shown in Figure 3.6 to illustrate where the *hyaline articular CEP* is normally situated within the ring epiphysis. The CEP is supported by porous subchondral bone and it serves as a

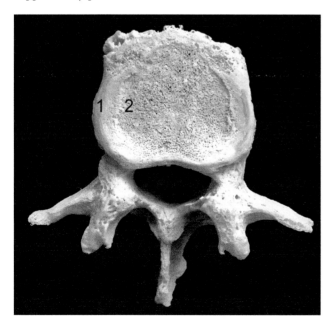

FIGURE 3.6 This figure shows a lumbar vertebra viewed from above to illustrate its narrow compact ossified *ring epiphysis* (1) around the subchondral bony *vertebral plate* of the vertebral body (2), with its many pores which are larger at the sides and less numerous centrally. The hyaline articular cartilage endplate normally exists within the ring epiphysis and covers the bony vertebral plate.

semi-permeable membrane to allow diffusive communication between disc nucleus cell and vertebral vasculature as well as to prevent large molecular weight proteoglycans from leaving the nucleus space (Bailey et al 2011).

The cortical *bone plate* possesses a marked porosity and is invaded by channels that provide a direct link between hyaline articular cartilage and the subchondral trabecular bone, and a high number of arterial and venous vessels, as well as nerves, penetrate through the channels and send tiny branches into the calcified cartilage (Li et al 2013; Madry et al 2010).

As the human IVD and the hyaline CEPs are inextricably linked anatomically and physiologically, they will now be presented together.

In adult males, the normal lumbar IVDs are approximately 5 cm wide and 1.25 cm thick and consist of a 'plate' of *fibrocartilaginous annulus fibrosus* sandwiched between two thin hyaline *CEPs* (Figure 3.2C) (approximately 1 mm thick centrally and thinner peripherally) that are surrounded by a smooth bony *epiphyseal* ring and the *bone plate* (Stockwell 1979) (Figure 3.6).

The disc is the largest avascular structure in the human body with some cells being up to 8 mm from the nearest direct blood supply (Urban et al 2004). However, small offshoots of spinal branches of arteries supplying the vertebral column form an anastomosis on the outer surface of the annulus fibrosus and supply its most peripheral fibres (Newell 2008).

The annulus fibrosus consists of concentric collagenous *lamellae* that interlace obliquely as they spiral between their upper and lower attachments in the hyaline *CEPs*; the *external* lamellae of the annulus fibrosus pass direct to the bone of the *bone plate* (ring epiphysis) or to ligaments, and the gelatinous nucleus pulposus is enclosed by the annulus (Stockwell 1979) (Figure 3.2C).

Fibrocartilage is a form of cartilage in which the matrix contains obvious bundles of thick collagenous fibres, and it is present in the IVD—it is a combination of dense connective tissue and cartilage with resistance to both compression and shear (Ross et al 1985). Fibrocartilage has small fields of cartilage blending almost imperceptibly with regions of fibrous tissue, and it has no perichondrium (Ross et al 1985). There are approximately 90 lamellae between the nucleus pulposus and the posterior margin of the lumbar IVD (Pope et al 1984), and these can tear due to trauma, resulting in a posterior disc bulge or protrusion.

The disc is a complex assembly of extracellular *proteoglycans* and *collagens* containing a relatively sparse population of disc cells for synthesizing water-trapping proteoglycans that contribute to the maintenance of disc hydration; annulus fibrosus cellularity reaches a plateau after the age of 50 years, whereas nucleus pulposus cell density reduces with age throughout life (Vernon-Roberts et al 2008).

The disc's principal function is to confer limited *mobility* on the spine and to act as a *shock absorber* (Urban et al 2007).

The biomechanical behaviour of the IVD ultimately depends on the viability and activity of a small population of resident cells that make and maintain the disc's extracellular matrix (Grunhagen et al 2011).

Elastic fibres are located only in the *lamellae* of the annulus fibrosus and the superficial zones of the nucleus pulposus from regions of the IVD that connect or interface with osseous vertebrae and penetrate bony *vertebrae* and the *hyaline cartilage* as Sharpey's fibres (Johnson et al 1982).

The IVD consists of three different structures: (i) a gelatinous core called the nucleus pulposus, (ii) an outer ring of fibrous tissue named the annulus fibrosus that surrounds the nucleus pulposus, and (iii) two hyaline CEPs that cover the upper and lower surface of both the annulus fibrosus and the nucleus pulposus and serve as an interface between the pliant IVD and the rigid vertebral body (Garcia-Cosamalon et al 2010). Thus the cranial and caudal *hyaline CEPs* separate the vertebral bone from the disc itself and prevent the highly hydrated nucleus from bulging into the adjacent vertebra (Moore 2006).

The thin layer of hyaline *CEP* (Joe et al 2015) in adults is comprised of layers of calcified and non-calcified cartilage (Roberts et al 1989; Bae et al 2013) with the bony endplate only containing relatively few vascular channels (Zhang et al 2014). Chemical analyses of the CEP show a change in composition through the CEP with that at the outer annulus i.e. *nearer the bone*, having *higher collagen* but *lower proteoglycan and water content* than the endplate nearest the disc at the nucleus (Roberts et al 1989). The CEP is composed of water, collagen, and proteoglycan (Raj 2008).

Using high-spatial-resolution MR imaging, Bae et al (2013) showed that the morphology of the CEP region on MR images had a *bilaminar* appearance, with a thicker upper layer and a thinner lower layer, that was consistent with the histologic appearance of layers of thicker uncalcified CEP (~ 1 mm thick) and thin calcified CEP (~ 0.1 mm thick).

An axial histological view (Figure 3.7) illustrates a section cut across the *lowest* level of the L4–5 IVD-endplate cartilage *interface*.

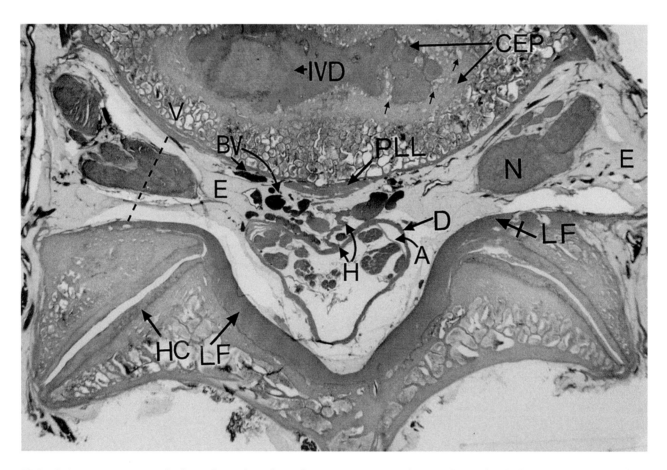

FIGURE 3.7   A 100-μm-thick axial view histological section cut across the very *lowest* level of the L4–5 intervertebral disc-cartilage endplate *interface* of a 46-year-old male illustrating the *vertebral body* (V) with its *cartilage endplate (CEP)* and a *sliver* of *intervertebral disc* (IVD). The staining uptake of the CEP appears to indicate that it is composed of *two* types of *chemically different material*, as the stained area of the CEP has two different colours within the thickness of this section. Note the small 'approximately circular' *vascular channels* (small arrows) seen in the CEP. A = arachnoid membrane; BV = Batson's venous plexus (*anterior internal vertebral (epidural) plexus*); D = dural tube containing *intrathecal cauda equina nerve roots*; E = epidural fat that occupies the space around all structures within the *vertebral foramen* (spinal canal) and the *intervertebral foramen* (dashed line); H = Hofmann's anterior epidural ligament; HC = hyaline articular cartilage on the facets of the zygapophysial joints with its characteristic tidemark (arrow); LF = ligamentum flavum along the length of the laminae bilaterally and extending anteriorly to wrap around the antero-medial region of the zygapophysial joints (LF tailed arrow); (N) = nerve root ganglion as part of the neural complex within the intervertebral foramen.

The CEP has fibres that are organized parallel to the vertebrae and nucleus pulposus that may contribute to large shear strains and delamination failure of the CEP commonly seen in herniated disc tissue (DeLucca et al 2016).

The endplates act as a biomechanical interface by playing an irreplaceable role in (i) *distributing loads* between the bony vertebral body and the compliant soft tissues of the IVD, (ii) providing a balance between conflicting *biomechanical* and *nutritional* demands, (iii) providing a unique physiological *mechano-electrochemical* environment inside the disc, and (iv) acting as a gateway impeding rapid solute diffusion through the disc (Wu et al 2017; Fields et al 2018).

Diffusion—or *solute transport*—is the solute motion that occurs when a membrane separates fluids that have the same hydrostatic pressure but a different solute concentration (*concentration gradient*) (Gumina et al 1999), and it is essential for the disc's cellular activity and viability (Urban et al 2004).

Diffusion through the CEP allows the *transport of small nutrients* (glucose, oxygen, amino acids) (Holm et al 1981), supplied by the endplate capillaries from *blood vessels and numerous marrow spaces* that *abut the cartilage layer*, to enter the disc and for waste products e.g. lactic acid to exit the disc by the reverse route (Urban et al 2004; Urban et al 2007; Lotz et al 2013) with venous drainage via the external and internal vertebral venous plexuses to the intervertebral veins, then to the larger named veins that drain the vertebral column (Newell 2008). Thus, the CEP plays a *critical role* in disc nutrition (Moon et al 2013), especially at its central region (Ito et al 2002) rather than the outer region of the CEP, and the outer portion of the annulus pulposus is entirely permeable (Gumina et al 1999). Nutrition of the disc is entirely dependent on this diffusion from the *subchondral bone plate* of the adjacent cancellous vertebral bodies (Hadley 1964; Epstein 1976; Newell 2008) that is *perforated by numerous marrow spaces* (Stockwell 1979) (Figures 3.6, 3.7, 3.8).

The low magnification histological section in Figure 3.8 was cut in the sagittal plane through the L5-S1 IVD of a younger cadaveric spine i.e. a 41-year-old male, in order to show the hyaline articular CEP appearance at this age.

Thus, the CEP plays an irreplaceable role in maintaining the unique physiological mechano-electrochemical environment inside the disc (Wu et al 2017), and this process of diffusion is essential for cellular activity and viability (Urban et al 2004). In addition, some blood vessels of the epidural space supply nutrition to the IVD (Gumina et al 1999).

CEP's consist of many vascular components, which provide vital nutrients for bone growth and regeneration, and subarticular collecting veins underlying the cancellous bony portion of the endplates branch and communicate and terminate in the *glomeruloid buds*, which are highly vasoactive (Rauschning 2016) (Figure 3.8). Thus,

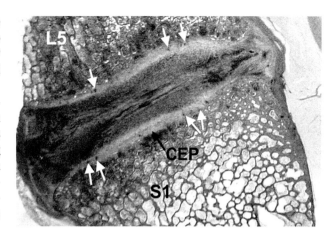

FIGURE 3.8 A lumbosacral disc histological section cut at 150 μm in the sagittal plane from a 41-year-old male. Note (1) the early internal disc disruption with small anterior and posterior bulges of the disc, (2) the fibrocartilaginous annulus fibrosus and the cartilage endplates (CEP) have a clear demarcation line between them, (3) the CEP contains numerous small *capillary vascular buds* (white arrows) associated with the arterial supply and venous drainage that takes place across the CEP (these capillary buds drain to the subchondral post capillary venous network), and (4) the *haematopoietic subchondral marrow contact channels* adjacent to the bone plate and CEP, respectively.

improving the supply of nutrients and blood to the disc, even if it is slightly degenerating or painful, provides better support and protection for the patient and remains the best treatment option (Rauschning 2016).

Because the lumbar spine carries significant forces and discs do not have a dedicated blood supply, endplates must balance conflicting requirements of being *strong* to prevent vertebral fracture and *porous* to facilitate transport between disc cells and vertebral capillaries (Lotz et al 2013). The bone marrow compartment adjacent to the bony endplate consists of hematopoietic cells, fat cells, sinusoids, thin-walled capillaries, and nerves (Lotz et al 2013).

The CEP and both the *periphery of the annulus* and the two *bone-cartilage interfaces* can act as nutrient sources (Stockwell 1979). Nonetheless, the nutritional conditions of the disc are precarious—it is possible that the diurnal fluctuation in disc thickness, caused by expulsion and imbibition of fluid (Inman et al 1947), might aid nutrition although, should the *marrow contacts at the centre of the endplate* become occluded, an inadequate supply of nutrient might cause deterioration of the disc tissue, as the *centre* of the disc apparently receives its nourishment only from the *marrow spaces* of the vertebra (Stockwell 1979).

As the IVD provides a balance between biomechanical and nutritional demands, it plays a key role in the development of disc degeneration and low back pain (Fields et al 2018). The incidence of IVD degeneration disease, caused by changes in the osmotic pressure of the nucleus pulposus cells, increases with age (Zhao et al 2020(a)).

Furthermore, aortic *atherosclerosis and stenosis* due to deposits in the posterior wall of the aorta (Kauppila et al 1997)—and in feeding arteries of the lumbar spine (Kauppila 2009)—are associated with disc degeneration and low back pain.

Using special MRI techniques with contrast, Bydder et al 2001 and Bydder 2002 demonstrated *solute transport* into the disc as well as within it (Figure 3.9).

It has been suggested that constantly changing body positions is important to promote flow of fluid (nutrition) to the disc (Wilke et al 1999).

Basivertebral Canal Nerve Bundle

The *basivertebral nerve* bundle, often in the form of paired nerves, originates from the *recurrent meningeal nerves* (Figure 2.8B) and enters the vertebral body posteriorly via the central vascular foramen (Fischgrund et al 2019) (Figures 3.10A and B) to course centrally within the vertebral body, generally following the basivertebral vessels and sending branches toward the endplates (Fischgrund et al 2019) (Figure 3.10A).

Brown et al (1997) found sensory and sympathetic innervation of the vertebral endplate in patients with degenerative disc disease, while Antonacci et al (1998) confirmed

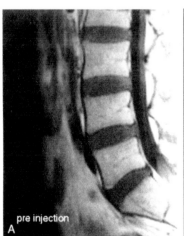
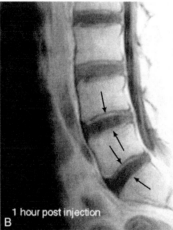
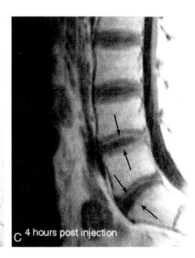

FIGURE 3.9   The lumbar spine is shown before contrast administration (**A**), one hour postcontrast injection (**B**), and 4 hours post injection (**C**). Transport of contrast into and within the disc is readily seen (arrows) as it crosses the *cartilaginous endplate interface* in the *postcontrast* administration images.

Source: Reproduced with permission from Bydder GM 2002 New approaches to magnetic resonance imaging of intervertebral discs, tendons, ligaments, and menisci. Spine 2002: 27(12): 1264–1268, DOI: 10.1097/0000 7632–200206150–00005.

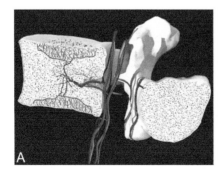
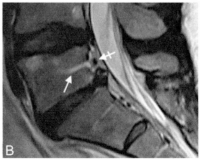

FIGURE 3.10   (**A**) Basivertebral nerve (red) and vasculature (blue) entering the basivertebral canal and extending into the vertebral body. (**B**) T2-weighted MRI sagittal scan of the lumbosacral region of a 34-year-old female (with low back pain) illustrates the L5 basivertebral canal (arrow) with the basivertebral neurovascular structures just posterior to the opening of the canal (tailed arrow) in a spine with L4–5 and L5-S1 disc degenerative changes.

Source: (A) Reproduced with permission from Fischgrund et al 2019 Intraosseous basivertebral nerve ablation for the treatment of chronic low back pain: 2-year results from a prospective randomized double-blind sham-controlled multicenter study. Int J Spine Surg.; 13(2):110–119. doi:10.14444/6015. ©2019 International Society for the Advancement of Spine Surgery.

the presence of neurovascular bundles and intraosseous nerves within the human vertebral body that may play a role in the clinical problem of back pain.

It is considered that, in some patients, the endplate is the source of most of the pathological innervation that occurs with disc degeneration and that this pain is transmitted by the basivertebral nerve (Fischgrund et al 2019; Lotz et al 2013). Recent studies have shown a *vertebrogenic model* that involves the basivertebral nerve (whereas historically the prevailing model of chronic low back pain followed a discogenic model), and this has led to convincing evidence that basivertebral nerve ablation can be beneficial (Kim et al 2020; Urits et al 2021).

In addition to vessels passing through the basivertebral canal, capillaries enter the small pores in the cortical shell of the vertebra to form an '*arterial grid*' at the vertebral centrum, before branching and terminating just adjacent to the CEPs (Lotz et al 2013).

An example of how significant *disc, endplate*, and *subchondral bone damage* can occur due to years of heavy manual labour involving *repetitive mechanical strain* and *overloading* of these structures may appear on T2-weighted MR imaging is illustrated in Figure 3.11. It has been reported that the presence of disc herniation with CEP herniation may be ascertained with the following MRI findings: posterior osteophytes, mid-endplate irregularities, heterogeneous low signal intensity of extruded disc material, Modic changes in posterior [vertebral body] corners and mid-endplates, and posterior marginal nodes (Joe et al 2015). Figure 3.11 shows some of these findings.

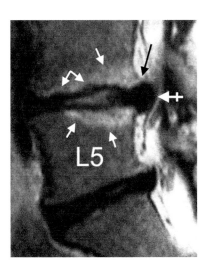

FIGURE 3.11 A T2-weighted MR image of the L4-S1 level from a 30-year-old female who had performed heavy manual work most of her life and which resulted in low back pain and right sided intermittent radiation as far as the knee is provided as an example of Joe et al's (2015) findings. Note the Modic changes (small white arrows), mid-endplate irregularities (conjoined arrows), heterogeneous low signal intensity of extruded disc material (tailed arrow), and the posterior osteophyte (black arrow).

Endplate damage, which can start as site-specific focal breaks, can result in a cascade of events resulting in degeneration; in such a case, a CEP becomes sclerotic and loses contact with blood vessels, providing less nutrition to the disc and the CEP itself (Joe et al 2015).

Vertebral Column Blood Supply

A brief overview will now be presented of the spinal column's extensive vascular system, which is closely connected with its surroundings and especially with the spinal canal and the spinal cord (Schmorl et al 1971). The various sized blood vessels *within* the spinal canal are derived from an *anterior* and *posterior arterial and venous arcade* that exists from the spinal arteries arising from the vertebral artery superiorly and then the thoracic and lumbar aorta—they anastomose with the *anterior spinal artery* running on the surface of the spinal cord, arising initially from the vertebral arteries of the circle of Willis (Richardson et al 2005). The vertebral venous plexus of Batson extends throughout the spinal canal and consists of valveless veins, so the direction of blood flow in these spinal veins is reversible (Schmorl et al 1971).

Schematic diagrams (Figure 3.12) show the *arterial* and *venous* vessels anterior to the lumbosacral spinal column, which supply and drain the lumbosacral spine; the primary function of the pelvic veins is to *drain deoxygenated blood* and to return it to the heart (Dao et al 2021).

The supply to the *fifth vertebral level* is from the *median sacral artery* (Crock et al 1977) that arises from the posterior aspect of the aorta, just proximal to its bifurcation, to descend close to mid-line over L4 and L5 vertebrae, sacrum, and coccyx and its distribution is to the inferior lumbar vertebra, sacrum and coccyx (Moore et al 2018).

In addition, it should be noted that small nerve fibres found in arteries and veins (*nervi vasora*) supply the adventitia (outermost wall of blood vessels) (Dorland's 1994) and trigger contraction of the smooth muscle in their walls (Betts et al 2019) and that small nutrient blood vessels in the walls of blood vessels (*vasa vasora*—literally vessels of the vessels (Ho et al 2017)) supply or drain the walls of the blood vessel (Dorland's 1994).

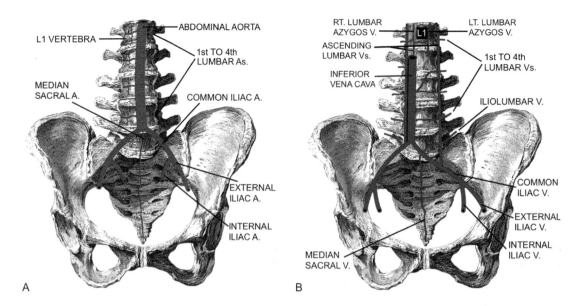

FIGURE 3.12 **(A)** *Four lumbar arteries* arise in pairs from the posterior wall of the abdominal aorta and pass laterally on each side, remaining closely applied to the centre of the front and side of each L1-L4 vertebral bodies, as the *lumbar segmental arteries*, until they reach the intervertebral foramina where each lumbar artery gives off the three main sets of branches shown in Figure 3.14. The *median sacral artery* arises from the back of the aorta, just above its bifurcation, and it gives rise to small paired *fifth lumbar arteries* that course across the L5 vertebra to the intervertebral foramina (Crock et al 1977) as illustrated. **(B)** The external *vertebral venous system* is shown (as described in Gray's Anatomy 38th ed.). The system is subject to many variations—in the lumbar region, the veins are known as the *ascending lumbar veins* and are connected by a variable series of longitudinally directed channels i.e. the *ascending lumbar veins* and *lumbar azygos veins* as shown. The lower lumbar veins drain into the *inferior vena cava* (Crock et al 1977).

Source: Lumbar spine and pelvis osseous structures courtesy of: Wellcome Library, London. Wellcome Images images@wellcome.ac.uk http://wellcomeimages.org Pelvis and base of spine. A set of anatomical tables William Smellie Published: 1754. Copyrighted work available under Creative Commons Attribution only licence CC BY 4.0 http://creativecommons.org/licenses/by/4.0/.

Lumbar vertebrae consist of a thin shell of *compact* [cortical] bone (Figure 3.13A) that covers the *internal spongy cancellous* bone (Figure 3.13D) and, as previously mentioned, it exhibits *epiphyseal rings* superiorly and inferiorly completely surrounding the hyaline CEP (Coventry et al 1945). The CEP has vascular channels in the first three decades of life (Coventry et al 1945), although they may be found in older individuals to some degree. In addition, the vertebra has numerous *vascular foramina*, some of which are shown in Figure 3.13B and C, that allow blood vessels to pass into the cancellous interior.

Red bone marrow lies entirely within the spaces of vertebral spongy bone and consists of blood vessels, specialized units of blood vessels called *sinuses* and a sponge-like network of haemopoietic cells (Ross et al 1985). The bone marrow is where circulating blood cells are produced—a process known as haematopoiesis (McLarnon 2021).

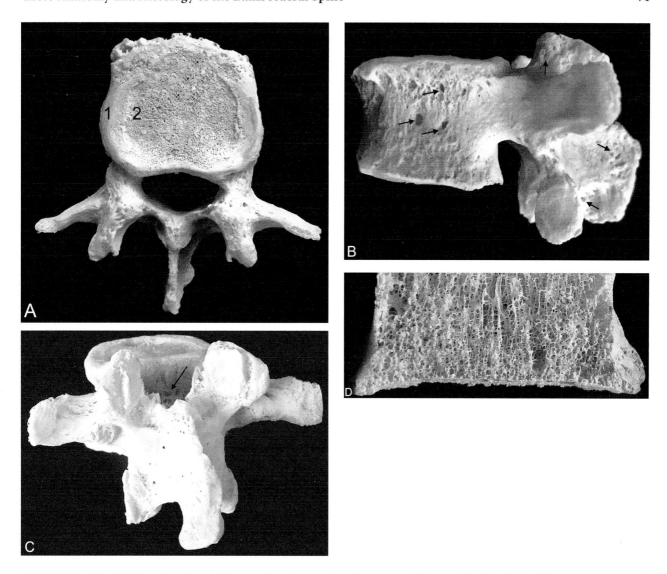

FIGURE 3.13 **(A)** An axial view of the previously mentioned macerated L4 vertebral body (VB) from a mature aged cadaver showing the narrow compact ossified *ring epiphysis* (1) around the bony *vertebral plate* (2) that shows many pores which are larger at the sides and less numerous centrally. (The epiphyseal ring may show calcification at ten years of age and ossification by adolescence (Hadley 1964)). A lateral view **(B)** shows some of the numerous *vertebral vascular foramina* that allow passage of blood vessels (arrows). **(C)** A somewhat oblique view showing further vertebral vascular foramina and the important *basivertebral canal* (arrow). Tzika et al (2021) found that 1 BVF occurs in 45.1% of specimens, 2 in 36.9%, 3 in 3.8% and 4 in 0.6%. Multiple small (< 1 mm) foramina occur in 10.1%, and asymmetry in 12.3%. The mean BVC depth is 12–21.8% of the VB anteroposterior diameter, and their distance was closer to the upper rim at T10-L4 and to the lower rim in L5. **(D)** A magnified view of a coronal plane section from the L4 vertebral body showing the interior of the bone's *spongy configuration*, consisting of numerous interconnecting *marrow spaces* of varying size bounded by bony trabeculae or spicules (Ross et al 1985) that are vertical and horizontal.

A highly simplified figure viewed from above (Figure 3.14), represents the basic *arterial* supply to an upper lumbar vertebra and shows how the arteries arise in pairs from the posterior wall of the abdominal aorta, the orifices for right-and-left sided branches at each level being separated by only a few millimetres for the *four upper lumbar vertebrae* (Crock et al 1977). These vessels pass laterally on each side while remaining closely applied to the centre of the front—and side—of each vertebral body, until reaching the intervertebral foramina before passing backward to the tip of the spinous process (Crock et al 1977).

Ratcliffe (1980), using fresh cadavers and contrast material described three types of *intra-osseous* arteries: *equatorial*, *metaphyseal*, and *peripheral*, each of which supplies a separate zone of the lumbar vertebral body—the *equatorial arteries* (Figure 3.14) supply the central core of the vertebral body subjacent to the nucleus pulposus and are the main nutrient arteries; the *metaphyseal arteries* supply an annular zone of the disc while the peripheral arteries supply the outer collar of the vertebral body.

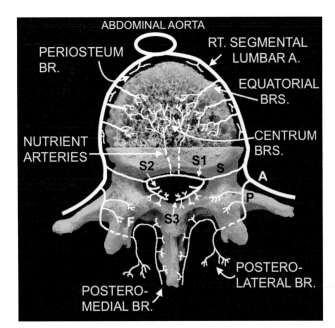

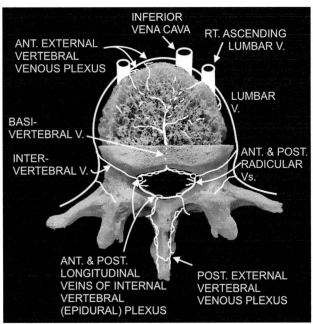

FIGURE 3.14 Schematic diagram illustrating the *segmental lumbar* arterial blood supply to an L4 lumbar vertebra from the abdominal aorta (just above the level of its bifurcation into the left and right common iliac arteries). The *segmental lumbar arteries*, in turn, give rise to the anterior *abdominal body wall branch* (A), *posterior spinal branch* (P), and the *spinal canal branch* S; S1 = *anterior vertebral spinal canal branch*; S2 = *nervous system branch*; S3 = *posterior spinal canal branch* (Crock et al 1977). Note the anastomoses between the nutrient and equatorial arteries to form centrum branches.

With respect to the vertebral body, each lumbar artery gives off *two sets of branches*—supplying networks on the front and sides of vertebral bodies (Figure 3.14)—and short *centrum branches* that penetrate the *vascular foramina* at regular intervals subjacent to the lumbar arteries (Crock et al 1977). Their terminal branches also penetrate the bone in the area *adjacent to each vertebral endplate*, while other branches form fine vertical networks on the surfaces of the longitudinal ligament and discs (Crock et al 1977). These penetrating vessels are arranged in constant basic patterns *within* the vertebral bodies (Figure 3.14), with most of their branches destined to be focused on the *vertebral endplate zones*, and an arterial grid is formed in the centre of the vertebral body from which vertical branches ascend and descend, in slightly tortuous paths, toward the respective endplates, forming a *brush border of arterioles* that pass *vertically into the vertebral endplate cartilage capillary beds* (Crock et al 1977) and provide *nutrition* to the vertebral body and endplate structures.

Veins of the vertebral column are divided into two main vascular systems: (i) the *internal* vertebral venous plexus and (ii) the *external* vertebral plexus. A schematic diagram of the lumbar spine's vertebral venous plexuses and their connections to the overall venous drainage is shown in Figure 3.15.

FIGURE 3.15 Schematic diagram illustrating the *segmental lumbar* venous blood drainage for an L4 lumbar vertebra.

A lateral lumbar diagram (Figure 3.16), illustrates the basic combined arterial and venous anatomy of the L1 to L3 lumbar spine structures.

Frymoyer et al (1989) illustrated the microvascular anatomy of cartilaginous end-plates with their capillary buds/tufts, and Crock et al (1973) showed a fine subchondral postcapillary venous network, draining by short vertical tributaries, to a horizontal collecting vein system communicating with the basivertebral vein.

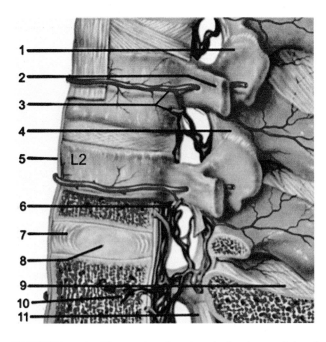

FIGURE 3.16 Illustration showing the basic arterial and venous anatomy of the lumbar spine vertebral bodies, intervertebral discs, vascular structures, and some ligaments.

FIGURE 3.16 (Continued)
1 = superior articular process; 2 = transverse process; 3 = lumbar artery and vein, respectively; 4 = inferior articular process; 5 = anterior longitudinal ligament; 6 = internal vertebral venous plexus; 7 = fibrous rings of intervertebral disc lamellae; 8 = nucleus pulposus; 9 = interspinous ligament; 10 = basivertebral vein; 11 = ligamentum flavum.

Source: Part of a colour plate by Professor Paul Peck. Modified and reproduced from Atlas of Normal Anatomy, Medical Student Edition, The Intervertebral Disks, Plate 2, 1956. Lederle Laboratories, American Cyanamid International, © 1974, Pearl River, N.Y.

To summarize the aforementioned arterial and venous systems of the vertebral bodies, a highly schematic one plane diagram, superimposed on a median sagittal plane anatomical specimen of the spine at the L3 and L4 vertebral levels, is shown (Figure 3.17). This illustrates the basic principle of *arterial supply to* and *venous drainage from* the vertebral bodies and the IVD CEPs.

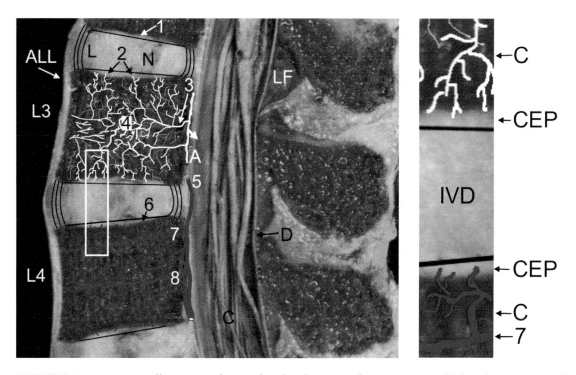

FIGURE 3.17 A sagittally sectioned L3 and L4 lumbar spine from a 70-year-old female, schematically representing part of the density of the vertebral intraosseous *arterial branching* within the spongiosa of the L3 vertebral body and the *venous drainage* at L4. Arterial supply is from an *anterior spinal canal branch* (A) that originates from the *segmental lumbar artery* and its *spinal canal branch*, with branches from the nutrient arteries (3) and the equatorial arteries to form the *centrum branches* (4) in the centre of the vertebral body. (See Figure 3.14 for a different schematic projection of the vertebral arteries using an L4 vertebra). 1 = cartilaginous endplate; (2) shows the arterial supply via capillary buds/tufts in the CEP. Small short arrow represents the beginning of the radicular segmental/medullary artery. Venous drainage is via the *anterior internal (epidural) vertebral venous plexus* (5) into which the *horizontal subarticular collecting vein* (7) and the *basivertebral vein* (8) drain. 6 = venous drainage through the CEP; ALL = anterior longitudinal ligament; C = cauda equina with its blood vessels (vasa nervorum); D = dural tube; LF = ligamentum flavum; N = nucleus pulposus situated within the annulus fibrosus lamellae (L) that are partly shown schematically as black curved lines on the intervertebral disc above and that attach as *Sharpey's fibres* to the *bone plate* (fused ring epiphysis and CEP). The white rectangle is enlarged in the insert to show an example of the extensive arterial and venous microcirculation of the vertebral body extending through its capillary bed within the hyaline cartilage endplate (CEP) and the subchondral cancellous bone (C) with its haematopoietic marrow contact channels through which capillary buds emerge (Ito et al 2002); the veins drain into the horizontal subarticular collecting vein (7) network as shown. (See Crock HV and Yoshizawa H 1976 Blood supply of lumbar vertebral column. Clin Orthop and Related Res 115: 6–21).

For explicit details of the arterial and venous circulation of the vertebral column and spinal cord, see, for example, the comprehensive text by Crock et al (1977) and, for microarteriographic studies of the adult human lumbar vertebral body, see Ratcliffe (1980).

A schematic diagram (Figure 3.18A) shows the plane (broken line) of a histological section cut *obliquely* across the centre of the lumbosacral disc (seen anteriorly) with the spinal canal posteriorly.

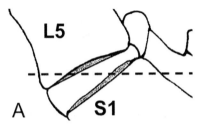

FIGURE 3.18(A)   Schematic diagram showing the axial plane of sectioning for Figure 18B.

The histological details of this section, with its disc-CEP-subchondral *haematopoietic marrow space relationship* at the body of the sacrum, is shown in Figure 3.18B.

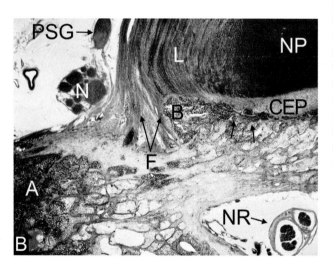

FIGURE 3.18(B)   A 100-μm-thick axial histological section, cut obliquely across the approximate centre of the intervertebral disc showing the spinal canal posteriorly at the L5-S1 level, from a 50-year-old male cadaver. This section illustrates how the intervertebral disc lamellae (L) and the nucleus pulposus (NP) are closely related to (1) the cartilage endplate (CEP) (that appears thicker because of the obliquity of the section across the endplate), and (2) the *haematopoietic marrow contact channels* of the sacrum (arrows). A = ala of sacrum; B = bone plate; F = fibres attaching the periphery of the disc to the sacral body; NR = nerve roots within the dural sleeve in the spinal canal, which passes through the adjacent foramen to emerge beyond the foramen as the neural complex (N); PSG = paraspinal sympathetic ganglion.

Morphological changes to the hyaline CEPs are usually seen with advancing age but are also evident in association with pathological changes of the nucleus and annulus (Moore 2006) resulting from degenerative changes, likely of mechanical origin. Figure 3.19 shows part of a magnified view of an IVD from an older male.

With respect to hyaline articular cartilage on *zygapophysial synovial joint surfaces*, this can effectively obtain nutrients from only two sources: (i) *synovial fluid* via the articular surface and (ii) *blood in the subchondral bone marrow*—in normal adult joints, the hyaline articular cartilage derives its *nourishment* mainly via the *articular surface* (Stockwell 1979). The cartilage discharges its *metabolites* via synovial fluid and the blood vessels of the adjacent bone marrow, as *perforations in the subchondral bone plate* allow capillaries from the marrow spaces to come into contact with 1–7% of the total osseous surface of the cartilage (Serafini-Fracassini et al 1974).

In *normal zygapophysial joints*, hyaline articular cartilage and the subchondral bone act as a functional unit (Imhof et al 1999; Menetrey et al 2010). However, *repetitive loading* leads primarily to lesions in the subchondral region (including vessels), which in turn impede flow of nutrition to the zygapophysial joint's articular cartilage, resulting in *degenerative joint disease*, and the subchondral region shows reactive enhanced vascularization and heightened metabolism with insufficient repair (Imhof et al 1999). In addition, *vascular pathology* plays a role in the initiation and/or progression of *osteoarthritis*, potentially due to episodically reduced blood flow through the small vessels in subchondral bone and associated with reduced interstitial fluid flow in the subchondral bone and *ischaemia* due to compromised nutrient and gas exchange into the articular cartilage, a potential initiator of degenerative osteoarthritic changes in the cartilage (Findlay 2007; Beckworth et al 2018) affecting the three-joint complex.

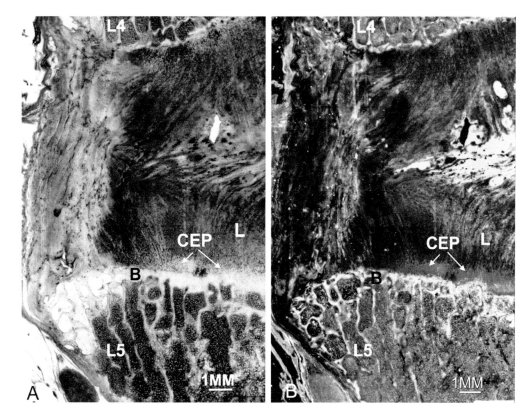

FIGURE 3.19 **(A)** A 100-μm-thick coronal section light microscope view, with corresponding darkfield view **(B)**, respectively, of part of a histological section from an L4–5 intervertebral disc between the vertebral bodies of a 76-year-old male cadaver. Note (1) the *subchondral bone plate* (B) and the CEP are in close proximity to numerous *haematopoietic marrow contact channels* below; (2) the lamellae (L) of the annulus fibrosus inserting into the cartilage endplate (CEP), and (3) the dark staining *chondrons* in the intervertebral disc that shows early internal disc disruption and degeneration.

Three-Joint Complex

The spinal column contains two series of joints i.e. *amphiarthrodial*, formed by the IVDs, and the bilateral *diarthrodial* or true joints, formed by the inferior pair of articular processes hooking down behind the superior segments below i.e. the encapsulated zygapophysial joints with their synovial lining and hyaline articular cartilage (Epstein 1976). Combined, these joints form the *'three-joint complex'*, also known as the *articular triad* (Inoue et al 2020), and together they transfer loads and guide and constrain spinal motions (Jaumard et al 2011).

The axial views in Figure 3.20 at the L5-S1 level show an X-ray with its corresponding anatomical block of tissue, from which the histological section was cut to illustrate the three-joint complex and its associated structures.

With respect to the term 'three-joint complex', it was first used by Dr H. F. Farfan (Kirkaldy-Willis 1999) to describe the *intervertebral joint* between the vertebral bodies (classified as a symphysis) (Newell 2008) and the adjacent two synovial *zygapophysial joints* between their articular processes. In the normal spine i.e. one without the effect of anomalies, such as (i) *facet joint tropism* (Giles 1987(b)), and (ii) *sacral obliquity* due to significant

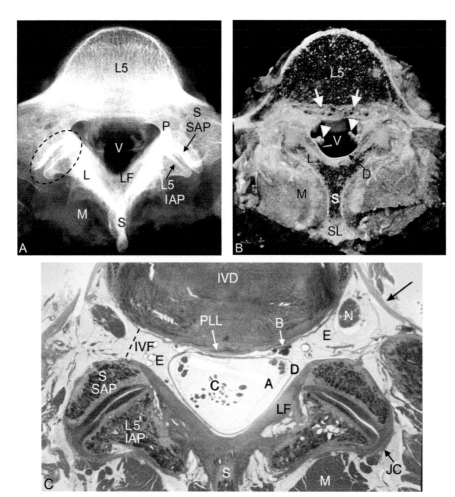

FIGURE 3.20 **(A)** Axial X-ray view of the lumbosacral *three-joint complex* (paired zygapophysial joints posteriorly and the vertebral body/disc joint anteriorly) from a 51-year-old female. Dotted oval = zygapophysial joint formed by the sacral superior articular process (S SAP) and the inferior articular process of L5 vertebra (L5 IAP); L = lamina; LF = ligamentum flavum; M = muscle; P = pedicle; S = spinous process; V = vertebral foramen forming part of the spinal canal. **(B)** Corresponding anatomical osteoligamentous specimen and its associated soft tissue structures. Small white arrows = epidural fat space containing the *anterior internal vertebral (epidural) plexus* i.e. *Baston's venous plexus veins* that are predominantly in the anterior spinal canal; arrow heads = nerve roots; D = dural tube; L = lamina; M = multifidus muscle as part of the posterior musculature; S = spinous process; SL = supraspinous ligament. **(C)** An axial plane 200-μm-thick histological section through the osteoligamentous block at the level of the intervertebral foramina. A = arachnoid mater; E = epidural fat surrounding the dural tube (D) and extending into the intervertebral foramina (IVF) containing the neural complex (N) on each side. Anteriorly, the epidural fat contains the anterior vertebral (epidural) plexus (B). The recurrent meningeal nerves of small diameter are not visible at this magnification. The zygapophysial joint capsule *anteromedially* is formed by the ligamentum flavum (LF) and postero-laterally the fibrous joint capsule (JC). The zygapophysial joint formation is by the sacral superior articular process (S SAP) and the inferior articular process (L5 IAP) of L5 vertebra. Black arrow = transforaminal ligament; C = cauda equina; IVD = intervertebral disc with internal disc disruption of some of its lamellae; M = muscle; PLL = posterior longitudinal ligament; S = spinous process adjacent to the junction of the laminae.

Source: Reproduced with permission from Giles LGF, Introductory graphic anatomy of the lumbosacral spine. In: Giles L G F, Singer K P (eds) Clinical anatomy and management of low back pain. Butterworth-Heinemann, Oxford, © Elsevier, 1997(a), p. 35–48.

(i.e. greater than 9 mm) LLI (Giles 1981; Giles et al 1981), to cause additional abnormal stresses on the three-joint complex, it seems clear that degeneration within the three-joint complex is a *multifactorial* pathological process including mechanical overloading stress (Imhof et al 1997) and that degeneration of one joint influences the two remaining joints (Kirkaldy-Willis 1999; Song et al 2019). Nonetheless, whether disc degeneration precedes zygapophysial joint facet degeneration or vice versa is not clear. The following have been proposed:

1. *Facet degeneration:* Using *skeletal* lumbar spines, facet *degeneration precedes disc degeneration* (Eubanks et al 2007(a)). Using *anatomical* specimens, Eubanks et al (2007(b)) concluded that facet arthrosis is a universal finding in the human lumbar spine and that it begins early with more than one half of adults younger than 30 years demonstrating arthritic changes in the facets, the most common level appearing to be L4-L5 with men having a higher prevalence and degree of facet arthrosis than women. In addition, when a facet joint anomaly is present i.e. facet tropism, it is significantly associated with lumbar disc degeneration (Song et al 2019).

2. *Disc degeneration*: Using CT and MRI scans Butler et al (1990) concluded that *disc degeneration precedes facet joint osteoarthritis.* According to Fujiwara et al (1999), who also used CT and MRI to examine spines of patients, in the *absence of disc degeneration* no facet joint osteoarthritis was found—most facet joint osteoarthritis appeared at the intervertebral levels with advanced disc degeneration.

However, the method of assessing lumbar spine degenerative processes in the three-joint complex is important as, from personal experience using CT or MRI (neither of which may have the resolving power to see *early* degenerative changes in patients), and examining skeletons, I believe these are not definitive methods. In addition, the Tesla strength of MRI units varies. Therefore, it appears that only post-mortem pathological examinations of the three-joint complex, using gross anatomical and histological studies, are likely to throw light on this complex issue. Thus, using post-mortem material for macroscopic and histological examination Farfan (1973) found that, concomitant with degenerative changes in the disc and vertebral body, there is early development of bilateral osteoarthritic degeneration in the facet joints, beginning with *fibrillation* of the articular cartilage and superficial *ulceration*. Li et al (2011) undertook a similar study to look at the prevalence of facet joint degeneration in association with intervertebral joint degeneration from L1 to L5 using a sample of *organ donors* i.e. 57 people aged 15 to 85 years (mean = 59 years) that were not part of a patient population. They found that MRI scans from only two spines (from 15- and 44-year-old males) showed no IVD degeneration but showed early fibrillation on the

facet articular surfaces when examined macroscopically and histopathologically; they concluded that facet joint degeneration is common, occurs early, and progresses with IVD degeneration.

Among all the factors leading to disc degeneration, lumbar CEP degeneration is considered a key factor (Zhao et al 2020(b)), and in disc degeneration, sclerosis of the adjacent bony endplate is considered to be responsible for decreased diffusion and disc cell nutrition (Wills et al 2018).

The degenerative process of a lumbar disc is a cascading event that is often attributed to cumulative damage to the various spinal motion segment components (Natarajan et al 2004) and probably any abnormal loading conditions upon discs can produce tissue trauma and/or adaptive changes that may result in disc degeneration (Stokes et al 2004).

An important chart showing the possible interaction of the three-joint-complex i.e. facet joints and disc changes was provided by Kirkaldy-Willis et al (1999) to illustrate the interactions between the facet joints and IVD during the three phases of degenerative spondylosis and stenosis. Postacchini et al (1999(b)) suggest that disc degeneration is related to the amount of functional stress to which the individual discs are subjected and that, in all likelihood, *overloading* an IVD will lead to the nucleus pulposus stressing its surrounding annular fibres and to some degree of excessive load-bearing upon the facets. In addition, Liang et al (2017) concluded that abnormal loading of discs was not only associated with disorders at the micro-scale but also alteration of the collagen fibrils at the nano-scale, possibly leading to changes in the mechanical and physiological environment around the cells of the annulus fibrosus.

To investigate degenerative spine changes Fields et al (2015) and Pang et al (2018) used an ultra-short time-2-echo (UTE) disc sign (UDS) and conventional 3-T MRI (T2W) to assess the UTE's association with disc degeneration and included pain and disability profiles (Oswestry Disability Index)—they concluded that UDS is a novel imaging biomarker that is highly associated with degenerative spine changes, chronic low back pain, and disability, over conventional T2W MRI. As gene expression circulating serum microRNA (ribonucleic acid) provides an insight into current disease states, Divi et al (2020) used whole blood samples from 69 patients with disc degenerative disease (DDD) and 16 healthy controls to identify serum microRNA and concluded that serum miR-155–5p is significantly downregulated in patients with DDD and may be a diagnostic marker for degenerative spinal disease as it was the sole miRNA that accurately predicted the presence of disc degeneration (P = 0.006).

Intervertebral disc changes have been given prominence by many authors. For example, Tomaszewski et al (2015) reported that the IVD undergoes changes with (i) *aging*, and (ii) *degeneration*, the latter having two types i.e. *'endplate-driven'*, involving endplate defects and inward collapse of the annulus fibrosus, and (2) 'annulus-driven', involving a radial fissure and/or an IVD prolapse.

In a study of the role of the vertebral *endplate* in low back pain, Lotz et al (2013) showed that *damaged endplate* regions can be sites of reactive bone marrow lesions that include *proliferating nerves*; for example, nerve fibre density across the L5-S1 level damaged endplates of a 63-year-old female was higher than in normal endplate regions, and thus can be a source of chronic low back pain; its role in patients is likely underappreciated because innervated damage is *poorly visualized* with diagnostic imaging (Lotz et al 2013). Using Dynamic Contrast-Enhanced MRI, Liu et al (2009) showed that in vertebral *marrow perfusion* of lumbar vertebral bodies between two *normal* discs, compared to perfusion of vertebral bodies between two *degenerated* discs, the blood perfusion was 14% less in the vertebral body marrow between two degenerated discs.

With aging, the decrease in the number of capillaries in the vertebral body and peridiscal tissue *impairs disc nutrition* and *favours degeneration* of disc tissue (Holm et al 1981).

In summary, with advancing age (approximately 60–73 years) the endplates consist of articular cartilage that *undergoes calcification* followed by *resorption* and *replacement by bone*—age changes occur in the arterioles, capillaries, and venules found in the nutrient canals or spaces of the bone adjacent to the cartilage or disc; thus, calcification of the articular cartilage and vascular changes seen in older vertebrae would *impede the passage of nutrients* from the blood to the disc proper (Bernick et al 1982; Grant et al 2016; Chen et al 2021), leading to IVD *degenerative processes* (Rudert et al 1993) because *CEP transport properties* dramatically affect nucleus pulposus cell survival/function (Wong et al 2019). The mechanism of low back pain caused by degeneration of lumbar IVDs and vertebral cartilaginous endplate is believed to be caused by the increased synthesis of pain-causing factors, such as calcitonin gene-related peptide and activation of the vertebral endplate trauma and aseptic inflammation (Chen et al 2021). *Degenerative endplate* marrow changes of the lumbosacral spine were examined by Savvopoulou et al (2011) using dynamic contrast-enhanced MRI profiles related to age, gender, and spinal level, and they found that degenerative endplate marrow changes differ significantly from normal marrow, regardless of the spinal level, age, or gender.

Excessive spinal loading and a lack of an appropriate nutritional supply may accelerate disc degeneration, in addition to genetic predispositions as studies clearly indicate that at high compressive forces *catabolic effect* and cell *apoptosis* (cell death) occur, whereas at more *physiologic compressions* cell *anabolic* activities are favoured (Ito et al 2002).

The previous review strongly suggests that *endplate degenerative change* would *adversely affect the three-joint complex* in time and may be the chief cause of degenerative IVDs and zygapophysial facet joints.

Plain Lateral X-Ray Images of the Lower Lumbosacral Level

Before presenting examples in Chapter 4 (Anatomical Atlas) illustrating anatomical and histological structures likely to be associated with pain arising from the IVDs, zygapophysial facet joints, and intervertebral foramina of the human lumbosacral spine, two lateral view plain X-ray images are shown. First, a lateral X-ray image of a 20-year-old male who experiences constant central low back pain (L4-S1 level), with left sided radiculopathy and left foot paraesthesiae and whose plain X-ray and MRI were reported as being *normal* (Figure 3.21A). However, one must remember that normal imaging reports do *not* mean the patient does not have low back pain or radiculopathy. Second, a cadaveric lower lumbar spine X-ray image showing *degenerative* changes at the L5-S1 level (Figure 3.21B). Plain X-ray images are used here as more sophisticated imaging scans, such as MRI or Computerized tomography (CT), are not normally the first line of imaging for spinal pain syndromes, unless there is a history of trauma or of a 'red flag' condition.

It is against this brief anatomical background that we now consider further histological/histopathological findings of the spine using histological sections.

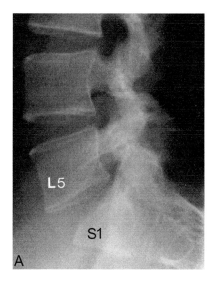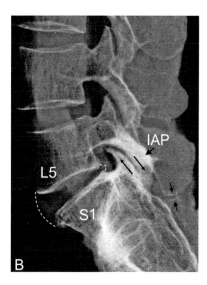

FIGURE 3.21 **(A)** An essentially *normal* lateral X-ray view of the lower, L3 to S1, spinal segments of a 20-year-old male with low back pain and left sided lower limb symptoms associated with radiculopathy, even though the L5-S1 disc space height and the intervertebral foramen appear normal. **(B)** An *abnormal* parasagittal X-ray view of the lower spinal segments of a 70-year-old female cadaver showing degenerative changes at *only* the L5-S1 level. Note: (1) thinning of the L5-S1 disc space height (compared to the disc space height at L4−5) due to anterior and posterior bulging of the L5-S1 disc (curved dashed lines), (2) imbrication/subluxation of the L5-S1 opposing zygapophysial joint facets (black lines) due to the disc space thinning causing the sacral superior facet osteophyte to project into the superior recess of the L5-S1 foramen (neural canal) and which will compromise the neurovascular structures within the epidural fat of the foramen, (3) the inferior articular process of L5 (IAP) approximates the posterior surface of the first sacral segment (S1), (4) sclerotic/eburnation changes seen as whitening of the subluxated opposing facet surfaces of the zygapophysial joint, and (5) minor sclerosis between the L5 somewhat enlarged (superior to inferior dimension) fifth lumbar spinous process and the adjacent sacral spinous tubercle (small arrows). Note that the L3−4 and L4−5 disc heights are normal with normal facet alignment at these levels.

Sectioning of Human Cadaveric Spines and of Fresh Surgical Specimens for Histological Examination

The cadaveric histological sections were cut as shown in Figure 3.22 in order to histologically examine various motion segment changes in the lumbosacral spine—large (7 × 8 cm) histological sections from osteoligamentous 'blocks' of human post-mortem spinal material were obtained for sectioning in the sagittal/parasagittal plane (Figure 3.22A) and approximately axial (horizontal) planes (Figure 3.22B); these large 'blocks' took up to seven months to prepare for each specimen, using a modification of the technique designed for smaller blocks by Giles et al (1983).

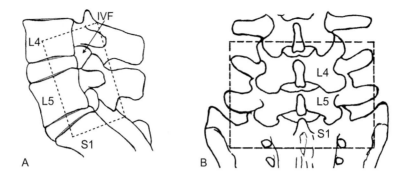

FIGURE 3.22 The majority of osteoligamentous blocks of tissue were cut approximately as shown for the lower lumbosacral spine for subsequent histological sectioning: **(A)** lateral view showing the intervertebral foramina (IVF) and adjacent areas retained for *sagittal/parasagittal plane* sectioning; **(B)** posterior view showing the lower lumbosacral blocks of tissue for sectioning across the spine in the axial plane. Smaller blocks were retained for particular areas, e.g. anterior IVD regions, kissing spinouses, etc.

Source: Reproduced with permission from Giles LGF 1992(b) Ligaments traversing the intervertebral canals of the human lower lumbosacral spine. Neuro-Ortho 13:25–38, Springer Nature.

The intervertebral foramen has three zones i.e. (i) *entrance zone* (containing the lumbar nerve roots, covered by dura mater and bathed in CSF), (ii) *mid-zone* (containing the PRG and the anterior motor nerve root (funiculus) covered by a fibrous connective tissue extension of the dura mater and bathed in CSF), and (iii) *exit zone* (containing the lumbar peripheral nerve which is covered by perineurium (Lee et al 1988)). Figure 3.23 diagrammatically shows the structures located within the intervertebral foramen where the nerve roots are covered by pia, arachnoid and dura mater as far as the spinal nerve, then the dura mater covering the roots gives rise to the dural sleeve. Therefore, depending on the position of each histological section cut through the block of osteoligamentous tissue, the structures within the intervertebral foramen zones vary.

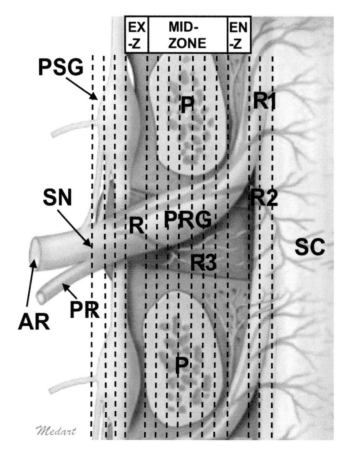

FIGURE 3.23 The vertical dashed lines represent the parasagittal plane of sectioning of the blocks that was performed at a thickness of 150–200 μm for all histological sections shown in this plane, depending on the overall size

FIGURE 3.23 (Continued)

of the block of spinal material. The approximate regions of the *entrance zone* (EN-Z), *mid-zone* (interpedicular zone), and *exit zone* (EX-Z) are shown. The spinal nerve (SN) gives rise to the anterior ramus (root) (AR) and the posterior ramus (PR). P = pedicle; PRG = posterior root (spinal) ganglion; PSG = paraspinal sympathetic ganglion; R = recurrent meningeal nerve of Luschka (sinuvertebral nerve) with branches R1—ascending branch, R2—descending branch, R3—direct branch to the intervertebral disc; SC = spinal cord lateral area.

Source: Modified from Kim HS, Wu PH, Jang I-T 2020 Lumbar degenerative disease Part 1: Anatomy and pathophysiology of intervertebral discogenic pain and radiofrequency ablation of basivertebral and sinuvertebral nerve treatment for chronic discogenic back pain: A prospective case series and review of literature. Int. J. Mol. Sci 21(4): 1483. License granted http://creativecommons.org/licenses/by/4.0/; Medart.

As a result of the serial sectioning, it was possible to visualize the neurovascular structures within the intervertebral foramen from which every fifth sequential section was stained for light microscopy. For example, the structures shown in Figure 3.24 show the sequential sections of the lumbosacral intervertebral foramen beginning, in this example, from the posterior nerve root ganglion (PRG) in the *mid-zone* beneath the pedicle (Figure 3.23) and progressing to the *exit zone*.

This series of sections from the left intervertebral canal of a 78-year-old female's spine illustrates that the *boundaries of the intervertebral foramina* are formed (1) *anteriorly* by the IVDs and adjacent vertebral bodies, (2) *posteriorly* by the synovial zygapophysial joints, and (3) *superiorly* and *inferiorly* by the vertebral notches of the pedicles of adjoining vertebrae (Berry et al 1995). In addition, the ligamentum flavum is illustrated as it forms part of the foraminal boundary. Each nerve is accompanied by a spinal artery, a small venous plexus, and its own recurrent meningeal branch or branches, together traversing the foramen (Berry et al 1995), but small structures are not visible at this magnification.

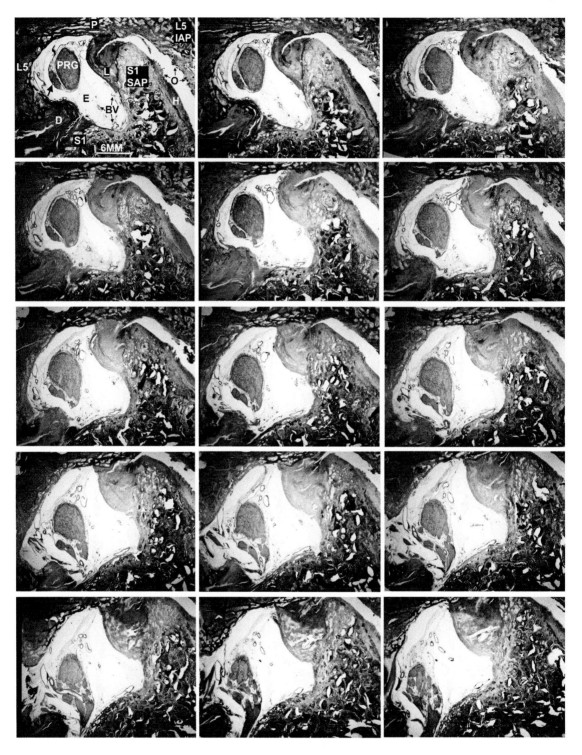

FIGURE 3.24 The first 200-μm-thick sequential section of the lumbosacral intervertebral foramen shows the boundaries of the bony canal, followed by its boundaries as the photomicrographs progress to the exit foramen. It can be seen that the neural complex in the lumbar region initially occupies the upper portion of the foramen, then gradually descends to the lower portion of the foramen. These sequential sections represent a distance of 15 mm from the first to the last histological section in this 78-year-old female's spine. D = intervertebral disc; L5 = fifth lumbar vertebral body; P = pedicle of L5 vertebra above with the sacrum (S1) shown inferiorly; S1 SAP = superior articular process of the sacrum with opposing inferior articular process (IAP) of fifth lumbar vertebra (L5 IAP); H = hyaline articular cartilage on the S1 facet surface; O = osteoarthrotic articular cartilage involving the facets; L = ligamentum flavum. Some of the contents of the foramen are shown e.g. the neural structures that occupy the upper portion of the lumbar canal—PRG = posterior root ganglion with cell bodies of first-order sensory neurons, and the associated anterior motor nerve root that lies anterior and below the PRG (arrow); BV = blood vessels; E = epidural fat.

In summary, the contents of the intervertebral foramen are the spinal ganglion, anterior spinal nerve root, recurrent meningeal nerve, spinal branch of the segmental artery or its branches, epidural fat, and numerous veins that connect the internal and external vertebral venous plexuses (Rickenbacher et al 1985). In addition, within the intervertebral foramen, there are lymphatics (Sunderland 1974), and it is interesting to note that latest research has established, beyond any reasonable doubt, that true lymphatic channels carry immune cells in meninges (Kumar et al 2019).

For simplicity, rather than describing the neural components of each intervertebral foramen seen in most of the following Atlas figures, whether the foramen is sectioned in the sagittal/parasagittal plane or in the axial (horizontal) plane, the smaller anterior motor nerve root, the larger posterior sensory nerve root and spinal ganglion together with their vascular and connective tissue

coverings will be referred to by the term *'neural complex'* as shown by 'N' in Figure 3.25B, whenever the structures are shown. In order to orientate the reader, all sagittal and parasagittal histological sections will be shown as depicted in Figure 3.25A and B where the *vertebral body* is always shown on the *left side* of each histological section.

The PRG shown magnified in Figure 3.25C consists of a group of cell bodies responsible for the transmission of sensory messages from various receptors to the CNS for a response (Pope et al 2013). It is surrounded by a thick protective layer of connective tissue (Haberberger et al 2019) i.e. the epineurium. The PRG neurons are considered to be pseudo-unipolar neurons, with a single axon that bifurcates into two separate branches resulting in a distal process and a proximal process (Ahimsadasan et al 2021).

The PRG serves as a vital link between the internal and external environment and the spinal cord, and it is

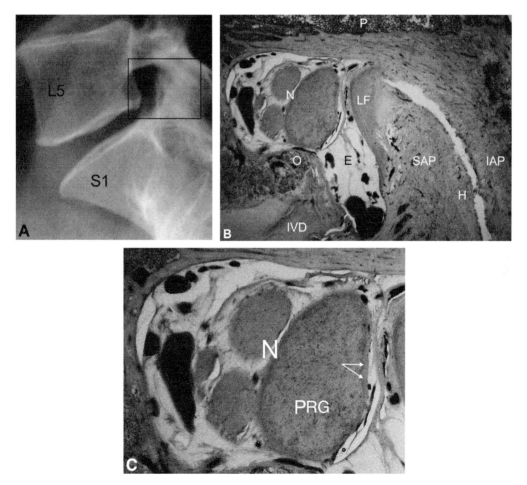

FIGURE 3.25 **(A)** A lateral view plain X-ray image of a 62-year-old-male cadaver, showing the L5-S1 intervertebral foramen. The rectangle represents the area deep within the foramen from which the 150 μm thick parasagittally sectioned histological specimen shown in (B) was obtained. **(B)** N = neural complex within the intervertebral foramen with associated extensive blood vessels in the epidural fat (E). H = hyaline articular cartilage within an osteoarthrotic lumbosacral facet joint; IAP = inferior articular process of L5 vertebra; IVD = intervertebral disc bulging posteriorly with an associated osteophyte (O); LF = ligamentum flavum; P = pedicle of L5 vertebra; SAP = superior articular process of the sacrum. **(C)** An enlargement of the intervertebral foramen to illustrate that the posterior root ganglion (PRG) consists of a group of sensory neuron *cell bodies* (appearing as various sized 'dots') enclosed within a thick outer connective tissue covering i.e. the *epineurium* (arrows).

an important site of neuropeptide production and may be considered as the 'brain' of the functional spinal unit (Grönblad et al 1991(b)). It controls pain perception (nociception) and temperature sensations and can be affected by trauma, degenerative disc disease, a herniated disc, or other spinal abnormalities (Krames 2014). *Nervi nervorum* located on the PRG, as well as peripheral nerves, are mechanically sensitive nociceptors themselves; therefore, the epineurium of the PRG may be directly activated by compression or mechanical stimulation of these nociceptors (Grönblad et al 1991(b)).

The blood supply to the posterior nerve root ganglion is by the spinal branch of the posterior trunk of the segmental arteries and blood flow to the ganglion is regulated by a muscular sphincter along the arterioles to meet the varying functional and metabolic demands of the current condition; the PRG is an exception to the otherwise restricted permeability of the PNS as, while most of the PNS has a low permeability between blood and nervous tissue, much like the blood-brain barrier, the PRG exhibits high permeability using its loose blood-nerve interface (Ahimsadasan et al 2021)

What then are some possible aetiological causes of mechanically induced spinal dysfunction and degenerative spinal changes with pain that may be helpful to '*lateral thinking*' in clinical decision making, once overt pathology has been considered and discounted?

As there are many putative causes of mechanical spinal pain syndromes, a gross anatomy and histology Atlas will provide large histological colour specimens from the human cadaveric lumbosacral spine to illustrate some possible causes of pain of mechanical origin (Chapter 4).

Chapter 4
ANATOMICAL ATLAS

Gross Anatomical and Histological Examples of Possible Causes of Non-Specific and Specific Spinal Pain Syndromes Due to Lumbosacral Spine Mechanical Dysfunction or Failure

Abstract: This chapter illustrates some human lumbar spine gross anatomical and histological examples of possible causes of non-specific, and specific, spinal pain syndromes due to lumbosacral spine mechanical dysfunction or failure. Some injuries affecting the three-joint-complex and the intervertebral foramen may result in mechanical low back pain with or without radiculopathy. The highly vascular and innervated synovial folds in the inferior zygapophysial joint recesses are demonstrated in detail using cadaveric specimens as well as fresh surgical specimens—the latter showed substance P antibody is present in the synovial folds, so pinching of the folds during movements may cause acute or chronic low back pain syndromes. A histological example of a joint capsule, beneath and separate from the ligamentum flavum, and enclosing the superior part of the zygapophysial joint, is presented. Examples of mechanical injury to blood vessels between moving bony parts such as the superior articular process of a zygapophysial joint and the pedicle above would likely cause pain as may early zygapophysial joint cartilage degenerative changes. Some of the histological structures illustrated, and which may cause pain, may not be seen on imaging. Histological examples of various parts of the three-joint complex, including some intervertebral foramina, are presented.

Key words: human lumbar spine, non-specific and specific spinal pain, spinal mechanical dysfunction, three-joint-complex, intervertebral foramen, radiculopathy, synovial folds, cadaveric specimens, surgical specimens, substance P antibody, joint capsule, ligamentum flavum, zygapophysial joint, facet joint, histopathology

Contents

DOI: 10.1201/9781003315964-4

The following Atlas represents a collection of lumbosacral spine anatomical and histological specimens illustrating some possible causes of non-specific and specific spinal pain syndromes due to mechanical dysfunction or failure. In some examples, only one of the joints from a given three-joint complex will be provided as a photograph in order to emphasize a particular degenerative change. Nonetheless, as previously mentioned, it is important to remember that degenerative processes in one joint will affect all three joints in the complex (Kirkaldy-Willis et al 1999; Song et al 2019). In addition, degenerative processes of the three-joint complex may also compromise the structures within the intervertebral foramen.

Each figure has detailed labelling to enable it to stand alone, so that the reader will not have to keep referring back to previous figures to identify structures.

Zygapophysial ('Facet') Joints

Chronic low back pain of facet joint origin represents a major healthcare problem as these joints constitute a common source of pain and remain a misunderstood, misdiagnosed, and improperly treated pathology (Perolat et al 2018). In a study of 320 patients (121 men and 199 women) the prevalence of facet joint pain based on double block injections was 38% in men and 43% in women

(Manchikanti et al 2002). These joints have a rich innervation with encapsulated, unencapsulated, and free nerve endings and contain substance P and calcitonin gene-related peptide, which are known pain mediators (Jadon 2016; Beaman et al 1993) and the clinical presentation of lumbar zygapophysial joint mediated back pain appears to overlap considerably with the presentation of low back pain due to other aetiologies (Dreyer et al 1996). Thus, it is important to understand the detailed anatomy of these joints. What is known is that lumbosacral facet joint degeneration, consistent with spinal osteoarthritis, is a prevalent condition that can be associated with dysfunction and low back pain; facet joint degeneration is a whole joint disease and involves many tissues that can contribute to pain including the synovium (Allison et al 2018).

There is a regular pattern of synovial fold structures within the zygapophysial joint capsules (ZJCs) of the human lumbosacral spine. In 1972 Tondury described these structures as various shaped 'meniscoids' although, according to Dörr (1958) they were first described as *synovial folds* by Friedrich Henle (Anatomist and pathologist 1809–1885). Having looked at these structures by dissection and histology, it is my experience that there are two types of *synovial lined folds* and these anatomical structures will now be shown in detail following an orientation diagram.

1. Lower Lumbar Zygapophysial Joints and Their Gross Anatomical and Histological Structures (Figures 4.1 to 4.5)

(A) Inferior Recesses

The largest synovial lined fat pads are found at the lumbosacral level, and Figure 4.1 diagrammatically represents anatomical dissections at this level.

Thus, zygapophysial joints have a *fibrous joint capsule* posterolaterally and the joint is surrounded by the *ligamentum flavum* anteromedially. These structures forming the capsule attach peripherally to the articular facets of adjacent zygapophyses (Soames 1995). The capsules contain two types of *synovial lined structures* i.e. (i) *large* fat pads in the *inferior joint recess* at L5-S1 level (smaller at higher lumbar levels), *smaller* fat or fibroadipose pads in the *superior joint recess*, and (ii) small *fibrous* structures of various shapes projecting a short distance towards the medial aspect of the joint from the ligamentum flavum at approximately the mid-level of the joint.

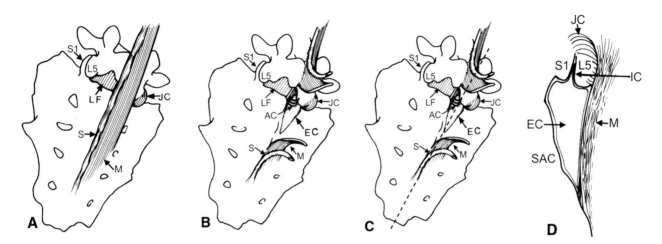

FIGURE 4.1 **(A)** Shows part of the *multifidus* muscle (M), the supraspinous ligament (S), the ligamentum flavum (LF), and the posterolateral fibrous joint capsule (JC). L5 = inferior articular process of L5 vertebra; S1 = superior articular process of the sacrum. **(B)** The multifidus muscle (M) and the supraspinous ligament (S) are reflected to show (i) the inferior joint recess ligamentous 'accessory' capsule (AC) bridging from the inferior articular process of L5 to the ligamentum flavum and (ii) the extent of the extracapsular *fat pad* (EC) below the accessory capsule. **(C)** The dashed line indicates the line of sectioning used to obtain the diagrammatic view shown in **(D)** and a similar histological view shown in (Figure 4.3). More laterally cut parasagittal sections will not show the large extracapsular fat pad but will show the joint capsule and the lateral part of a zygapophysial joint.

Source: Modified from: Giles LGF, Anatomical basis of low back pain. Baltimore, Williams and Wilkins, © Wolters Kluwer, 1989, p. 34.

Images of the structures in the *inferior joint recess* are shown in Figure 4.2. This gross anatomical dissection shows a large synovial lined fat pad in situ at the lumbosacral joint level of a 33-year-old male.

A histological parasagittal section from the region of the 'dashed' line in Figure 4.1C showing the extent of the synovial lined *intracapsular* part of a synovial fold, with its long *extracapsular* extension including its blood vessels, is shown in Figure 4.3. (See Figures 4.1C and D for orientation.)

An axial view diagram to show the *capsular anatomy* at the L5-S1 level (Figure 4.4) is followed by histological axial sections from the right lumbosacral zygapophysial joint to illustrate this anatomy (Figure 4.5A and B).

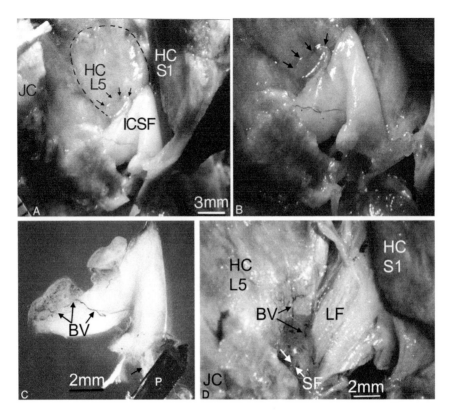

FIGURE 4.2 **(A)** The left L5-S1 zygapophysial joint from a 33-year-old male cadaver that has been opened out to display most of the large intracapsular *synovial lined fat pad* (ICSF) in situ in the inferior recess of the joint; the hyaline articular cartilage on the inferior facet of the fifth lumbar vertebra (HC L5) and on the sacral articular process (HC S1) can be seen. Small arrows = a fringe of the synovial lined fat pad projecting into the lower region of the joint. **(B)** A magnified view of this structure. **(C)** The synovial lined intracapsular part of the fat pad following its excision. BV = some blood vessels; arrow = part of the intracapsular synovial lined fat pad region of attachment where it was excised; P = probe. **(D)** The joint recess is shown following removal of the synovial lined fat pad—part of the remaining portion of the synovial fold is shown (SF) as well as part of the vascularity (BV) of the synovium lining the inner aspect of the capsule inferior to the L5 facet. Some of the vessels extend into the ligamentum flavum (LF). The posterolateral fibrous joint capsule (JC) is reflected.

Source: **Modified from Giles LGF, Anatomical basis of low back pain. Baltimore, Williams and Wilkins, © Wolters Kluwer, 1989, p. 27.**

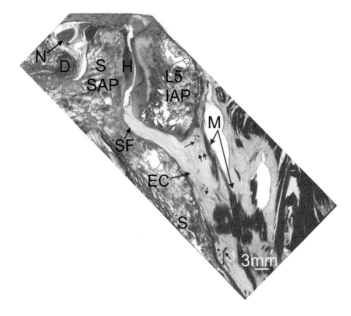

FIGURE 4.3 A 150-μm-thick parasagittal histological section of an L5-S1 zygapophysial joint of a 74-year-old male cadaver to show the *intracapsular synovial lined* part of the fat pad (SF) that extends below the inferior joint recess as

FIGURE 4.3 (Continued)

extracapsular adipose tissue (EC); it is limited posteriorly and inferiorly by multifidus muscle fibres (M). Small arrows indicate some of the numerous blood vessels seen throughout the fat pad; D = intervertebral disc posterolateral protrusion into the intervertebral foramen; H = hyaline articular cartilage; L5 IAP = inferior articular process of the 5th lumbar vertebra; N = neural complex within the intervertebral foramen; S = sacrum; S SAP = sacral superior articular process.

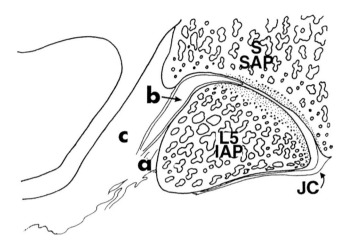

FIGURE 4.4 Diagram of a zygapophysial joint with its associated soft tissue structures. (a) = the ligamentous accessory capsule at L5-S1; (b) = synovial fold; (c) = ligamentum flavum. JC = posterolateral fibrous joint capsule; L5 IAP = inferior articular process of L5; S SAP = sacral superior articular process.

Source: **Modified from: Giles LGF, Anatomical basis of low back pain. Baltimore, Williams and Wilkins, © Wolters Kluwer 1989.**

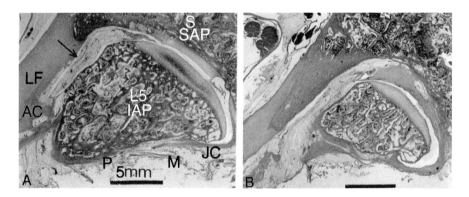

FIGURE 4.5 **(A) and (B)** Two 'sequential' cephalad to caudad 100-μm-thick axial view sections of the lower pole of the right lumbosacral zygapophysial joint of a 54-year-old male cadaver. **(A)** Shows a section where the ligamentous *'accessory'* joint capsule (AC) passes *above* the large synovial lined fat pad that passes beneath it. JC = fibrous joint capsule; LF = ligamentum flavum; L5 IAP = inferior articular process of L5; M = muscle fibres; P = periosteum; S SAP = sacral superior articular process; arrow = *intra-capsular* synovial lined fat pad. **(B)** A lower section that shows how the synovial fold passes through a gap in the capsule at this level. Black line represents 5 mm.

Source: **This article was published in JMPT 7(1), Giles LGF, Lumbar apophyseal joint arthrography, 21–24. Copyright Elsevier, 1984(b).**

(B) Intra-Articular Synovial Folds—Their Histological Structure Including Their Innervation (Figures 4.6 to 4.10)

Clinical relevance: Synovial fold nipping or pinching between bony surfaces can cause traumatic synovitis (Giles 1986(a), Giles 1987(a), Giles et al 1987(b) with pain, as synovial folds have nociceptive nerves (Giles et al 1987(a); Grönblad et al 1991(a)). Spinal manipulation in such cases may free a synovial fold that has been trapped between the facets of a zygapophysial joint (Giles 1987(a)).

A slightly oblique axial view of a histological section cut across the L5-S1 level of a cadaveric spine showing a large adipose synovial fold in its right inferior recess is shown in Figure 4.6A, with enlargement of the synovial fold in Figure 4.6B.

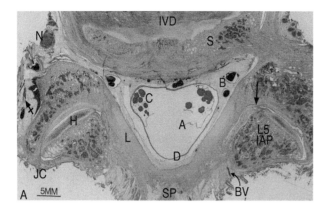
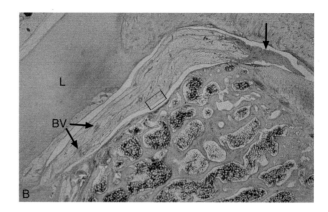

FIGURE 4.6 **(A)** A 100-μm-thick slightly oblique axial histological section of the lumbosacral zygapophysial joints at the level of the inferior joint recesses from a 54-year-old male cadaver. This shows a highly vascular intra-articular synovial fold (black arrow) with a fibrotic tip. A = arachnoid mater; B = Batson's venous plexus (anterior internal vertebral (epidural) plexus); BV = blood vessel; C = cauda equina; D = dura mater; H = hyaline articular cartilage; L5 IAP = inferior articular process of L5 vertebra; IVD = intervertebral disc; JC = posterolateral fibrous joint capsule; L = ligamentum flavum; N = neural complex; S = sacrum; SP = spinous process. A neurovascular bundle close to the left zygapophysial joint is shown by the tailed arrow. **(B)** Magnified view of the synovial fold with its numerous blood vessels (BV). The rectangle represents an area of the synovial fold from which small sections of synovial fold tissue were resected for microscopy from surgical specimens. The histological anatomy of such an area is shown greatly magnified in Figures 4.7 to 4.10.

Source: **Modified from Giles LGF, Taylor JR, Intra-articular synovial protrusion in the lower lumbar apophyseal joints. Bulletin of the Hospital for Joint Diseases Orthopaedic Institute 42(2): 248–255, 1982. With permission of the publisher.**

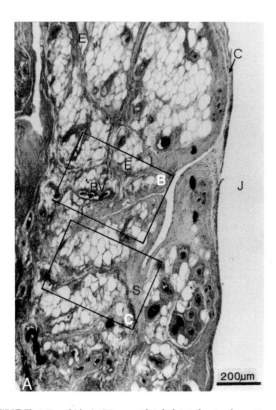
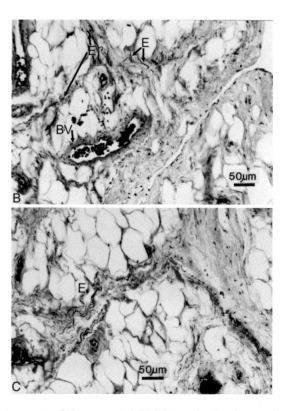

FIGURE 4.7 **(A)** A 30-μm-thick histological section showing part of the synovial fold from the lumbosacral zygapophysial joint of a 45-year-old female patient who underwent a partial facetectomy during surgery to remove a protruded intervertebral disc. Note the irregularly spaced synovial lining cells (C) in the synovial lining (intimal) layer. BV = blood vessels containing blood cells; J = joint 'cavity'; S = interlocular fibrous septum in the subsynovial (subintimal) layer. There is a rich blood supply and the unilocular fat cells indicate that synovial folds consist of *white* adipose tissue in adults. The rectangles highlight areas where numerous elastic fibres (E) run in various directions in the subsynovial

FIGURE 4.7 (Continued)

tissue within interlocular fibrous septa. **(B and C)** High-power magnifications of the rectangles in (A) show the intra-locular fibrous septa containing black-stained elastic fibres (E). Some of the blood vessels (BV) also show elastic fibres. (Modified Schofield's silver impregnation and Verhoeff's haematoxylin counterstain).

Source: **Reproduced with permission from Giles LGF Human zygapophyseal joint inferior recess synovial folds; a light microscope examination. Anat Rec 220: 117–124, 1988. © A.R. Liss, New York.**

An example of paravascular nerves from fresh synovial fold surgical material is shown in Figure 4.8.

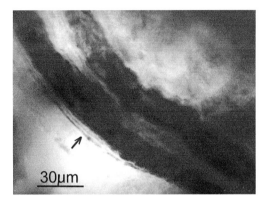

FIGURE 4.8 Two paravascular axons (arrow) accompany a blood vessel that is seen as a non-uniformly stained structure in the sub-synovial tissue from a 50-year-old female (L4–5 level) who underwent a partial facetectomy. The average diameter of the lumen of the blood vessel is 15 μm. (Modified gold chloride impregnation technique of Zinn DJ and Morin LP: The use of commercial citric juices in gold chloride staining of nerve endings. Stain Technol 37: 380–382, 1962).

Source: **Reproduced with permission from Giles LGF Human zygapophyseal joint inferior recess synovial folds; a light microscope examination. Anat Rec 220: 117–124, 1988. © A.R. Liss, New York.**

Fresh surgical specimens that showed examples of small diameter nerve fibres not associated with blood vessels in synovial fold lining membranes are shown in Figure 4.9 using silver impregnation and gold chloride impregnation, respectively.

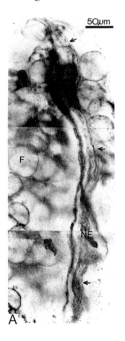
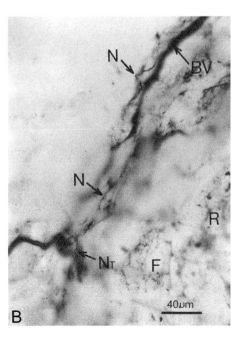

FIGURE 4.9 **(A)** A montage of a 30-μm-thick section from the synovial fold of a 25-year-old male (L4–5 level) showing a free ending nerve fasciculus remote from blood vessels (arrows). F = fat cell; NF = nerve faciculus from near the tip of the synovial fold. **(B)** Montage of the L4–5 zygapophysial joint synovial fold from a 49-year-old male

FIGURE 4.9 (Continued)

who underwent a partial facetectomy, showing the small nerve fibre (N) that appears to terminate as a 'free ending' nerve (NT) in the synovial lining membrane. The average diameter of the nerve fibre between N and N is 1.1 μm. BV = blood vessel; F = fat cell; R = reticular fibres. (Modified Schofield's silver impregnation). There are both paravascular and non-paravascular nerves in the synovial fold's lining membrane (Giles et al 1987(b); Grönblad et al 1991(a)). The small diameter non-paravascular nerves are considered to have a putative function of nociception (Giles et al 1987(a)).

Source: (A) **Reproduced with permission from Giles LGF, Taylor JR 1987. Human zygapophyseal joint capsule and synovial fold innervation Br J Rheumatol 26: 93–98 Copyright Oxford University Press—Journals, Oxford. (B) Reproduced with permission from Giles L G F 1988 Human zygapophyseal joint inferior recess synovial folds; a light microscope examination. Anat Rec 220: 117–124. © A.R. Liss, New York.**

Nerves with a putative function of nociception in synovial folds, obtained during routine facetectomy surgery, were demonstrated using an immuno-fluorescent Substance-P antibody technique (Figure 4.10A and B).

important role in causing low back and leg pain, although the synovial folds cannot be seen in great detail, if at all, on routine MR imaging.

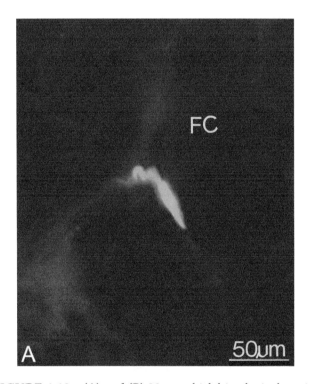

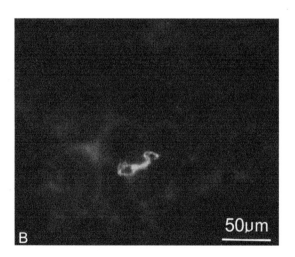

FIGURE 4.10   **(A) and (B)** 80-μm-thick histological sections from the synovial fold of a 25-year-old male obtained at surgery. The fluorescent nerves illustrated have an approximate average diameter of 6.3 μm (Figure A) and 3.1 μm (Figure B).

Source: (A) **Reproduced with permission from Giles LGF and Harvey AR Immunohistochemical demonstration of nociceptors in the capsule and synovial folds of human zygapophyseal joints. Br. J Rheumatol 26: 362–368, 1987. Copyright Oxford University Press—Journals, Oxford. (B) Reproduced with permission from Giles LGF, Anatomical Basis of Low Back Pain. Williams and Wilkins, Baltimore, © Wolters Kluwer, 1989 p. 67–82.**

Using radiographically localized injection of steroids and local anaesthetic precisely into the facet joint as a diagnostic therapeutic procedure, Mooney et al (1976) demonstrated that structures related to the facet joint can be a persistent contributor to chronic pain complaints of individuals with low back and leg pain. This supports the concept that synovial fold pinching most likely plays an

In addition, when a zygapophysial joint's capsule is mechanically torsioned between moving bony parts thus leading to joint effusion and distension, this may cause *nerve root pain* due to pressure on the nerve root (Ghormley 1933) or due to direct diffusion of chemical mediators of inflammation arising from irritation of the posterior facets (Haldeman 1977).

Zygapophysial Joint Synovial Cysts (Figure 4.11)

A further zygapophysial joint structure that may develop due to the joint structures being subjected to mechanical forces is an *intraspinal synovial cyst* associated with a degenerative facet joint (Hsu et al 1995). This can cause low back pain, with or without radiculopathy. Once it enlarges, it should be seen on MR imaging (Figure 4.11). This patient had experienced mild low back pain, of unknown aetiology, for approximately five years, with periodic left or right lower limb radicular pain.

Synovial cysts can be shown particularly well using 3D CISS gradient-echo MRI sequencing (Li et al 2019).

(C) Mid-to-Upper Region of Lumbosacral Zygapophysial Joint Recesses and Their Histological Structure (Figure 4.12)

An axial section from the upper half of a cadaveric lumbosacral zygapophysial joint (at the intervertebral foramen level) of a 54-year-old-male is shown in Figure 4.12 to illustrate the fibrous type of synovial lined structures, at approximately the mid-joint level, projecting from the ligamentum flavum to the lumbar zygapophysial joints.

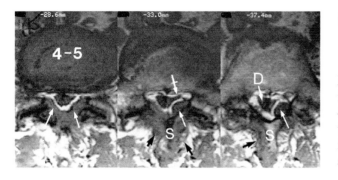

FIGURE 4.11 A 68-year-old male's MRI axial T1-weighted series of images of the L4–5 zygapophysial joints. Note the hypertrophy of the *ligamentum flavum* bilaterally (white arrows) causing a degree of trefoil stenosis of the central canal and the lateral recesses, and the *intraspinal synovial cyst* on the left side that bulges into the spinal canal, *compressing* the dural tube (D) and, to some extent, the left nerve root at this level (small tailed arrow).

Source: Reproduced with permission from Giles LGF 100 Challenging Spinal Pain Syndrome Cases, Churchill Livingstone Elsevier, Edinburgh, 2009, © Elsevier.

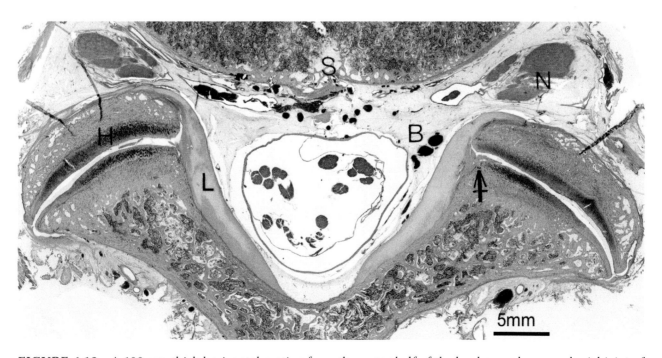

FIGURE 4.12 A 100-μm-thick horizontal section from the upper half of the lumbosacral zygapophysial joint of a 54-year-old male cadaver cut through the intervertebral foramina. Tailed arrow shows a fibrous synovial lined

FIGURE 4.12   (Continued)

intra-articular inclusion projecting a short distance from the ligamentum flavum into the right zygapophysial joint. B = part of Batson's epidural venous plexus; H = hyaline articular cartilage on the sacral superior articular process; L = ligamentum flavum; N = neural complex; S = sacrum.

Source: **This article was published in Clin Biomech 2, Giles LGF Lumbo-sacral zygapophyseal tropism and its effect on hyaline cartilage p. 2–6, 1987(b), © Elsevier.**

(D) Upper Pole of a Lumbosacral
Zygapophysial Joint Recess (Figure 4.13)

A parasagittal section cut through the L5-S1 joint of a cadaver shows a synovial lined fibrous intra-articular structure in the upper pole of the joint (Figure 4.13).

A *capsule* bridging across the upper pole of the joint, in close proximity to the ligamentum flavum, has also been noted by Sato et al (2002) who found difficulty in separating the ligamentum flavum from the joint capsule during their dissections—they did not illustrate the actual anatomical relationship between the capsule and the ligamentum flavum that is shown in Figure 4.13.

Lowis et al (2018) noted that the anatomical features of the facet joint recesses do not have a direct communication between the facet joint cavity and the retrodural space.

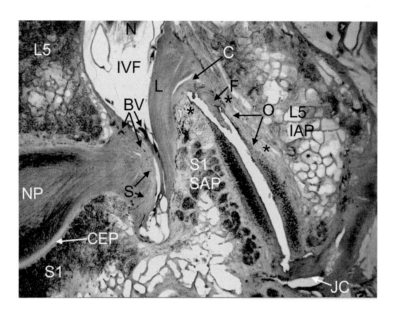

FIGURE 4.13   A 150-µm-thick *far lateral* parasagittal plane histological section from a 40-year-old male cadaver's spine, cut vertically. This illustrates (1) the cartilage endplates (CEP) adjacent to the L5-S1 intervertebral disc's lamellae surrounding the nucleus pulposus (NP); (2) the lower region of the intervertebral foramen (IVF), with part of its neural complex (N); (3) the ligamentum flavum (L) that encloses the superior pole of the zygapophysial joint where there also is a distinct capsule (C) bridging across the upper pole of the joint (from the sacral superior articular process (S1 SAP) to the L5 inferior articular process (L5 IAP), a synovial lined *fibrous* intra-articular structure (F) projecting from the capsule a short distance into the upper pole of the joint. JC = fibrous joint capsule inferiorly. The section has been cut beyond the region of the large intracapsular fat pad that is normally seen in the inferior joint recess. The postero-lateral disc herniation, with posterior extrusion of part of the nucleus pulposus (NP), has resulted in some thinning of the disc space height, causing some degree of imbrication/subluxation of the L5-S1 articular processes, leading to early *osteoarthrotic* degeneration (O) in the upper regions of the opposing facets and their hyaline cartilage. In addition, note the small blood vessels within the posterior part of the herniation and part of the adjacent Sharpey fibres (S). The postero-lateral disc herniation compresses some small blood vessels (BV) between it and the ligamentum flavum. Thus, there are several potential causes of low back pain generators in this specimen.

While routine MR imaging would show the posterolateral disc herniation and early subchondral sclerosis, it would not be likely to show the remaining pathological changes that may cause low back pain.

---

2. Lumbar Ligamentum Flavum
   (Figures 4.14 and 4.15)

(A) Axial Section

An axial view through the intervertebral foramen level of the lumbosacral zygapophysial joints shows that *bilateral vascular channels* pass into the ligamentum flavum a short distance from the joints (Figure 4.14). In addition, there are blood vessels on the lateral sides of the ligamentum flavum. These blood vessels show that the ligamentum flavum has a limited vascular supply due to a few small vessels with an average diameter of 10 microns in the superficial part.

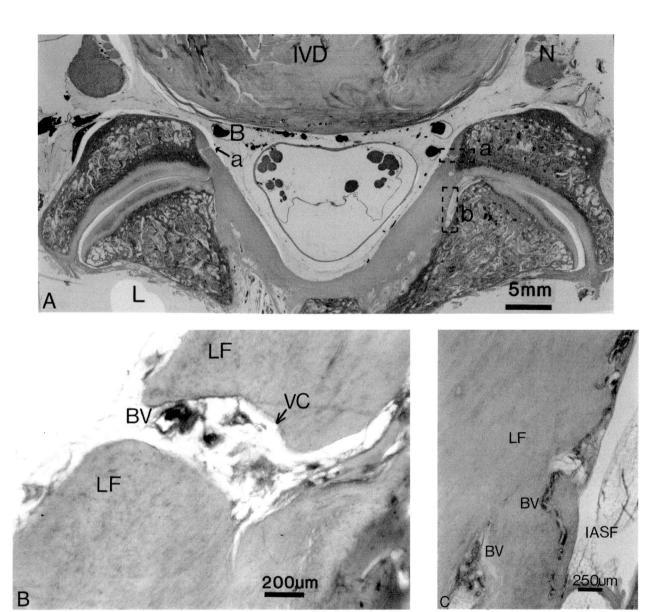

FIGURE 4.14 **(A)** A 100-μm-thick axial view section from the lower half of the lumbosacral zygapophysial joints of a 54-year-old male cadaver showing regions of bilateral vascular channels (dashed rectangles). a = bilateral vascular channels; b = blood vessels in the ligamentum flavum laterally. N = neural complex; B = part of Batson's venous plexus; IVD = intervertebral disc; L = left side of specimen. **(B) and (C)** represent magnification of the rectangles (a) and (b), respectively. **(B)** Zone 'a'—vascular channel in the ligamentum flavum on the spinal canal side of the ligamentum flavum. BV = blood vessel; VC = vascular channel; LF = ligamentum flavum. **(C)** Zone 'b'—blood vessels (BV) in the lateral part of the ligamentum flavum (LF) adjacent to the inferior joint recess. IASF= intra-articular synovial fold adjacent to the ligamentum flavum.

Source: Modified from: Giles LGF, Anatomical basis of low back pain. Baltimore, Williams and Wilkins, © Wolters Kluwer, 1989.

(B) Coronal Section

An anatomical model (Figure 4.15A) shows the location of a histological section cut in the coronal plane (Figure 4.15B) illustrating the zygapophysial joints in this plane.

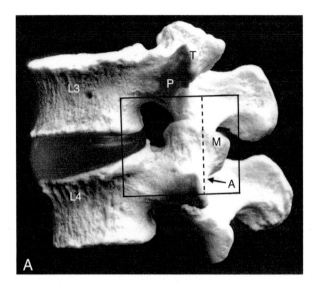

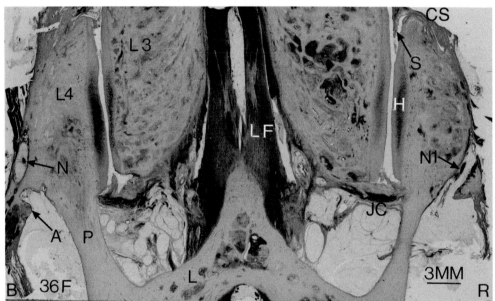

FIGURE 4.15 **(A)** L3-L4 vertebral model. The rectangle represents the block of tissue that was cut for histological processing. The dashed line shows the plane of coronal serial sectioning, which represents the approximate position of the histological section through the facets in (B). A = accessory process; M = mammillary process; P = pedicle; T = transverse process. **(B)** A 100-μm-thick histological section cut in the coronal plane, as shown by the dashed line on (A), from a 36-year-old female cadaver. The section is slightly oblique as the mamillo-accessory ligament is clearly seen enclosing the medial branch of the posterior primary ramus (N) on the left side of the specimen, whereas the mamillo-accessory ligament is not present on the right side where the medial branch of the posterior primary ramus (N1) is seen. A = accessory process; JC = fibrous capsule inferiorly. LF = ligamentum flavum. The ligamenta flava join at the junction of the laminae, but the left and right ligaments are partly separated between the spinous processes; CS = fibrous capsule superiorly with an adjacent small fibrous synovium lined structure (S); H = hyaline articular cartilage on the superior articular process of the L4 vertebra forming part of the zygapophysial joint; L = lamina of the L4 vertebra; P = pars interarticularis of the L4 vertebra.

Source: This article was published in J Manipulative Physiol Ther. 14, Giles LGF, The relationship between the medial branch of the lumbar posterior primary ramus and the mamillo-accessory ligament, 189–192, © Elsevier 1991.

Having examined the anatomy of the lumbosacral zygapophysial joints and their synovial folds in this chapter, and the sacroiliac joints in Chapter 2, both from different anatomical planes in cadavers, the following collection of specimens is used to provide further examples illustrating why mechanical lumbosacral spine pain may occur in some individuals without there being obvious imaging findings.

3. Multifactorial Degenerative Changes at One Level of the Spine (Figures 4.16A and B)

Clinical relevance: It has been known for many years that pain of vascular origin is a recognized clinical phenomenon, but the blood vessels vary in sensitivity within relatively wide limits (Kuntz 1953). The sympathetic nervous system primarily innervates blood vessels (Tucker et al 2021) and the *recurrent meningeal* nerves are distributed to the contents of the spinal canal including blood vessels (Moore et al 2018). Thus, trauma due to pinching of the blood vessels between the superior articular process of the sacrum and the pedicle above (Figures 4.16A and B) would most likely result in pain. In addition, pressure upon blood vessels may cause pain due to venous stasis and ischaemia (Sunderland 1975; Hoyland et al 1989; Jayson 1997). It is unlikely that this potential source of mechanical lumbosacral pain would be seen on MRI.

Furthermore, such pinching could cause *traumatic haemarthrosis* that has been observed during surgery following zygapophysial joint injuries (Dr Ian Macnab, Personal communication 1983) resulting in pain. It

should be noted that haemarthrosis is known to lead to cartilage damage, perhaps within two days of injury (Jansen et al 2007).

An example of (i) trauma to blood vessels between moving bony parts, (ii) posterolateral disc protrusion into the intervertebral foramen, and (iii) perineurial fibrosis surrounding the neural complex within the intervertebral foramen is shown in Figure 4.16A.

Figure 4.16B presents another example of likely trauma to blood vessels between moving bony parts. It shows a highly vascular connective tissue adhesion, between the neural complex and the fibrotic synovial fold, that is vulnerable to pressure between the superior articular process of the sacrum and the pedicle of the L5 vertebra above—this may well result in pain of ischaemic origin (Sunderland 1975).

It is unlikely that compression of the small blood vessels between the adjacent L5 and S1 bony surfaces would be seen on routine MR imaging, and this compression may generate pain due to vascular stasis and ischaemia (Sunderland 1975; Hoyland et al 1989; Jayson 1997).

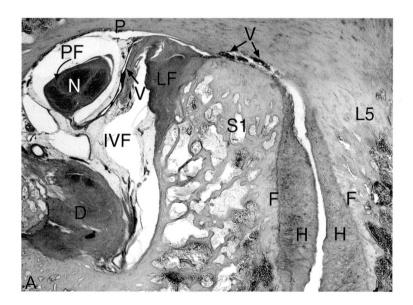

FIGURE 4.16 **(A)** A 150-μm-thick parasagittal histological section at the lumbosacral level showing the intervertebral foramen (IVF) containing the neural complex (N) within its upper region and an *associated blood vessel* (V). There appears to be perineurial fibrosis (PF) surrounding the neural tissue. Note the blood in the small blood vessels (V) in the upper pole of the zygapophysial joint that are vulnerable to being pinched between the adjacent L5 and S1 bony surfaces; such pinching could lead to bleeding within the zygapophysial joint; D = disc protruding posterolaterally into the intervertebral foramen, possibly causing discogenic pain (Shayota et al 2019). The narrowing of the foramen causes deformation of some blood vessels may result in pain of ischaemic origin (Sunderland 1975). H = hyaline cartilage on the imbricated L5 and S1 facet (F) surfaces of the zygapophysial joint; LF = ligamentum flavum; P = pedicle of the L5 vertebra.

Source: **Reproduced with permission from Giles LGF, 100 Challenging Spinal Pain Syndrome Cases, Edinburgh, Churchill Livingstone Elsevier, © Elsevier, 2009.**

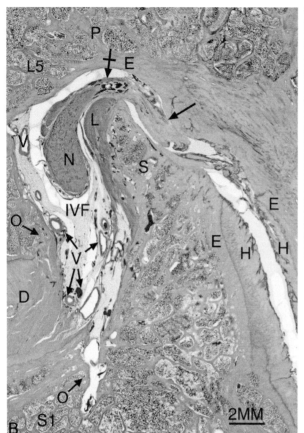

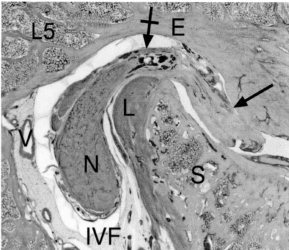

FIGURE 4.16 **(B)** A 100-μm-thick parasagittal histological section of the left lumbosacral intervertebral foramen from an 82-year-old female cadaver showing how the neural complex (N) (enlarged on the right) and the fibrous intra-articular synovial fold (arrow) in the superior joint recess have become attached to each other via a highly vascular connective tissue adhesion (tailed arrow). Pinching of this highly vascular structure would most likely cause pain. D = degenerating intervertebral disc with adjacent small osteophytic spurs (O) superior and inferior to the disc margins posterolaterally; E = eburnation (sclerosis) of the inferior aspect of the pedicle (P) of the L5 vertebra; H = hyaline articular cartilage on the subluxated/imbricated facet surfaces on each side of the zygapophysial joint shows osteoarthrotic changes of cartilage fibrillation (particularly on the inferior articular process of L5), with subchondral eburnation (E) due to abnormal biomechanical stresses resulting from the subluxation of the joint facets where the superior articular process of the sacrum has ridden up towards the pedicle above; L = ligamentum flavum on the superior articular process of the sacrum (S). Note the numerous blood vessels (V) within the intervertebral canal's foramen (IVF).

Source: Reproduced with permission from Giles LGF, A review and description of some possible causes of low back pain of mechanical origin in homo sapiens. Proc Aust Soc Hum Biol 4: 193–212, 1991(b).

A plain X-ray examination would not be likely to reveal the neurovascular adhesion, so the report may well not reflect the true extent of pathology causing a patient's low back pain. Sophisticated MR imaging may show the neurovascular adhesion.

4. Blood Vessels Mechanically Tractioned by Zygapophysial Joint Osteophytes (Figure 4.17)

Clinical relevance: Mechanical irritation of nerve endings located in the walls of the vertebral vessels, as a result of excessive distention of the vessel, may cause vascular pain (Wyke 1980), as the sympathetic nervous system primarily innervates blood vessels (Tucker et al 2021) and the *recurrent meningeal* nerves are distributed to the contents of the spinal canal including blood vessels (Moore et al 2018) and the intervertebral foramen blood vessels.

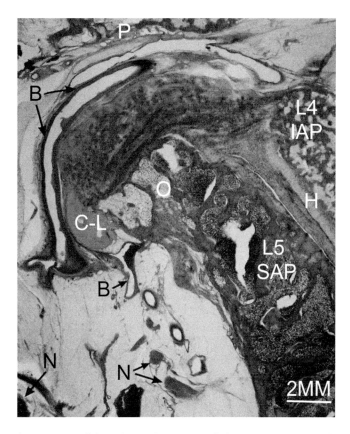

FIGURE 4.17 A far lateral parasagittal histological section of the L4–5 intervertebral foramen of a 79-year-old male cadaver. The blood vessel (B) is deformed and tractioned by an osteophytic spur (O) projecting from the superior articular process of the L5 vertebra (L5 SAP). The blood vessel conforms to the contour of the osteoarthrotic joint. C-L = joint capsule-ligamentum flavum junction; H = hyaline articular cartilage; L4 IAP = inferior articular process of L4 vertebra; N = neural structures within the intervertebral foramen.

A plain X-ray examination may show the osteophytic spur but not the soft tissue structures.

5. Zygapophysial Joint Facet Hyaline Articular Cartilage Early Degeneration (Figure 4.18)

Before considering cartilage early degeneration, it is important to understand the histological anatomy of virtually normal hyaline articular cartilage (Figure 4.18 A).

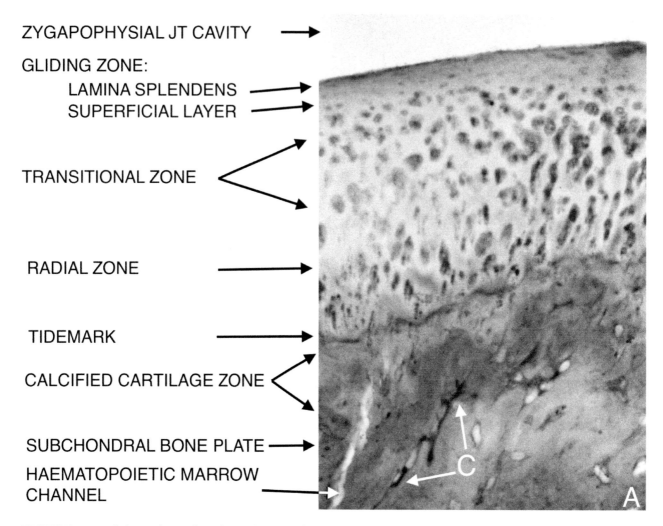

ZYGAPOPHYSIAL JT CAVITY ⟶

GLIDING ZONE:
    LAMINA SPLENDENS ⟶
    SUPERFICIAL LAYER ⟶

TRANSITIONAL ZONE

RADIAL ZONE ⟶

TIDEMARK ⟶

CALCIFIED CARTILAGE ZONE

SUBCHONDRAL BONE PLATE ⟶

HAEMATOPOIETIC MARROW CHANNEL

FIGURE 4.18   (A) Axial view histological section from an L5-S1 zygapophysial joint of a 50-year-old female illustrating its approximate histological zones. C = subchondral capillary. Magnification ×8.

Clinical relevance: Early changes in the facet's hyaline articular cartilage, as demonstrated by a loss of metachromasia (Dick 1972) indicates the onset of early osteoarthrosis, which may cause pain. Figure 4.18 (B–D) illustrates axial plane histological sections with early hyaline articular cartilage and subchondral bone degenerative changes as seen using light and darkfield microscopy.

The bones and periosteum are well innervated by nociceptive fibres (Haldeman 1999), so osteoarthrosis is a common cause of spinal pain (Beers et al 2006) and,

when advanced, would be seen on imaging. Beaman et al (1993) implicated osteoarthrotic lumbar facet joints in facet pain, having found Substance-P nerve fibres within the subchondral bone of degenerative facet joints. In addition, venous stasis occurs in osteoarthrotic bone marrow, resulting in increased pressure and pain (Bland 1983), supporting the work of Arnoldi (1976, 1994) and that of Kirkaldy-Willis (1999) that *venous hypertension* may produce pain by causing pressure on small nerves in bone.

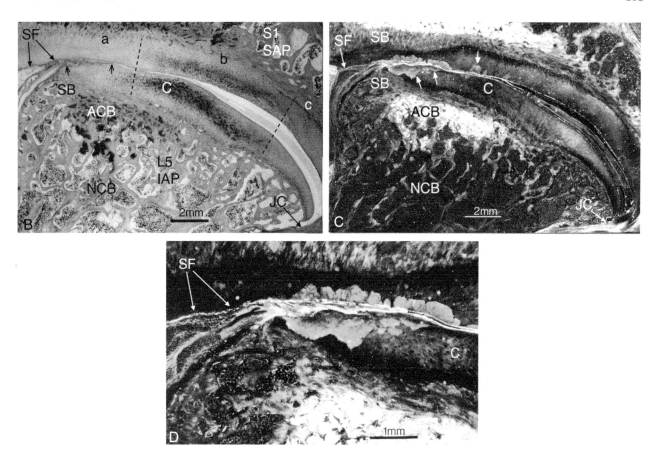

FIGURE 4.18 **(B)** A 100-µm-thick axial view light photomicrograph of the right lumbosacral zygapophysial joint's opposing hyaline articular cartilages from a 54-year-old male cadaver, showing part of an intra-articular synovial fold (SF) fat pad with its fibrotic tip (arrows) projecting between the hyaline cartilages (H) medially in Zone 'a' where the cartilage surfaces are in contact. The remaining part of the paired joint cartilages, where the cartilages are not adjacent to each other, is relatively normal. In the approximately central region of the joint, i.e. Zone 'b', the cartilage exhibits relatively normal chondrocytes. Beyond this in Zone 'c' the remaining portion of the cartilage appears to be normal, apart from a lack of a normal chondrocyte population. ACB = abnormal cancellous bone above normal cancellous bone NCB in the region of pressure between the cartilages in Zone 'a' and to some degree in part of Zone 'b'; C= chondrocytes; L5 IAP = inferior articular process of L5; S1 SAP = superior articular process of the sacrum; SF = synovial fold; SB = subchondral bone. **(C)** A dark-field light photomicrograph of the same histological section in (A) illustrating matrix changes in the hyaline cartilage on each side of the fibrotic tip of the intra-articular synovial fold (short white arrows) and a small isolated area just beyond this region. The regions of abnormal cancellous bone (ACB) on either side of the areas of different staining of the cartilages is seen. This medial region is where the joint surfaces have been in greater contact and, presumably, been under greatest pressure during life (arrows). NCB = normal cancellous bone; SB = subchondral bone; SF = synovial fold; **(D)** A high-powered dark-field photomicrograph of (C) clearly shows the areas of abnormal hyaline cartilage on each side of the joint. C = chondrocytes; SF = synovial fold exhibiting blood vessels.

Source: Reproduced from Giles LGF, Pressure related changes in human lumbo-sacral zygapophyseal joint articular cartilage. The Journal of Rheumatology 13: 1093–1095, 1986(b).

There are many diverse opinions concerning the cause and development of osteoarthritis (Tirgari 1978). According to Bland (1983), four theories of the pathogenesis of osteoarthritis are (i) the initial event occurs in cartilage because of a change in the microenvironment of the chondrocytes (most investigators hold this view); (ii) the initial event occurs in subchondral bone with *mechanical* factors being the primary cause; (iii) micro-osteonecrosis occurs in the subchondral bone as a result of vascular disease; and (iv) a proteolytic enzyme from type A synovial cells (phagocytes), which is normally neutralized by an inhibitor from type B synovial cells, digests the protein core of chondroitin sulphate if the inhibitor is absent (Glynn 1977).

> These early cartilage changes may not be seen on MRI, but the subchondral bone changes should be seen.

6. Tropism of Zygapophysial Joints Causing Mechanical Low Back Pain (Figures 4.19 and 4.20)

Facet joint tropism appears to have first been referred to by Brailsford (1929) in his paper on *Deformities of the lumbosacral region of the spine* in which he defined facet tropism as asymmetry between the left and right vertebral facet joint angles, with one more sagittally oriented than the other. A difference *of 5 degrees or more* between the horizontal planes of the left and right zygapophysial joints represents tropism (Cihák 1970). The incidence of tropism in the lumbar spine is 40–70%, with L4-L5 level being the most commonly afflicted level, and it leads to unequal biomechanical forces on the facet joint and IVD during rotation and other physiologic movements (Garg et al 2021). For investigating the alteration of lower lumbar facet joint angles in *patients* Karacan et al (2004) used a method of measuring tropism on CT images. Using the method of Karacan et al (2004), Tisot et al (2018) found a statistical relationship (p = 0.023) between facet joint tropism and the side where the lumbar disc herniation occurred, while Deepak et al (2020), in a smaller study, did not find a statistically significant association of facet tropism with lumbar disc herniation.

As LLI with pelvic obliquity or sacral anomalies can contribute to zygapophysial joint facet cartilage changes (Giles et al 1984), a small study was conducted to examine tropism between left and right, i.e. paired joints, at a given level in 13 lumbosacral spines from cadavers following orthoradiography and an antero-posterior plain X-ray of the pelvis and lumbar spine (Giles 1987(b)). Of the 13 cadavers radiographed, 8 met the inclusion criteria of having only LLI with or without tropism: four (35–83 years; mean 61) exhibited tropism of greater than 4 degrees; four (46–73 years; mean 59.5) exhibited no tropism, and the latter were used as a control group.

For measuring the degree of facet joint tropism and its effect on hyaline articular cartilage in the *cadaveric* material, anatomical blocks of spinal tissues were cut in the horizontal plane (Figure 4.19A), then radiographed in the same plane for measurement of paired joint angles to determine the degree of tropism (Figure 4.19B). The blocks were then processed (Giles et al 1983) for histological sectioning and examination of the paired joints (Figure 4.19C).

The histological findings appear to confirm the hypothesis of Cyron et al (1980) that, in tropism, there are greater inter-facet forces in the more *sagittally* oriented facets, which may predispose these facets to osteoarthritis. For another example of tropism, see Figure 4.20A.

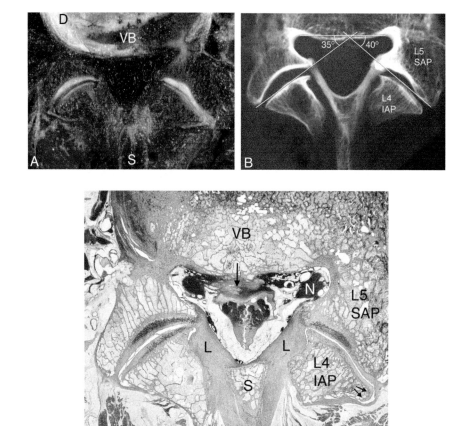

FIGURE 4.19 (A) Axial view of a block of cadaveric spinal material from a 56-year-old male at the L4–5 level showing the paired left and right articular facet joint cartilages. D = intervertebral disc; S = spinous process; VB =

FIGURE 4.12 (Continued)

vertebral body. **(B)** An X-ray of the block of material for measurements to determine whether tropism is present. It can be seen that there is a 5-degree difference between the paired joints. L5 SAP = superior articular process of L5; L4 IAP = inferior articular process of L4. **(C)** A 200-μm-thick histological axial view section cut across the block of material shows that there is an obvious difference between the planes of the paired joints in that the *left joint* is in the more *coronal* plane, whereas the *right joint* is in a more *sagittal* plane. Approximately the *posterior half* of this sagittal plane joint exhibits (1) less thickness of the cartilage, on each facet, (2) less cellular cartilage on both sides of the facets, and (3) fibrocartilage bumper wrapping around the L4 inferior articular process (L4 IAP) (arrows) within the fibrous joint capsule. In contrast, the left joint shows approximately only *one-third* of its posterior cartilages have less cellular cartilage and there is no fibrocartilage bumper. There is a small midline posterior disc bulge/protrusion (arrow) indenting the dural tube. L = ligamentum flavum; L5 SAP = superior articular process of L5; N = neural structure; S = spinous process; VB = vertebral body.

Source: (C) Reproduced with permission from Giles LGF Zygapophyseal (Facet) Joints. In: Giles L G F and Singer K P (eds) Clinical anatomy and management of low back pain. Edinburgh, Butterworth-Heinemann, © Elsevier, 1997(d), p. 72–96.

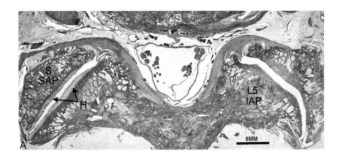

FIGURE 4.20 **(A)** A 100-μm-thick histological axial view section from a 73-year-old female cadaver that clearly shows that in the right, more *sagittal* facing joint, virtually all the hyaline articular cartilage has been eroded, with some osteoarthrotic subchondral sclerosis on both sides of the joint. On the left side, the more coronal facing joint exhibits early osteoarthrotic changes with cartilage fibrillation and a loss of normal metachromasia of the cartilage, as well as some subchondral sclerosis, particularly on the L5 IAP. Both left and right joints show small areas of fibrocartilage bumper posteriorly. H = hyaline articular cartilage; S = sacrum; L5 IAP = inferior articular process of L5; S SAP = superior articular process of the sacrum.

Source: This article was published in Clin Biomech 2, Giles LGF Lumbo-sacral zygapophyseal tropism and its effect on hyaline cartilage p. 2–6. © Elsevier (1987(b).

It is important to conduct a tropism study using a large number of cadavers with a LLI of 9 mm or more—and an equal leg length control group—to determine whether LLI affects the results of histological measurements of any joint degenerative changes.

Clinical relevance: An important part of the three-joint complex of the spine, i.e. the lumbar facet joint, has a far-reaching influence on the spine (Gao et al 2017). It was also suggested by Cyron et al (1980) that spines with asymmetrical facet planes, i.e. tropism, produced instability, manifesting itself as rotation of the lumbar spine, which put the ligaments of one facet joint under extra strain. In addition, instability due to tropism of the affected motion segment may cause strain on the innervated joint capsule or pinching of the intra-articular synovial folds, which have small nociceptive nerves (Giles et al 1985). Furthermore, Noren

et al (1991) concluded that the risk of disc degeneration is increased in the presence of facet joint tropism while Schleich et al (2016) found that facet tropism and sagittal orientation of the facet joint represent risk factors for the development of *early biochemical alterations* of intervertebral lumbar discs. Tropism strongly suggests mechanical instability and susceptibility to ligamentous injury (Willis 1959; Schmorl et al 1971) and Yang et al (2020) concluded that there was a significant correlation between facet tropism and chronic low back pain and suggested that a loading imbalance due to tropism may accelerate degeneration of the facet joints and IVDs.

If the clinician is aware of the possibility of tropism causing low back pain, tropism may be recognized in some antero-posterior plane X-ray images as shown in Figure 4.20B.

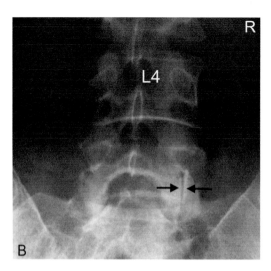

FIGURE 4.20 **(B)** Anteroposterior plane X-ray image of a 35-year-old female with intermittent low back pain during the last six months. On examination, there were no clinical signs except for aggravation of symptoms on lumbar spine extension. The X-ray shows that the right L5-S1 joint plane is in the *sagittal* plane (arrows), whereas the joint on the left is more *coronally* orientated. This represents a case of tropism with associated sclerosis of especially the more sagittally facing right L5-S1 joint plane in keeping with degenerative change.

Tropism may be present, but its extent may not be identified unless an MRI (or CT) axial image is obtained to define its degree of asymmetry. Nonetheless, it is an important cause of mechanical low back pain that may initially be missed unless the clinician specifically looks for tropism in its early stages i.e. before sclerosis develops.

---

7. Zygapophysial Joint Facet Degenerative Fibrocartilage Bumper Formation (Figure 4.21)

Clinical relevance: Pain may be generated in the pain sensitive fibrous capsule due to joint cartilage forming a *bumper* region between the cartilage and the capsule, as shown in the histological specimen (Figure 4.21A). This may cause mechanical friction against the pain sensitive joint capsule leading to low back pain and inflammatory changes.

Fibrocartilage bumper is not the hyaline type of cartilage that normally covers the facet surfaces (Hadley 1964).

Advanced facet lipping and overgrowth (Figure 4.21B) will result in significant zygapophysial joint fibrocartilage bumper formation and bony lipping between two points of bony pressure within the joint (Hadley 1964). This may well restrict motion between adjacent vertebral bodies, resulting in abnormal biomechanics and low back pain at this level that may radiate to the posterolateral thigh (rarely below the knee) (Jadon 2016).

Fujiwara et al (1999) suggest that wrap around bumper osteophyte formations provide an additional stabilizing effect in segmental degenerative disease and that MRI tends to underestimate the severity of osteoarthritis of the facet joints compared to CT.

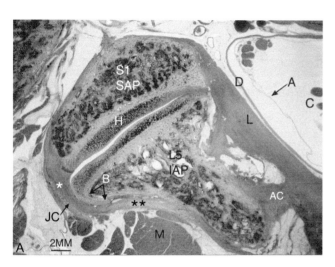

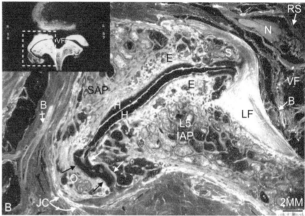

FIGURE 4.21 (A) This 100-μm-thick axial histological section through the left L5-S1 joint of a 51-year-old female cadaver illustrates the formation of a fibrocartilage bumper (B) wrapping around the L5 inferior articular process (L5 IAP) facet laterally, against the inner surface of the fibrous joint capsule (JC). It appears from the stain uptake in the fibrous joint capsule, lateral to the joint (*), that there is a difference in stain colouration compared to that of the capsule region further away from this area (**). This different stain uptake, combined with the adjacent fibrocartilage bumper, suggests that there has been mechanical lateral thrusting of the L5 facet margin against the innervated and pain sensitive tough fibrous capsule. A = arachnoid mater; AC = ligamentous accessory capsule; C = cauda equina; D = dural tube; H = hyaline articular cartilage with its narrow strip of acellular *lamina splendens* forming its surface (Giles 1992(a)) (also see Figure 4.18A); L = ligamentum flavum; M = muscle; S1 SAP = superior articular process of the sacrum.

FIGURE 4.21 (B) A 200-μm-thick axial histological darkfield photomicrograph section through the L5-S1 zygapophysial facet joint of a 65-year-old male cadaver, with corresponding axial CT scan. The rectangle on the scan shows the approximate region of the histological section. Note the blood vessel (B tailed arrow), the hyaline articular cartilage (H) on the facet surfaces, and how the cartilage has developed around the lateral margins of the facets to form fibrocartilage bumpers (arrows), with the development of a large hypertrophied osteophytic spur (O) beneath the fibrous joint capsule (JC). A smaller osteophytic spur (S) is adjacent to the ligamentum flavum (LF) that constitutes the joint capsule on the medial side of the joint (Hadley 1964). E = eburnation (sclerosis) in the subchondral regions on each side of the joint. L5 IAP = inferior articular process of the L5 vertebra; SAP = sacral superior articular process; VF = vertebral foramen containing blood vessels (B arrow) and nerve roots (N) in their nerve root sleeve (RS).

This degree of pathological change may well not be seen on plain X-ray imaging or on CT or MRI in spite of patient experiencing low back pain. Diagnostic positive facet joint block can indicate facet joints as the source of pain (Perolat et al 2018).

This degree of zygapophysial joint degeneration and lipping should be visible on plain X-ray images, and the CT insert axial view shows that CT imaging easily demonstrates the degenerative changes.

8. **Zygapophysial Joint Facet Imbrication/
   Subluxation Causing Osteoarthrotic Changes
   between the Subjacent Articular Process
   and the Pedicle Above (Figure 4.22)**

   Clinical relevance: Noxious stimulation of the periosteum—or bone marrow—can cause pain as sensory neurons are known to innervate periosteum and bone marrow (Nencini et al 2016). Therefore, impingement of the *periosteum* due to the sacral superior facet impinging upon the pedicle above could cause pain. In addition, pain could also result from the *bony eburnation* that is due to the localized bony pressure contact between both sides of the impingement areas (Hadley1964).

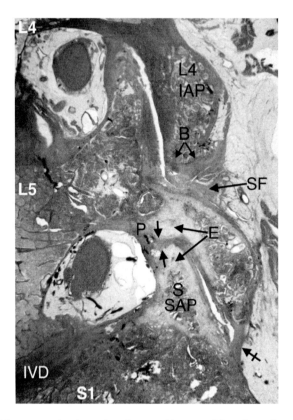

FIGURE 4.22 A 150-μm-thick parasagittal section from a 41-year-old male cadaver. Due to thinning of the L5-S1 intervertebral disc (IVD), which may well cause pain, there is imbrication/subluxation of the L5-S1 joint facets with the sacral articular process (S SAP) pressing upon the inferior aspect of the L5 pedicle (P) above, resulting in flattening of the sacral facet superiorly (arrows). This has resulted in eburnation (E) between these two bony structures, and it extends particularly into the subchondral region of each facet. There is thinning of the articular cartilage on both facet surfaces at this L5-S1 level. At the L4–5 level, where the intervertebral disc only has minor thinning, the zygapophysial joint is relatively normal apart from a small degree of facet imbrication and minor fibrocartilage bumper (B) formation at the tip of the L4 inferior articular process (L4 IAP). A fibrotic synovial fold (SF) due to traumatic pinching over the years between its adjacent bony structures is present. These pathological findings suggest abnormal biomechanical stresses have taken place over the years and that these could also result in pain. Tailed arrow = L5-S1 fibrous joint capsule inferiorly.

The bony eburnation in Figure 4.22 at the L5-S1 level and the IVD thinning would be seen on radiography but not the fibrotic synovial fold at L4–5 or the tractioning of the L5-S1 fibrous joint capsule inferiorly.

9. Multifactorial Degenerative Changes Affecting the 'Three-Joint Complex' As Well As the Neurovascular Structures within the Intervertebral Foramen (Figures 4.23 and 4.24)

Clinical relevance*: Mechanical low back pain, with or without radicular symptoms, may be multifactorial in origin (Haldeman 1977), as several soft tissue and bony structures may be involved at one spinal level where degenerative changes have occurred. Examples of such multifactorial degeneration at one level are provided in Figures 4.23 and 4.24, respectively.

The importance of the constricted foramen is that it *reduces the space containing the reserve cushion* of adipose and other soft tissue structures that surround neurovascular structures in a normal foramen; this predisposes to root pressure in the event of oedema and haemorrhage (Hadley 1950).

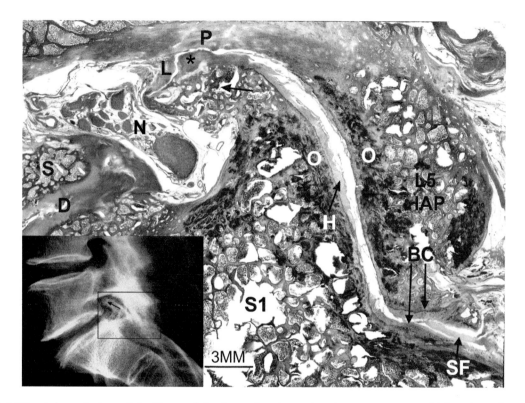

FIGURE 4.23   A lateral view plain X-ray of the lower lumbar spine from an 83-year-old female cadaver is shown as an insert. Due to disc space thinning, the L5-S1 zygapophysial joint has a subluxation of its opposing facet surfaces, with an osteophytic spur having developed superiorly on the sacral facet that approximates the pedicle above that shows sclerosis/eburnation. A small spur projects posteriorly from the inferior margin of the L5 vertebral body, encroaching upon the inferior region of the foramen. The superior sacral facet spur, combined with the small spur projecting into the lower region of the foramen from the L5 body inferiorly, have resulted in an 'hourglass' configuration of the foramen (Meschan 1959). The rectangle shows the L5-S1 intervertebral foramen and its associated structures illustrated histologically. The 100-μm-thick parasagittal histological section cut across the foramen that contains blood vessels, lymphatics, fat, and areolar tissue (Hadley 1950) illustrates the pathology involving the foramen and its associated structures i.e.: (1) osteophytic spur (arrow) at the superior pole of the sacral facet that approximates the sclerotic pedicle (P) above that has developed a fibrocartilage bumper superiorly (asterisk) that articulates with the pedicle; (2) the sacral facet spur and the spur (S) adjacent to the contained 3 mm deep postero-lateral disc herniation (D) combine to create a 'pincer' effect by encroaching upon the neurovascular structures (N) within the hourglass shaped foramen i.e. the intervertebral foramen exhibits a degree of antero-posterior stenosis; (3) tractioning and deformation of the ligamentum flavum (L) is present; (4) osteoarthrotic sclerosis (O) involves each facet's subchondral areas; (5) the S1 superior facet hyaline articular cartilage (H) is sparse and stains poorly, while there is very little cartilage remaining on the L5 inferior articular process (L5 IAP); (6) a fibrocartilage bumper (BC) has developed between the L5 inferior articular process (L5 IAP) and the posterior aspect of the first sacral segment (S1); (7) a synovial fold (SF) projects between the fibrocartilage bumper surfaces and has become fibrotic due to being pinched between the mobile bony surfaces during joint movement.

Source: **Reproduced with permission from Giles LGF, Kaveri MJP, Some osseous and soft tissue causes of human intervertebral canal (foramen) stenosis. J Rheumatol 17: 1474–1481, 1990.**

A lateral view radiograph showing *more advanced* multifactorial degenerative changes of the three-joint complex, with significant disc degeneration and much greater imbrication/subluxation of the L5-S1 facets, is shown in Figure 4.24A.

Osteoarthrosis is primarily a disease of the articular cartilage and early changes are *focal softening of cartilage* with loss of *metachromasia* and of affinity for haematoxylin; following surface flaking and 'fibrillation' in the superficial layers, deep clefts [fissuring] develop and chondrocytes cluster around the margins of these defects (Dick 1972). It is postulated that exposure to synovial fluid lysosomal enzymes—and enzymes from the chondrocytes themselves—thereafter accelerates cartilage destruction, which is seen radiologically as loss of joint space (Dick 1972). In a comprehensive description of the properties of lumbar facet cartilage O'Leary et al (2017) suggested that the human facet joint is highly susceptible to pathology and they graded degenerative changes as follows: Grade 1—minor fibrillation with the cartilage *surface* largely intact and the middle and deep zones are well preserved and cellular arrangement and density appear relatively normal; Grade 2—greater surface discontinuity and disruption of the structure is observed as far as the *middle zone*; Grade 3—the presence of surface erosion and loss of cartilage with multiple vertical fissures that almost stretch to the *deep zone*; Grade 4—complete denudation of unmineralized cartilage is observed, leaving only calcified cartilage and/or bone present.

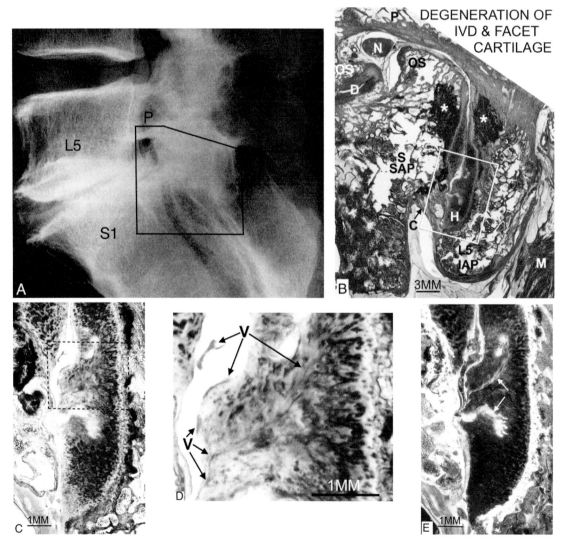

FIGURE 4.24 **(A)** Lateral view radiograph from the lower lumbosacral region of a 73-year-old male cadaver's spine illustrating multifactorial degenerative changes of the three-joint complex. L5 = fifth lumbar vertebra; P = pedicle of L5 vertebra; S1 = first sacral segment. **(B)**, **(C)**, **(D)**, and **(E)** are 100-μm-thick histological sections cut from the

FIGURE 4.24 (Continued)

approximate area indicated on the X-ray. **(B)** Advanced subluxation of the L5-S1 facets is due to the considerable disc thinning (D) and posterolateral herniation. In addition, tractioning of the pain sensitive inferior part of the joint capsule (C) is present due to the facet subluxation. The posterior herniation of the disc, with associated osteophytic spur (OS) encroaches upon the anterior side of the foramen, and there is encroachment upon the foramen posteriorly due to the osteophytic spur (OS) at the tip of the superior articular process of the sacrum (S SAP). In the subchondral bone, particularly above the rectangle shown, there are areas of advanced degenerative bone marrow changes (asterisks). The rectangle illustrates the area magnified in Figures **(C)** and **(E)** that show *deep fissuring* of the hyaline articular cartilage (H) by both light microscopy **(C)** and darkfield light microscopy **(E)** (white arrows), respectively, indicating that this cartilage shows Grade 3 degenerative changes (using O'Leary et al's (2017) grading). **(D)** Greater magnification of part of the cartilage from the dashed rectangle on Figure **(C)** shows blood vessels (V) between the opposing facet surfaces and in the region of deep fissuring. M = muscle; N = neural complex within the intervertebral foramen.

Source: Reproduced from: Giles LGF, Kaveri MJP, Lumbosacral intervertebral disc degeneration revisited: a radiological and histological correlation. Manual Medicine 6: 62–66, 1991a, Springer Nature.

10. Multifactorial Degeneration Occurring at Two Adjacent Spinal Levels (Figure 4.25)

Clinical relevance: Degenerative changes at the L4–5 and L5-S1 three-joint complex levels with encroachment upon the neural complex in the L5-S1 intervertebral foramen independently and collectively can cause low back pain, with or without radicular symptoms.

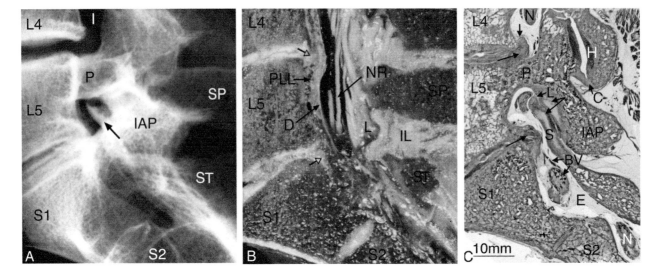

FIGURE 4.25 The lateral view plain X-ray extending from L4 to S2 from a 59-year-old female cadaver (A) with its corresponding sagittally bisected cadaveric spine (B) and a parasagittal histological section (C) all show the intervertebral disc thinning at L4–5 and L5-S1 levels. **(A)** I = intervertebral foramen; IAP = inferior articular process of L5 vertebra; P = pedicle of L5 vertebra; SP = spinous process; ST = sacral tubercle (median crest) of the sacrum. The superior articular process of S1 (arrow) *projects into the L5-S1 foramen* due to the very thin disc and facet subluxation at this level that is confirmed histologically in (C). **(B)** The L4–5 and L5-S1 intervertebral discs show degeneration with *posterior protrusions* (open headed arrows) and *loss of disc height*. Note the posterior longitudinal ligament (PLL), dural tube (D), nerve roots (NR), and spinous process (SP). IL = interspinous ligament that extends from the supraspinous ligament posteriorly (not shown) to the ligamentum flavum (L) anteriorly; ST = spinous tubercle (median crest) of the sacrum. **(C)** A 200-µm-thick histological section cut in the *parasagittal* plane from the specimen shows parts of the L4 to S2 spinal segments. N = neurovascular complexes within the L4-L5 and L5-S1 intervertebral foramina and within the sacral canal—they are surrounded by epidural fat (E) and are highly vascular (BV). Posterolateral intervertebral disc *protrusions* (arrows) with *thinning* of the L4–5 and L5-S1 discs is demonstrated; this has resulted in approximation of the vertebral bodies with *imbrication (subluxation)* (Hadley 1950, 1951) of the opposing facets of the zygapophysial joints and their hyaline articular cartilage lined surfaces (H). The zygapophysial joint imbrication has caused some *tractioning of the L4-L5 joint capsule* (C) inferiorly, and, at the L5-S1 level, the subluxation has caused 'buckling' of the ligamentum flavum (L). This buckling, together with early osteophytosis of the superior articular process (S) of the sacrum, has caused *deformation and compression* of the adjacent posterior aspect of the neural complex with its vascular supply. Pressure upon the neural complex and its blood vessels can cause vascular congestion that could impair the circulation through the neural complex to a degree that could be responsible for the earliest neurological signs and symptoms associated with intervertebral disc thinning (Sunderland 1980). There is *subchondral sclerosis/eburnation* (conjoined arrows) of each facet at the L5-S1 level, in particular, with *osteoarthrotic* changes. IAP = inferior articular process of L5 vertebra; P = pedicle of L5 vertebra.

Source: Reproduced with permission from Giles LGF, 100 Challenging Spinal Pain Syndrome Cases, Edinburgh, Churchill Livingstone Elsevier, © Elsevier, 2009.

Routine plain X-ray images would show the loss of IVD space height and the osseous degenerative changes. MR imaging should provide insight into the L5-S1 foraminal compromise of the neural complex but may well not show the stretching of the L4–5 joint capsule.

11. Adhesions within a Zygapophysial Joint Capsule and Bridging across Joint Surfaces (Figure 4.26)

Clinical relevance: Such adhesions may cause pain as the fibrous joint capsule is innervated by nociceptors (Kim et al 2011). In addition, spinal manipulation may, in all likelihood, result in slight post-manipulation pain or discomfort due to breaking down of the adhesions while restoring normal function to the three-joint complex.

Cramer et al (2013) have shown that spinal manipulation causes gapping between the facet surfaces of zygapophysial joints.

As the joint capsule contains nociceptors, the adhesions would be a source of back pain during any movements that tractioned them, and therapeutic manipulation would be aimed at breaking down intra-articular joint or capsular adhesions (Mennell 1960).

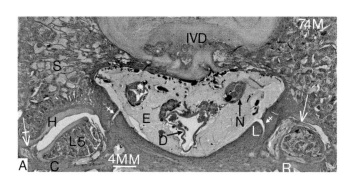
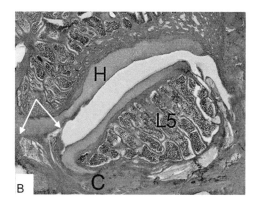

FIGURE 4.26   (A) A 100-μm-thick histological section cut in the axial plane, below the L5-S1 intervertebral foramina, of a 74-year-old male cadaver. Part of the left zygapophysial joint's fibrous capsule (C) fibres have become *attached to the surface of the hyaline articular cartilage* (H) on the sacral facet's cartilage surface (long tailed arrow), between the articulating surfaces laterally; see enlargement in **(B)** to visualize the width of the adhesions (white arrows). The right (R) zygapophysial joint shows a large highly vascular intra-capsular synovial fold, with a partly fibrotic tip projecting between the osteoarthrotic hyaline articular cartilage surfaces (arrow). This intra-articular part of the fat filled synovial lined structure's fibrotic change is probably due to 'nipping' between the joint surfaces during life. D = dural tube containing the cauda equina within the CSF. E = epidural fat; IVD = intervertebral disc with a small midline posterior bulge/protrusion; L = ligamentum flavum with a neuro-vascular channel bilaterally (small tailed arrows); L5 = inferior articular process of the fifth lumbar vertebra; N = nerve roots in their dural sleeves (see Figure 4.27B for the development of nerve roots and their root sleeves); S = sacral ala.

Source: Reproduced with permission from Giles LGF, A review and description of some possible causes of low back pain of mechanical origin in homo sapiens. Proc Aust Soc Hum Biol 4: 193–212, 1991(b).

Plain X-ray examination would not be likely to show such adhesions. In addition, the detail of such adhesions would most likely not be seen on routine MR imaging.

---

12. Nerve Roots and Their CSF Relationship
     (Figures 4.27 and 4.28)

  Clinical relevance: As mechanical pressure upon nerve roots can cause circulatory disturbance of the nerve root resulting in radicular pain (Yoshizawa et al 1991), the formation of these important structures within the normal spinal canal is illustrated in Figures 4.27A and B where the

anterior and posterior roots exit the subarachnoid space in which the rootlets are immersed in CSF. As previously mentioned, nerve roots derive some of their nutritional supply via diffusion from the surrounding CSF (Rydevik et al 1990) that is also involved in CNS tissue *drainage* and *detoxification* (Thomas et al 2019).

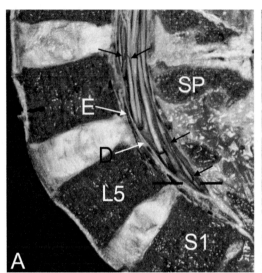
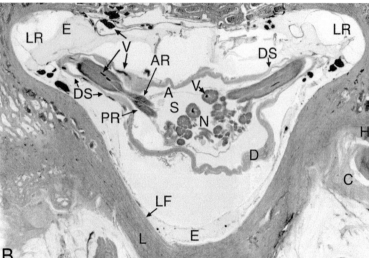

FIGURE 4.27   **(A)** Lower lumbosacral spine bisected in the sagittal plane. Cauda equina nerve roots descend with their small diameter blood vessels i.e. vasa radiculorum (black arrows) within the dural tube (D) that is surrounded by epidural fat (E), then pass out of the dural tube, enveloped within *root sleeves*, as shown in (B). SP = spinous process. **(B)** This 100-μm-thick axial histological section has been cut approximately at the lumbosacral level represented by the broken black line in (A) from a 55-year-old male cadaver. The dural tube (D) surrounds the arachnoid mater (A) that contains the *cerebrospinal fluid* and the cauda equina nerve roots (N) with their small diameter blood vessels (V). In this section, the left dural sleeve (DS) illustrates how blood vessels are normally seen in these structures. Within the subarachnoid space, the *sacral* roots occupy a more posterior position than do the *lumbar* roots that are more anterior (see Figure 2.9B); E = epidural fat within the spinal canal that surrounds the dural tube and the nerve root sleeves. The anterior nerve root (AR) and the posterior nerve root (PR) pass from the dural tube, within the dural sleeve (DS), to the *lateral recess* (LR) of the vertebral foramen before entering the IVF. C = fibrous capsule of the L5-S1 zygapophysial joint; H = hyaline articular cartilage on the sacral superior articular process; L = lamina; LF = ligamentum flavum. Some blood vessels are seen in various regions of the epidural fat.

  Furthermore, axial histological sections shown in the following three examples (Figures 4.28A, B, and C) illustrate the close relationship between the epineurium of the *neural complex* and its adjoining *vascular structures* within the intervertebral foramen.

  An axial view (Figure 4.28C) of a left intervertebral foramen at the lumbosacral level of another specimen, again indicating a possible vascular channel connection between Batson's vertebral venous plexus and the adjacent neural complex.

  This topic was raised under CSF drainage around nerve roots in Chapter 2—*Neuroanatomy Summary of the Lumbosacral Spine* (Figures 2.28–2.30).

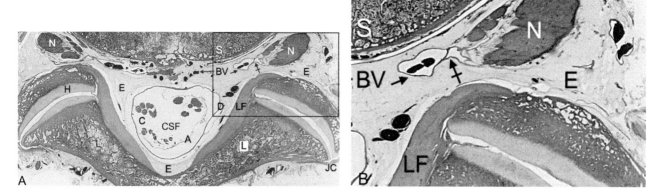

FIGURE 4.28 **(A)** A 100-μm-thick axial lumbosacral section at the level of the left and right intervertebral foramina of a 54-year-old male cadaver. A = arachnoid mater surrounding the CSF with its cauda equina nerve roots (C); BV = Batson's venous plexus (anterior internal vertebral (epidural) plexus) that also communicates with the external vertebral venous plexuses on the external surface of the vertebrae (Moore et al 2018); D = dura mater; E = epidural fat space; H = hyaline articular cartilage; JC = joint capsule (fibrous) of the zygapophysial joint; L = lamina; LF = ligamentum flavum; N = neural complex; S = sacrum. Tailed arrow indicates a possible vascular channel connecting Batson's venous plexus with the neural complex. Rectangle shows that area magnified in Figure **(B)**.

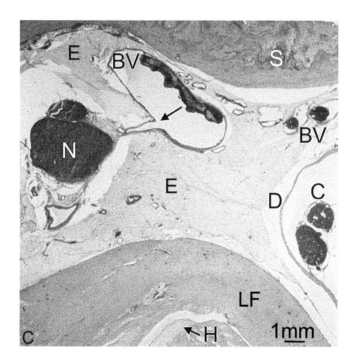

FIGURE 4.28 **(C)** Axial histological view of the left intervertebral foramen at the lumbosacral level of a 35-year-old female cadaver that exhibits a possible vascular connection (arrow) between the neural complex (N) and one of the internal vertebral venous plexus blood vessels (BV) as seen at this magnification for this 100-μm-thick section; C = cauda equina; D = dural tube; E = epidural fat; H = hyaline articular cartilage on the adjacent facet joint surface; LF = ligamentum flavum; S = sacrum.

Intervertebral Disc Joints

1. Intervertebral Disc Protrusion Anteriorly and Posteriorly with Internal Disc Disruption at Only One Spinal Level (Figure 4.29)

Clinical relevance: Internal disc disruption can cause low back pain (Cooke et al 2000). Protruding IVD

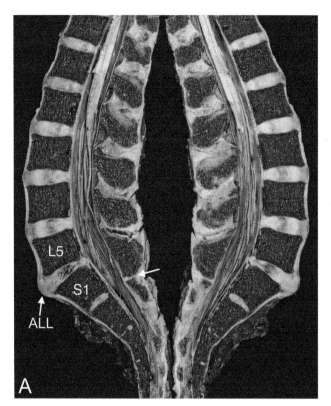

pressure upon the pain sensitive anterior surface of the dural tube (Figure 4.29), the intervening blood vessels and the recurrent meningeal nerves can cause low back pain, as discogenic low back pain is mediated by the recurrent meningeal nerves (Zhao et al 2020(c)). In addition, pressure is being exerted upon the innervated anterior longitudinal ligament and this may generate pain. It should be noted that this disc injury at only one level is highly unlikely to be a 'constitutional' condition—a term that I have frequently seen in medico-legal reports where only one disc shows degenerative changes.

As an IVD degenerates, the peripheral nerve tissues have corresponding structural reorganization, and series of nerve cells become involved in progression of discogenic back pain (Yang et al 2018).

Tissue samples from lumbar disc operations studied immunohistochemically suggest that *pressure* and *chemical irritation* of nociceptive nerves associated with degenerated discs excite sensory neural elements, especially in the posterior longitudinal ligament and possibly in the peripheral parts of the annulus fibrosus, while the disc itself, at least if not penetrated by vascular granular tissue, is painless and neuroanatomically lacks a structural basis for pain perception (Konttinen et al 1990).

An axial view L5-S1 histological example (Figure 4.29B) shows an IVD bulging posteriorly, with internal disc disruption and some disruption of the outer annulus fibrosus fibres (curved white arrow).

FIGURE 4.29 (A) Anatomical specimen of a sagittally sectioned lumbosacral spine of a 70-year-old female cadaver. Note the approximation (arrow) of the somewhat enlarged (superior to inferior dimension) fifth lumbar spinous process and the adjacent sacral spinous tubercle, in spite of the normal lumbar lordosis. This can cause Baastrup's disease i.e. mechanical low back pain arising from the close approximation of adjacent posterior spinous processes with resulting degenerative changes of the interspinous ligament and sclerotic changes of the opposing spinous processes. It is important to note that, in this elderly specimen, *only* the L5 intervertebral disc shows degenerative changes. These changes include (i) anterior protrusion of the disc, causing pressure upon the innervated anterior longitudinal ligament (ALL) and (ii) posterior protrusion of the disrupted nucleus pulposus and annulus fibrosus causing elevation of the posterior longitudinal ligament with resulting pressure upon the pain sensitive dural tube.

Source: Reproduced with permission from Giles LGF, Miscellaneous pathological and developmental (anomalous) conditions. In: Giles L G F, Singer K P (eds) Clinical anatomy and management of low back pain. Butterworth-Heinemann, Oxford, © Elsevier, 1997(c) pp. 196–216.

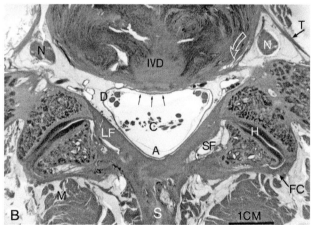

FIGURE 4.29 (B) A 200-μm-thick axial histological section from a 51-year-old female cadaver. Note the *internal disc disruption* within the intervertebral disc (IVD) with some radial tears seen as white spaces, and there is some disruption of the outer annulus fibrosus lamellae (curved white arrow). There is some central posterior bulging of the disc that *indents* (small black arrows) the anterior part of the dural tube (D), which contains the cauda equina (C) that is immersed in cerebrospinal fluid within the arachnoid mater (A). The neural complex (N) passing through the lateral part of the intervertebral foramen is in close proximity to transforaminal

FIGURE 4.29 (Continued)

ligaments (T). S = remains of spinous process. SF = synovial lined fat pad adjacent to the ligamentum flavum (LF). H = hyaline articular cartilage on the surfaces of the facets of the zygapophysial joints. FC = fibrous joint capsule posterolaterally. M = muscle.

Source: Reproduced with permission from Giles LGF, 100 Challenging Spinal Pain Syndrome Cases, Churchill Livingstone Elsevier, Edinburgh, © Elsevier, 2009.

> **An axial view MRI or CT scan should show this central disc posterior bulging-dural tube abnormality.**

A sagittal view lumbar spine MRI of a patient illustrating annular tears is shown in Figure 4.29(C).

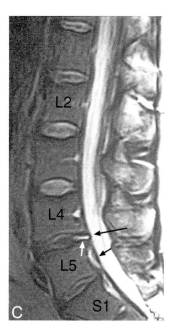

FIGURE 4.29 (**C**) A lumbar spine MRI sagittal T2-weighted image of a 35-year-old male showing that, at the L4–5 level, there is a moderate sized posterior disc bulge (long black arrow), due to a tear in the posterior fibres of the intervertebral disc represented by a *high signal intensity zone* (white arrow) (Haldeman et al 2002) and a degree of desiccation of the disc. The disc bulge presses upon the pain sensitive anterior surface of the dural tube. The discs above the L4 level show *intranuclear clefts* of varying thickness across the centre of these discs, with thinner intranuclear clefts above L2. The intranuclear cleft is an area within the disc where there is a relative absence of glycosyl amino glycans (GAG) and a relative increase in hydroxyproline or collagen content i.e. it is not a gross, morphologic structure but rather a *zone of different biochemistry* (MT Modic, MD, FACR, Personal communication, 2002). According to Theodorou et al (2020), in individuals after the third decade of life, nuclear clefts form in the setting of dehydration of the nucleus pulposus.

Source: Reproduced with permission from Giles LGF, 100 Challenging Spinal Pain Syndrome Cases, Churchill Livingstone Elsevier, Edinburgh, © Elsevier, 2009.

2. Intervertebral Disc *Central* Posterior Protrusion (Figure 4.30)

Clinical relevance: A central protrusion is likely to cause low back pain due to pressure upon the pain sensitive anterior surface of the dural tube, intervening blood vessels, and the associated recurrent meningeal nerves. However, there would *not be* associated radicular symptoms as the nerve roots are not compressed (Figures 4.30 A and B). Therefore, the straight leg raising test would likely not cause further pain, in spite of the protrusion, as illustrated by the following very briefly outlined case as an example. A 29-year-old female presented with intermittent central low back pain since jumping out of an army truck approximately 15 months prior to consultation. There was no radiation to the lower limbs. The straight leg raising test did not aggravate the low back pain. Imaging showed a central IVD protrusion (Figure 4.30A).

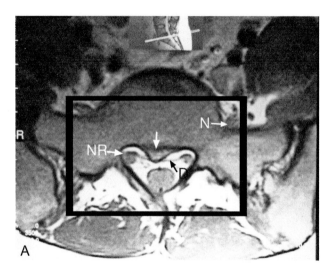
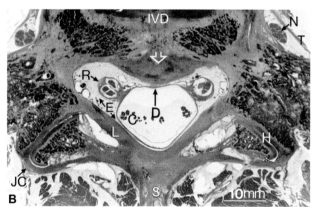

FIGURE 4.30 **(A)** L5-S1 level axial MRI Intermediate Weighted Spin Echo image showing a *central* disc protrusion (arrow) that does *not abut* the adjacent nerve roots (NR) but indents the pain sensitive anterior surface of the dural tube (D). N = spinal nerve. **(B)** In order to complement the MR image, a 200-μm-thick axially cut histological section from a cadaver with a central posterior disc (IVD) protrusion (open white arrow) that indents the dural tube (D) but does *not* affect the nerve roots is presented. R = nerve root sleeve budding off from the dural tube that contains small nerve roots arising from the cauda equina (C). E = epidural fat space; H = hyaline articular cartilage on the zygapophysial joint facet surfaces; JC = joint capsule (fibrous); L = ligamentum flavum; N = spinal nerve; S = spinous process; T = transforaminal ligament.

Source: Reproduced with permission from Giles LGF, 100 Challenging Spinal Pain Syndrome Cases, Churchill Livingstone Elsevier, Edinburgh, © Elsevier, 2009.

Thus, clinically, the patient's low back pain may not be understood until an MRI is performed to illustrate the reason for low back pain symptoms when the straight leg raising test is negative. It is important for such a patient's condition to be taken seriously and thoroughly investigated in order to prevent psychological sequelae.

3. **Intervertebral Disc** *Broad-Based*
   Posterior Protrusion (Figure 4.31)
   Clinical relevance: Several aetiologies of lumbosacral spine pain and radiculopathy exist:

1. It has been known for many years that IVD posterior or posterolateral protrusion with *nerve root compression* will cause low back pain with some degree of radicular symptoms (Mixter et al 1934; Crock 1976; Paksoy et al 2004; Summers et al 2005), and it is most common origin of lumbar radiculopathy (Dydyk et al 2020). Also, lumbar radicular pain can be caused by irritation of the sensory root ganglion (Govind 2004).

2. Mechanical compression of a spinal nerve or nerve root ganglion, altering root microcirculation, will lead to ischaemia (Rydevik et al 1984; Olmarker et al 1989; Yoshizawa et al 1991) and markers of nerve tissue injury have been found in the CSF of patients with lumbar disc herniation and sciatica (Brisby et al 1999). Impairment of intraneural circulation in the nerve roots caused by chronic compression, *even at low pressures*, may induce intra- and extraneural fibrosis that leads to dysfunction of nerve fibres (Yoshizawa et al 1991).

3. The acute localized pain associated with an IVD herniation also undoubtedly emanates from the disrupted posterolateral annulus fibrosus and impingement on the posterior longitudinal ligament—pain is conveyed initially by the meningeal branches of the spinal nerves (Moore et al 2018).

4. The dural pain concept was first defined by Cyriax in 1945, and it is known that IVD herniation pressure upon the pain sensitive anterior surface of the dural tube (Summers et al 2005) with its recurrent meningeal nerves—or on a dural sleeve—can result in pain (Wyke 1980).

5. Intervertebral disc herniation pressure upon blood vessels, causing pain of ischaemic origin (Sunderland 1975) due to vascular damage (Hoyland et al 1989; Jayson 1997) between the herniation and the dural tube may result in pain.

6. Symptoms due to herniated nucleus pulposus can ultimately be attributed to the significant inflammatory response it generates inside the spinal canal; disc injury results in an increase in the pro-inflammatory molecules interleukin (IL)—1, IL—8, and tumour necrosis factor alpha (TNF alpha), an anti-inflammatory cytokine produced by macrophages/monocytes during acute inflammation and is responsible for a diverse range of signalling events within cells, leading to necrosis or apoptosis (Idriss et al 2000).

The anatomical and histological appearance of a large posterior herniation due to mechanical failure, as a result of abnormal stresses, is shown in Figure 4.31.

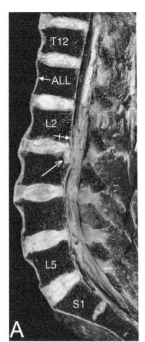
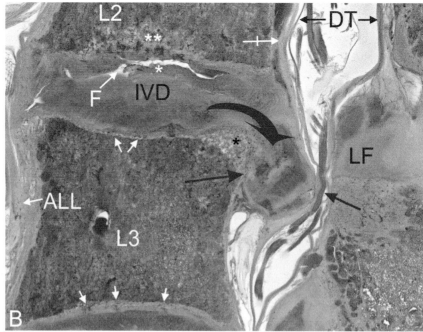

FIGURE 4.31 **(A)** Part of a spinal column extending from T12 disc to S2 is shown bisected in approximately the sagittal plane. The intervertebral discs appear to be relatively normal for this 62-year-old male cadaver's spine apart from the L2–3 internal disc disruption with large posterior herniation (arrow) that causes compression of the anterior epidural space, dural tube, and cauda equina, resulting in some stenosis of the spinal canal at this level. ALL = anterior longitudinal ligament; tailed arrow = posterior longitudinal ligament. **(B)** A 200-µm-thick parasagittal histological section showing the L2–3 intervertebral disc (IVD) herniation magnified. The large arrow shows the herniated disc material with inferior migration that disrupts the posterior longitudinal ligament (white tailed arrow) and compresses the dural tube (DT). Note the nerve root (small black arrow) between the protrusion and the ligamentum flavum (LF) and adjacent bone. As the section is 200 µm thick (1/5th of a millimetre), only one nerve root is seen to be compressed. However, in a broad-based disc protrusion a number of nerve roots would be compressed, causing the cauda equina syndrome. ALL = anterior longitudinal ligament. Apart from the large posterior herniation, the superior CEP interface between the vertebral body and the disc shows degenerative changes with some avulsion of the CEP (*) and a small fracture (F) in the CEP, with a degree of subchondral bony sclerosis (**) in the adjacent vertebral body. In addition, the L3 vertebral body's superior and inferior CEPs appear to show hyperaemia of their capillary tufts (small white arrows). Black asterisk represents early Modic changes.

Source: Reproduced with permission from Giles LGF, 100 Challenging Spinal Pain Syndrome Cases, Churchill Livingstone Elsevier, Edinburgh, © Elsevier, 2009.

MRI should provide an appropriate diagnosis for such a case.

4. Endplate Injury/Microfracture with Associated Posterolateral Disc Herniation and Examples of Schmorl's Nodes (Figures 4.32 and 4.33)

Clinical relevance: Although endplate sub-acute traumatic failures (microfractures) may not be visible on plain radiographs, they may well be a source of acute low back pain (Hansson et al 1981; Hamanishi et al 1994; Lotz et al 2013) and lead to accelerated spinal degeneration (Hilton et al 1976; Fraser et al 1997) (Figure 4.32). In vitro studies revealed that the most likely cause of an endplate fracture is as a result of compression (van Dieen et al 1999).

It is known that the posterior longitudinal ligament may be a source of low back pain (Lin et al 2020), and this may occur due to pressure from a protruding disc pressing against the posterior longitudinal ligament.

Schmorl's nodes are described as a rupture of IVD tissue into the underlying spongiosa of the vertebral body (Rickenbacher et al 1985). They are defined histologically as a focal herniation of IVD material through the endplate into the vertebral body (Kim et al 2018), and Lotz et al (2013) showed that damaged endplate regions can be the sites of reactive bone marrow lesions that include *proliferating nerves* that can be a source of chronic low back pain by irritating nociceptors (Kim et al 2018). These acute 'cartilaginous nodes' are perhaps an under-recognized entity that can cause intense localized spinal pain (Ghuman et al 2014).

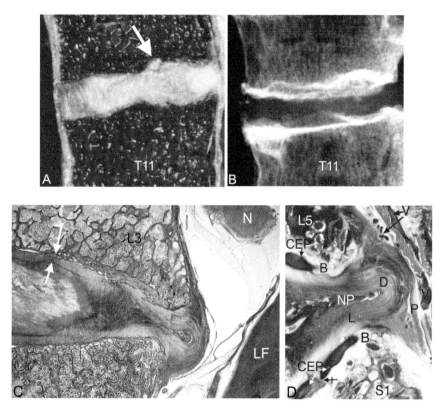

FIGURE 4.32 **(A)** An anatomical specimen from a 78-year-old male cadaver. Note: (1) the T10 inferior endplate shows some irregularity as does the superior endplate of T11, (2) a small Schmorl's node (arrow) that is due to a CEP mechanical injury. The corresponding plain X-ray **(B)** does not clearly demonstrate the small Schmorl's node itself but shows the overall irregularity of the endplates. This provides an example of the limitation of plain X-ray imaging. **(C)** A 150-μm-thick parasagittal histological section from the L3–4 spinal level of a 75-year-old male cadaver illustrating an endplate fracture (arrows), which could cause pain, and yet the fracture would not be seen on routine imaging. Note the posterolateral disc herniation, ligamentum flavum (LF), and neural complex (N). **(D)** A 200-μm-thick sagittally cut histological darkfield section from a 70-year-old female cadaver showing a cartilage endplate (CEP) microfracture (tailed arrow) of the caudal (inferior) endplate of the L5-S1 disc (D). The intervertebral disc shows degeneration with *internal disc disruption* and posterior protrusion of part of the annulus fibrosus. This causes the protruding disc's lamellae (L) to arch around the posteriorly migrating nucleus pulposus (NP) toward the spinal canal, thus elevating the posterior longitudinal ligament (P). The annular lamellae attach to (1) the CEP and (2) the bone plate (B) (fused ring epiphysis) as Sharpey's fibres. Note the proximity of the CEP to the bone plate, both of which are associated with haematopoietic marrow elements, particularly the CEPs (see Figure 3.19). The bulging disc with the posterior longitudinal ligament press upon the adjacent blood vessels (V). L5 = fifth lumbar vertebral body; S1 = first sacral body.

Source: (D) Reproduced with permission from Giles LGF, 100 Challenging Spinal Pain Syndrome Cases, Churchill Livingstone Elsevier, Edinburgh, © Elsevier, 2009.

Lateral view images of a 27-year-old male's lumbosacral spine, following a fall off a ladder onto his low back on a hard surface, resulting in low back pain, are shown in Figure 4.33A to D. The plain X-ray was taken four months post injury (Figure 4.33A) and only just gives an outline of a possible Schmorl's node in the superior surface of the sacrum that went unreported at the time. Due to continuing significant low back pain, a CT scan was performed six months following the fall (Figure 4.33B and D) and was followed by an MR examination shortly thereafter (Figure 4.33C). The CT and MRI images showed a Schmorl's node type compression fracture in the superior surface of the sacrum, with typical early sclerotic changes; these also went unreported.

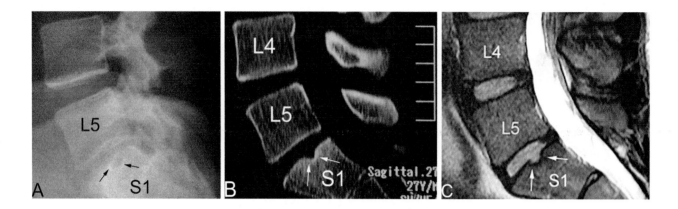

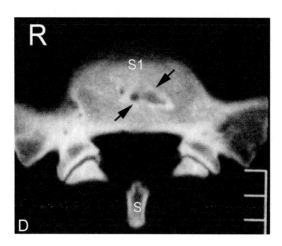

FIGURE 4.33 **(A)** Lumbosacral spine plain X-ray lateral view showing the suspicion of a Schmorl's node type compression fracture in the S1 superior endplate (black arrows). **(B)** Lumbosacral spine sagittal CT bone window scan showing a Schmorl's node compression fracture in the superior endplate of the S1 body (white arrows). **(C)** Lumbosacral spine MRI sagittal T2-weighted image showing a typical Schmorl's node type compression fracture of the superior endplate of S1 body (small white arrows). The lumbar discs have normal hydration. **(D)** Axial CT scan of the first sacral segment (S1) through the Schmorl's node (arrows) shown in (B). R = right side of patient; S = spinous process.

The characteristic appearance of a Schmorl's node is a well-circumscribed rounded lucency in a vertebral body, with associated endplate defect and a thin sclerotic rim (Carr et al 2012), and anatomical studies have repeatedly shown that there is more extensive pathology than is visualized upon radiography (Hadley 1964).

In a study of Schmorl's nodes and low back pain using MRI, Takahashi et al (1995) found the following: in all symptomatic cases, the vertebral body marrow surrounding the Schmorl's node was seen as low signal intensity on T1-weighted images and as high signal intensity on T2-weighted images; it was confirmed by histological examination that the MRI finding indicated the presence of inflammation and oedema in the vertebral bone marrow; these MRI findings were not seen in asymptomatic individuals—inflammatory changes in the vertebral body marrow induced by intraosseous fracture and biological reactions to intraspongious disc material might cause pain; MRI is not only useful in detecting a recently developed Schmorl's node but also in differentiating between symptomatic and asymptomatic Schmorl's nodes. Furthermore, in the treatment of symptomatic

Schmorl's nodes using percutaneous vertebroplasty, this was found to be an effective and safe procedure when the nodes were refractory to medical or physical therapy (He et al 2017).

5. Posterior Migration and Leakage of Nuclear Material (Figure 4.34)

Clinical relevance: A nucleus pulposus displacement due to an annular tear (or fissure) allowing nuclear material to leak out of the disc (Giles 1992(b)) (Figure 4.34B) can cause *discogenic back pain* and sciatica (Grönblad et al 1997) due to chemical irritation of adjacent neural structures, i.e. *chemical radiculopathy* (Marshall et al 1973; Marshall et al 1977; Goupille et al 1998, 2006; Slipman et al 2002; Byun et al 2012) with the involvement of leakage of chemical mediators or inflammatory cytokines, which are produced in the painful disc (Peng et al 2007). Unfortunately, annular tears may not be seen even on sensitive imaging such as MR (Giles 2003(b)) and Eriksson et al (2022) confirm that, although MRI is a sensitive method, fissures are sometimes unobservable in T2-weighted MR images.

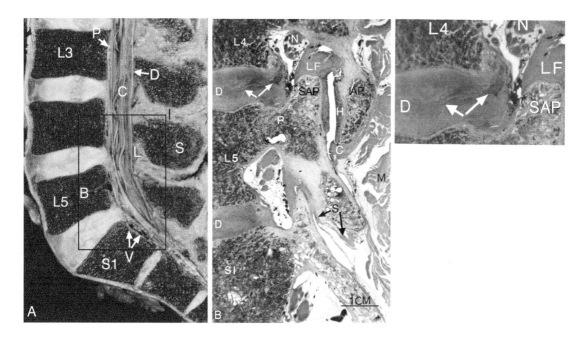

FIGURE 4.34 **(A)** Part of a spinal column extending from L3 to S2 is shown bisected in the sagittal plane. The intervertebral discs appear to be relatively normal for a 78-year-old male cadaver. B = basivertebral vein canal; C = cauda equina; D = dural tube; I = interspinous ligament; L = ligamentum flavum; P = posterior longitudinal ligament; S = spinous process; V = veins of the anterior internal vertebral (epidural) plexus within the spinal canal. **(B)** A 200-μm-thick parasagittal histological section from the rectangular area shown on (A) and cut through the pedicles, viewed by light microscopy, showing a *tear* within the L4–5 intervertebral disc with retrograde movement of nuclear material in this disc (white arrows). The tear region of the disc is enlarged on the right. C = capsule (inferiorly) of the L4–5 zygapophysial joint; D = intervertebral disc; H = hyaline articular cartilage on the facet of the inferior articular process (IAP) of the L4 vertebra; L4 = part of the fourth lumbar vertebral body; L5 = part of the fifth lumbar vertebral body; LF = ligamentum flavum; M = muscle; N = neural complex within the nerve root sheath located in the pear-shaped intervertebral foramen; P = pedicle of the L5 vertebra; S = synovial fold projecting into the inferior recess of the zygapophysial joint at the L5-S1 level; S1 = first sacral segment; SAP = superior articular process of the L5 vertebra.

Source: **(B) Reproduced with permission from Giles LGF, Ligaments traversing the intervertebral canals of the human lower lumbosacral spine. Neuro-Ortho 13:25–38, 1992(b), Springer Nature.**

Briefly, a clinical example to emphasize the important issue of a disc tear follows. A 20-year-old male who presented with central 'moderate' low back pain with some radiation down the lateral aspect of his left leg and paraesthesias in the left foot that followed heavy lifting at work six months before consultation. He said previous consultations had included referrals for MR imaging (reported as being 'normal') and that the consultations had not explained the cause of his 'genuine' symptoms. He had subsequently been told that he did not have an injury enabling him to claim for Workers' Compensation. He was disillusioned and depressed as he had pain that prevented him from working. In view of this, a CT myelogram (Figure 4.34C) was requested and it showed a *"full thickness left posterolateral tear in the annular fibres (arrows) with some internal disc disruption centrally"*.

When the substance of the nucleus pulposus comes into contact with sensory nerves of the epidural tissues including the outer annulus it: (i) induces degeneration of nerve fibres, (ii) increases discharge of nerve fibres, (iii) attracts inflammatory cells (cellular mediators of pain), and (iv) induces increased intraneural capillary permeability (di Zerega et al 2010) resulting in low back pain.

The patient was very pleased to finally have a diagnosis made and to be told that he had a genuine organic condition!

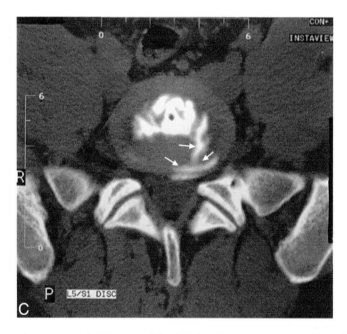

FIGURE 4.34 **(C)** Post-myelogram axial CT scan of the L5-S1 disc in a 20-year-old male.

Source: **Reproduced with permission from Giles LGF, 100 Challenging Spinal Pain Syndrome Cases, Churchill Livingstone Elsevier, Edinburgh, © Elsevier, 2009.**

6. Blood Vessels Associated with Intervertebral Disc Degenerative Changes and Accompanying Vascular Ingrowth (Figures 4.35 and 4.36)

Clinical relevance: Annulus fissures provide a low-pressure microenvironment that allows focal proteoglycan loss, leaving a matrix that is mechanically and chemically conducive to the ingrowth of nerves and blood vessels (Stefanakis et al 2012), i.e. these degenerative changes allow the *nerves and blood vessels* in the peripheral annulus of adult IVDs to grow inwards and to become associated with discogenic pain (Lama et al 2018; Binch et al 2021). In addition, degenerative disc disease with disc protrusion and osteophytic proliferation may lead to *compression of epidural veins*, with dilation of non-compressed veins and venous obstruction, resulting in hypoxia that leads to nerve root damage (Jayson 1992).

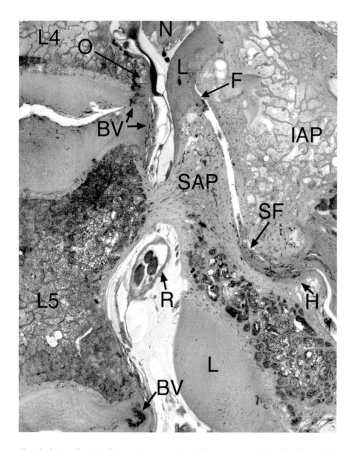

FIGURE 4.35 A 200-μm-thick histological section cut in the para-sagittal plane through part of the right L4–5 and L5-S1 intervertebral foramina, and the L4–5 zygapophysial joint of a 62-year-old male cadaver. IAP = inferior articular process of the L4 vertebra and the adjacent superior articular process of the L5 vertebra; L = ligamentum flavum; L4 = fourth lumbar vertebral body; L5 = fifth lumbar vertebral body; N = neural complex in the respective intervertebral foramina; R = root sleeve containing neural and vascular structures. Blood vessel (BV) ingrowth into the posterior parts of both the degenerating discs is present. The L4–5 level disc bulge is accompanied by osteophytes (O). An L4–5 zygapophysial joint fibrous intra-articular structure (F) projects from the ligamentum flavum (L) into the upper pole of the degenerating zygapophysial joint that shows loss of facet hyaline cartilage. A large synovial fold (SF) is noted in the inferior pole.

Source: Reproduced with permission from Giles LGF, 100 Challenging Spinal Pain Syndrome Cases, Churchill Livingstone Elsevier, Edinburgh, © Elsevier, 2009.

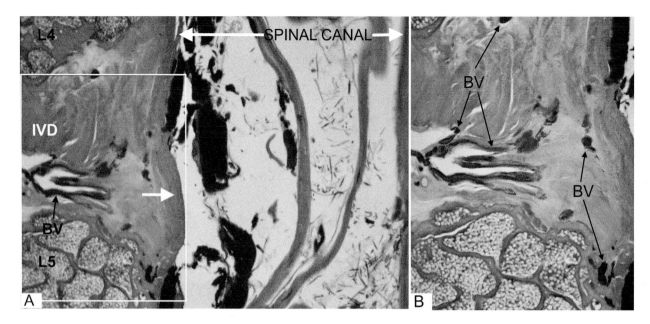

FIGURE 4.36 **(A)** A 150-μm-thick histological section from a degenerating L4–5 intervertebral disc (IVD) of an 82-year-old female cadaver showing blood vessel (BV) ingrowth within the degenerating disc that has a *minor* posterior intervertebral disc bulge (white arrow). **(B)** Represents an enlargement of the area in the rectangle in (A), showing part of the disc that has several blood vessels (BV) within it.

Sophisticated contrast MR imaging would be necessary to show blood vessels within an IVD to best advantage.

7. Vertebral Body Posterolateral Osteophytes (Figure 4.37)

Clinical relevance: Osteophytes projecting from the vertebral body postero-laterally and mechanically pressing upon adjacent neural structures will cause pain (Kobayashi et al 2005).

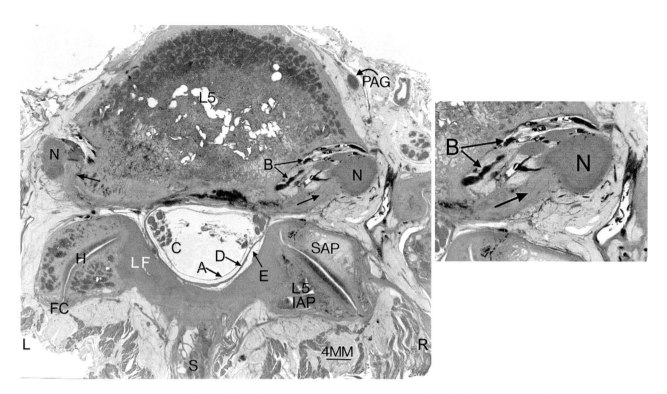

FIGURE 4.37 A 200-μm-thick axial histological section from the L5-S1 level of a 60-year-old female cadaver. On the left (L) and right sides (R) there are posterolateral osteophytes (arrows) abutting the adjacent neural complexes (N) that are being deformed by the osteophytes (enlarged on the right side). Note the extensive blood vessels (B) around the neural complex on the right side and, to a lesser extent, on the left. A = arachnoid mater of the dural tube (D), containing the CSF; C = cauda equina nerve roots within the lumbar dural tube; E = epidural fat in the epidural space; FC = fibrous capsule posteriorly of the zygapophysial joint; H = hyaline articular cartilage on the zygapophysial joint facet surfaces; L5 IAP = inferior articular process of the L5 vertebra; LF = ligamentum flavum that covers the medial aspect of the zygapophysial joint; L5 = body of the L5 vertebra; PAG = paraspinal autonomic ganglion; SAP = superior articular process of the sacrum; S = spinous process.

This type of posterolateral osteophytic lipping should be seen on CT or MRI axial scans. However, the best way to obtain good detail of such neural distortion would be to use the technique of high-resolution 3D-CISS MR images.

8. Intervertebral Disc Protrusion with Vertebral Body Lateral Osteophytes (Figure 4.38)

Clinical relevance: The osteophytes cause mechanical pressure upon—and traction of—the *paravertebral autonomic ganglia* (Nathan 1962, 1968, 1987) and have been implicated in the *vertebrogenic autonomic syndrome* (Jinkins et al 1989; Jinkins 1997). This far-reaching perplexing combined somatic autonomic neurogenic syndrome stems from spinal disease that includes varying degrees of (i) local somatic pain, (ii) centripetally (afferent)/centrifugally (efferent) referred pain, (iii) *local and referred sympathetic reflex dysfunction* (diaphoresis, piloerection, vasomotor changes,

somatic muscle spasm), (iv) somatic reflex dysfunction, (v) somatic muscle weakness, (vi) peripheral somatic dysesthesias, and (vii) generalized alterations in *viscerosomatic tone* (blood pressure, heart rate, respiratory rate, alertness) (Jinkins 1997).

The plain X-ray anteroposterior view (Figure 4.38A) illustrates the principle that neurological tissues of the spine cannot be seen on plain X-ray images. Therefore, the neurological implications of the lateral osteophytes on the vertebral bodies would be overlooked if the clinician treating a patient is not aware of the possible neuroanatomical structures being mechanically deformed.

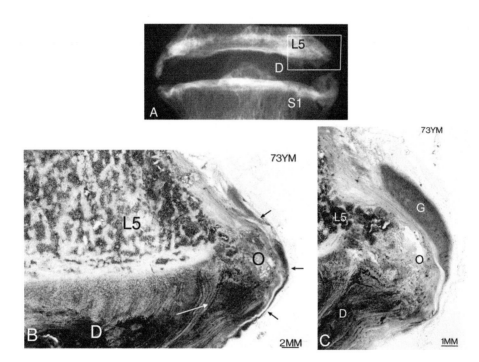

FIGURE 4.38 **(A)** Radiograph showing the L5-S1 intervertebral disc space (D) of a 73-year-old male cadaver. Note the lateral osteophytes on the vertebral bodies adjacent to the intervertebral disc, but the X-ray view cannot illustrate the mechanical pressure upon, or traction of, the deformed paraspinal autonomic nervous system chain. **(B)** A 100-μm-thick coronal plane histological section from the approximate area shown in the rectangle in (A) that illustrates the degenerating intervertebral disc (D) with lateral intervertebral disc protrusion (white arrow) and associated osteophyte (O) on the L5 body. The paraspinal autonomic chain (black arrows) being *mechanically tractioned and deformed* by the large osteophyte on the inferolateral margin of the body of the L5 vertebra is illustrated. **(C)** A magnified view of a paraspinal autonomic ganglion (G), containing cell bodies, that appears to be deformed and tractioned by the large osteophyte (O).

Source: From Taylor JR, Giles LGF, Lumbar intervertebral discs. In: Giles LGF, Singer K P (eds) **Clinical anatomy and management of low back pain**, Butterworth-Heinemann, Edinburgh, © Elsevier, 1997, p. 49–71.

> The paravertebral ganglia and their left and right sympathetic chains (or trunks) can be identified on high-resolution 3D-CISS MR imaging to visualizing structures not typically seen with standard spine MR imaging techniques (Chaudhry et al 2018).

9. Adhesion Formation between a Nerve Root Sleeve and an Intervertebral Disc Protrusion (Figure 4.39)

Clinical relevance: Acute discal herniation accompanied by non-specific inflammation and venous stasis (Breig 1978) in which the pH is lowered (Nachemson 1969) may be accompanied by oedema of the dura and root sheath, with vasodilation and consequent scarring that may then anchor the dural root-sheath to the herniated disc (Breig et al 1963; Ido et al 2001). Adhesions between dural sleeves and an IVD protrusion are a known source of pain (Wilkinson 1986; Ido et al 2001).

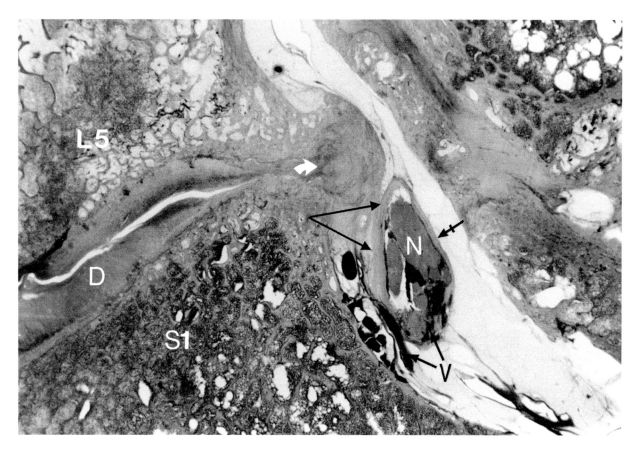

FIGURE 4.39 A 200-μm-thick histological section, cut in the parasagittal plane through the lumbosacral intervertebral disc of a 59-year-old female cadaver, showing a disc protrusion (small curved white arrow) with *perineural adhesions* (black arrows) between the protrusion and the adjacent dural sleeve (tailed arrow) containing neural structures (N). D = intervertebral disc showing internal disc disruption; L5 = fifth lumbar vertebral body; S1 = first sacral segment. Note the *extensive Batson's venous plexus vascularity* (V) posterior to the sacrum and blood vessels within and around the neural structures.

Source: Reproduced with permission from Taylor JR, Giles LGF, Lumbar intervertebral discs. In: Giles LGF, Singer KP (eds) Clinical anatomy and management of low back pain, Butterworth-Heinemann, Edinburgh, © Elsevier, 1997, p. 49–71.

Plain X-ray examination would show disc space thinning and the associated lipping of the vertebral bodies but not the nerve root adhesion—the latter would require an MRI investigation.

10. Pressure upon Neural Structures within the Intervertebral Foramen (Figure 4.40)

Clinical relevance: Deformation of the nerve root or nerve root ganglion can be related to clinical symptoms such as pain and neurological deficit in the back and legs (Olmarker 1991). Pressure upon neural structures such as a nerve root or nerve root ganglion will cause pain (Rydevik et al 1984; Kobayashi et al 2005) as nerve fibres (especially those of large diameter) are exquisitely vulnerable to localized pressure differences (Schaumburg et al 1975). In the intervertebral foramen, a condition that may render a peripheral sensory nerve susceptible to compressive effects can occur due to osteophytosis, which alters the course of a nerve, serving as a point of friction (Lam et al 2020) (Figure 4.40). Both ischaemic and mechanical factors are involved in the development of compression neuropathy, and it is likely that the greater the duration and amount of pressure, the more significant is neural dysfunction (Mackinnon 2002). Furthermore, disc protrusion may lead to compression of epidural veins with dilation of non-compressed veins (Jayson 1992). Histopathologic findings of fibrosis, with thickening of the external epineurium and perineurium would interfere with blood flow as the vessels pass through the epineurium and perineurium and produce dynamic ischaemia to the nerve fibres (Mackinnon 2002). Intra-foraminal fibrosis may cause foraminal neuropathy (Choi 2019).

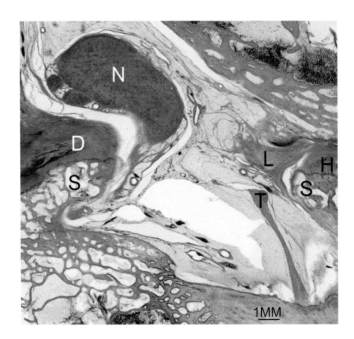

FIGURE 4.40   A 100-μm-thick parasagittal histological section across the lumbosacral intervertebral foramen of a 73-year-old male cadaver. Note the large osteophytic spur (S) and the associated lumbosacral intervertebral disc protrusion (D). This disc-osteophyte complex projects 5 mm into the posterolateral region of the intervertebral foramen and deforms the adjacent neural complex (N) that includes part of the dorsal root ganglion, resulting in some epineurial fibrosis. The ligamentum flavum (L) is seen adjacent to an osteophytic spur (S) on the superior articular process of the first sacral segment that shows some hyaline articular cartilage (H). This spur and the intervertebral disc protrusion with adjacent bony spur, considerably lessen the anteroposterior diameter of the central part of the intervertebral foramen. T = part of a transforaminal ligament.

Source: **Reproduced with permission from Giles LGF, Kaveri MJP, Some osseous and soft tissue causes of human intervertebral canal (foramen) stenosis. J Rheumatol 17: 1474–1481, 1990.**

A plain X-ray would show the disc thinning and the associated osteophytes but not the neural structures—the latter would require MR imaging.

11. Transforaminal Ligaments Traversing the Intervertebral Foramen and Their Innervation (Figure 4.41)

Clinical relevance: Transforaminal ligaments are considered normal structures (Amonoo-Kuofi et al 1997) but, under altered conditions such as structural variations or pathological change, they may be predisposed to pain or produce pain due to direct mechanical pressure on the neural complex (Amonoo-Kuofi et al 1997; Giles 1992(b); Cramer et al 2002) giving rise to severe pain and paraesthesiae along the distribution of the nerve (Amonoo-Kuofi et al 1997).

The transforaminal ligament in Figure 4.41A was resected and examined by high power light microscopy using thin sections stained with Richardson's stain (Giles et al 1991) to show its structure in greater detail (Figure 4.41B).

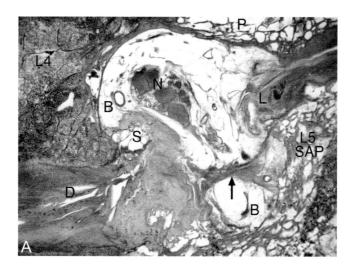

FIGURE 4.41 **(A)** A 200-μm-thick histological section cut in the parasagittal plain across the left L4–5 intervertebral foramen of a 69-year-old male cadaver. The arrow shows a ligament within the foramen that traverses the lower part of the intervertebral canal, thus bisecting it. The width and thickness of the ligament within the intervertebral foramen is 4 mm. B = blood vessel; D = intervertebral disc with posterolateral protrusion due to internal disc disruption and fissuring; L = ligamentum flavum (buckled); L4 = fourth lumbar vertebral body; N = neural complex; P = pedicle of L4 vertebra; S = spur posterolaterally on the inferior margin of the L4 vertebral body adjacent to the disc protrusion; L5 SAP = fifth lumbar superior articular process.

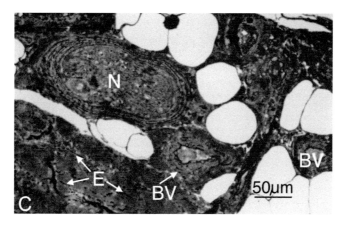

FIGURE 4.41 **(B)** A 1-μm-thick section of the transforaminal ligament shown in **(A)** that contains elastic fibres (E), a small myelinated nerve (N), and blood vessels (BV).

Source: Reproduced with permission from Giles LGF, Ligaments traversing the intervertebral canals of the human lower lumbosacral spine. Neuro-Ortho 13:25–38, 1992(b), Springer Nature.

> **Transforaminal ligaments may be seen and reported on by experienced MRI radiologists.**

12. Interspinous Ligament Injury Due to 'Kissing Spinouses' i.e. Baastrup's Disease or Syndrome (Figure 4.42)

Clinical relevance: Lumbar interspinous ligaments consist of thin and short fibres connecting adjacent spinous processes—they are well vascularized and contain sensory nerves (Iwanaga et al 2019) as they are innervated by branches of the posterior ramus of the spinal nerve (Jinkins 2004(b)). They form a continuous band with the supraspinous ligament posteriorly (Wong et al 2007) and the ligamenta flava anteriorly.

Intermittent mechanical compression of the interspinous ligaments, due to '*kissing spinouses*' destroys the ligament, and a fibrocartilage bumper can develop on the opposing spinous processes i.e. on each side of the joint space; normally the spinous processes are only covered with periosteum, and there is no fibrocartilage bumper but, due to the intermittent compression, an adventitious bursa may develop (Hadley 1964). The trauma to the interspinous ligaments causes degenerative changes, which are a common cause of low back pain syndrome (Schmorl et al 1971; Epstein 1976; Jinkins 2004(b); Philipp et al 2016). In due course, degenerative changes can be seen radiologically as *sclerosis* and *osteophytosis* (Kellgren 1939) and the most commonly affected level is at L4–5 (Philip et al 2016).

A plain X-ray example of kissing spinouses and a histological section are shown in Figure 4.42A and B, respectively.

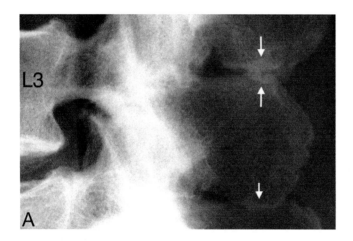

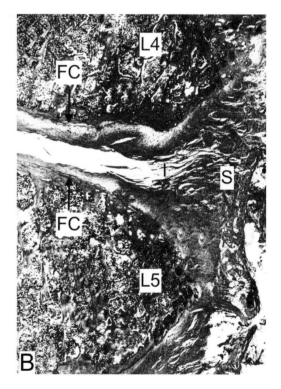

FIGURE 4.42 **(A)** Plain X-ray of an 83-year-old female cadaver's spine showing sclerotic changes (arrows), particularly at L3–4—and to some extent at L4–5—spinous processes due to 'kissing' spinouses. **(B)** Sagittal plane histological section cut at 150 μm thickness from a 72-year-old female cadaver's spine at the L4–5 interspinous (I) region showing that a *fibrocartilage bumper* (FC) has developed on opposing spinous process surfaces. In addition, this section shows some disruption of the supraspinous ligament (S) that can also be a source of pain due to its free nerve endings near the attachment to the spinous processes (Yahia et al 1988).

Source: (B) Reproduced with permission from Giles LGF, Anatomical Basis of Low Back Pain. Williams and Wilkins, Baltimore, © Wolters Kluwer, 1989 p. 105, 106.

> Plain X-ray images would not show early mechanically induced degenerative changes of an interspinous ligament being compressed; later sclerotic changes become visible. Therefore, if the clinician is suspicious of low back pain being due to interspinous soft tissue compression, in order to see the interspinous ligament by imaging requires T2-weighted fast spin echo, fat-suppressed images in the sagittal, axial, and coronal planes as this will allow the visualization of interspinous ligament degeneration (Jinkins 2004(b)).

13. Spondylolysis Due to Isthmus Mechanical Stress Fracture—X-Ray and a Histological Example (Figure 4.43)

Clinical relevance: Pars interarticularis (*isthmus*) fractures can cause low back pain and should be promptly diagnosed (Duarte et al 2021); when they are symptomatic, the low back pain frequently radiates to the buttock or proximal lower limb (Syrmoue et al 2010).

The intact pars interarticularis (or isthmus) is illustrated anatomically in a partly oblique view of an L4 vertebra (Figure 4.43A) and radiologically in Figure 4.43B, which shows normal pars interarticulares above L5 vertebra where there is a bilateral fracture of the Scotty dog's neck.

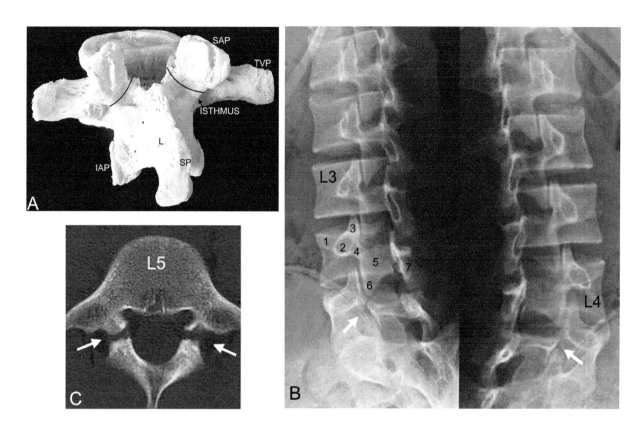

FIGURE 4.43 **(A)** A pars interarticularis defect may be unilateral or bilateral. The black lines represent the approximate region of fracture of the isthmus. IAP = inferior articular process; L = lamina; SAP = superior articular process; SP = spinous process; TVP = transverse process. **(B)** Left and right 45-degree oblique (i.e. position of the patient's body to the X-ray film) plain X-ray radiographs of the L1 to S1 spinal levels showing normal 'Scotty dogs' of Lachapelle (1880–1934) above the L5 vertebral level. Normal 'Scotty dog' anatomy is illustrated at the L4 level: 1 = snout (transverse process); 2 = eye (pedicle); 3 = ear (superior articular process); 4 = neck (pars interarticularis or isthmus); 5 = body (lamina); 6 = front leg (inferior articular process); 7 = back leg (arch and inferior process of the opposite side of the vertebra). At the L5 level the Scotty dog has a broken neck (arrows) on each side, which represents spondylolysis bilaterally i.e. a mechanical stress fracture of each isthmus. **(C)** Axial CT scan of the L5 vertebra to show the left and right pars interarticularis defects (arrows).

Source: (B) and (C) reproduced with permission of Morimoto M et al, **Is the Scotty dog sign adequate for diagnosis of fractures in pediatric patients with lumbar spondylolysis?** Spine Surg Relat Res 3(1): 49–53, 2019, doi: 10.22603/ssrr.2017–0099 © Japanese Society for Spine Surgery and Related Research. Figure B has been modified in that numbers 1–7 have been added as well as L3 and L4.

This mechanical *stress* or *fatigue fracture* of the pars interarticularis (Baker et al 1956; Wiltse et al 1975; Jackson 1979) may later result in forward slipping of the vertebral body to cause spondylo*listhesis* (Panteliadis et al 2016). Lumbo-sacral spine radiographs of 143 patients (av. age = 27 years) who had never walked and who had *no isthmus defects* support the theory that spondylolysis and isthmic spondylolisthesis (with a combined incidence of 5.8% in the general population) represent a *fatigue fracture* resulting from activities associated with ambulation (Rosenberg et al 1981).

Advanced imaging procedures, such a MRI are recommended in the early stage of lumbar spondylosis in paediatric patients requiring conservative treatment to achieve bony healing (Morimoto et al 2019).

The isthmus defect should be seen in a lumbosacral spine lateral view of a patient but requires the patient to be *correctly positioned* for plain X-ray imaging (i.e. without rotation) and the X-ray *exposure* needs to be optimal in order to penetrate the L5 interarticularis area, because the iliac crests can be superimposed over the defect and obliterate part of the isthmus (Figure 4.43D). A histological section from a cadaver showing a pathological lesion of spondylolysis is shown in Figure 4.43E.

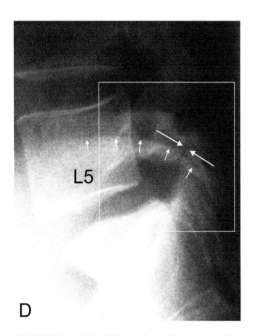
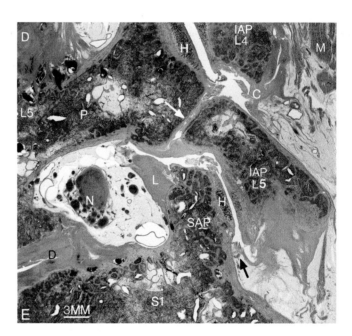

FIGURE 4.43 **(D)** A plain X-ray lateral view of the lumbosacral region of a 30-year-old male patient who suffers from low back pain due to slipping on steps and sitting down heavily, resulting in immediate central to left lower L5-S1 pain, 18 months before consultation. On examination there were no positive signs except for aggravation of his localized L5-S1 pain on full lumbar spine flexion and extension. X-ray examination was reported as being 'normal'. However, there is a pars interarticularis defect of the L5 isthmus (large white arrows). This briefly mentioned case is to illustrate the issue that, because the iliac crests (small white arrows) can partly obliterate the pars interarticularis region, it is important to carefully examine the X-ray images. **(E)** A 200-μm-thick parasagittal histological section from a 78-year-old male cadaver cut to include the *isthmus defect* (white arrow), which has developed *fibrocartilaginous* type tissue on both bony surfaces i.e. not hyaline articular cartilage—some of the fibrocartilaginous tissue crosses the isthmus defect in an attempt to repair the fracture. There is a distinct bony cortex on each side of the defect. C = fibrous joint capsule (disrupted); D = intervertebral discs; H = hyaline articular cartilage; IAP L5 = inferior articular process of the fifth lumbar vertebra (L5); L = ligamentum flavum (presumably disrupted due to an injury that caused the isthmus defect); IAP L4 = inferior articular process of the 4th lumbar vertebra; M = muscle; N = neural complex within the intervertebral foramen; P = pedicle of L5; S1 = first sacral segment with its superior articular process (SAP). Black arrow shows a synovial fold.

Source: **Reproduced with permission from Giles LGF, Miscellaneous pathological and developmental (anomalous) conditions. In: Giles LGF and Singer KP (eds) Clinical anatomy and management of low back pain. Butterworth-Heinemann, Edinburgh, © Elsevier, 1997(c).**

Miscellaneous Conditions

1. Ossicles of Lumbar Vertebra Posterior Elements (Figures 4.44 and 4.45)

Background:Primary ossification centres start appearing at nine weeks *in utero* and complete primary ossification by one year (Knipe et al 2021). A typical lumbar vertebra is ossified from three primary ossification centres i.e. one in each half vertebral arch and one in the centrum (Soames 1995; Knipe et al 2021). *Secondary* ossification centres, of which there are seven (Prakash et al 2007) to nine (Meschan 1962), are a normal finding and appear at puberty and fuse by 25–30 years of age (Carr et al 2012; Matesan et al 2016; Knipe et al 2021) although occasionally these centres may remain unfused

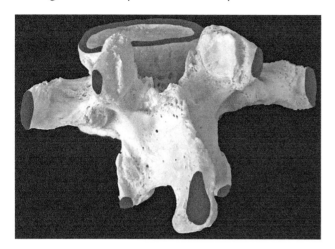

FIGURE 4.44 The approximate location of the secondary ossification centres of a lumbar vertebra are illustrated. There is a ring (or annular) epiphysis at the upper and lower surfaces, respectively, of the vertebral body (Knipe et al 2021), one at the tip of the spinous process, one at the tip of each transverse process (Soames 1995; Knipe et al 2021), and one on each *mammillary process* of the superior articular processes of the vertebra (Rothman et al 1992). In addition, Meschan (1962) shows two ossification centres at the inferior articular process tips.

until later into adulthood (Carr et al 2012). The ossification centres are located as shown in Figure 4.44.

The secondary ossification centres may represent potential sites for unfused ossicles of the lumbar spine (Pech et al 1985).

Clinical relevance: Variations and anomalies of the neural arch result from alterations in the ossification process, but these conditions usually remain asymptomatic, although a small number of these variations and anomalies may *result in painful syndromes* and/or fractures (Basara et al 2015) that may be readily identified on multi-detector computed tomography (MDCT) studies (Mellado et al 2011(a)). (MDCT refers to a reformatted MDCT procedure (Stöppler 2021)). Their most

common location is the inferior articular processes of L2 or L3 (Pech et al 1985). Although the size of the ossicle varies, it always has *well corticated smooth margins*, unlike fractures, which are irregular and often multiple—they are bilateral or multiple in approximately 20% of cases (Pech et al 1985) and the incidence of lumbar unfused ossicles is 0.5–1.5% (Fulton et al 1934). Unfused lumbar ossicles rarely have any clinical significance although, when subjected to trauma, the ossicle may cause persistent low back pain (Hipps 1939; Pech et al 1985).

Basara et al (2015) report a case of a 47-year-old male with lower back pain who was examined before being referred for radiological evaluations where plain X-ray imaging indicated, at the bilateral inferior articular process of the L2 vertebra, two 8 mm 'ossicles' that were seen and confirmed by MDCT examination and diagnosed as 'Oppenheimer's ossicles'—following excision of the ossicle, the patient recovered.

'Oppenheimer's ossicles' were first described as nonfusion remnants of secondary ossification centres of articular processes by Oppenheimer (1942); they originate from a *horizontal cleft* through the inferior articular process (Mellado et al 2011(b)) and may be mistaken for a facet fracture (Keats et al 2007). Mellado et al (2011(b)) presented an example of an Oppenheimer's ossicle located at the caudal aspect of the left inferior L3 articular process (in a 39-year-old man who presented with low back pain and sciatica), using (i) an anteroposterior *plain X-ray* image, followed by (ii) a coronal reformatted *MDCT* image.

It should be noted that ossicles of lumbar articular facets (OLAF) can be overlooked on reversed gantry angle CT scans and that MDCT is the most reliable investigation in the diagnosis of OLAF (Kumar et al 2012).

Young athletes with backache due to mechanical induced trauma of articular facets may benefit from MDCT examination to investigate the possible presence of ossicles of lumbar facets (Kumar et al 2012).

An example of ossicles at the L2–3 spinal level is illustrated in a plain X-ray image (Figure 4.45A). The specimen's corresponding histological structure is shown in Figure 4.45B).

The opposite side of the bisected spine did not exhibit any ossicles.

The three ossicles presented in Figure 4.45 are not of traumatic origin as they have smooth and corticated margins. The pseudo-joints may well be generators of pain under certain movements or mechanical stresses, as they appear to be synovial type joints lined by a fibrocartilage bumper.

There has to be a clinical awareness of possible ossicles, and it is important for imaging to be of good quality to enable the clinician to visualize such ossicles, should a patient present with unexplained low back pain of mechanical origin.

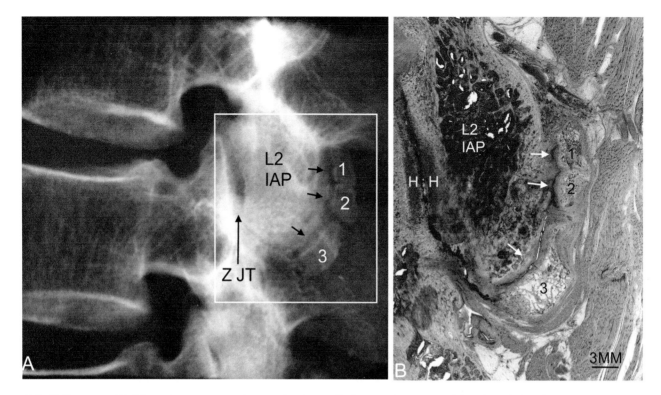

FIGURE 4.45 **(A)** Plain X-ray image of part of a sagittally bisected 62-year-old cadaver's lumbar spine, in which the height of the associated intervertebral disc spaces appears to be normal, suggesting no injury to the discs. The L2 inferior articular process is shown with the zygapophysial joint (Z JT) anteriorly and three smoothly corticated bony ossicles posteriorly. **(B)** A corresponding (but enlarged) photomicrograph of this spine's L2–3 zygapophysial joint with its hyaline articular cartilage and the L2 inferior articular process (L2 IAP) is shown, as well as three posterior corticated ossicles (1, 2, 3) posterior to the inferior articular process. H = hyaline articular cartilage on opposing facets of the zygapophysial joint shows some osteoarthrotic changes. The three white arrows indicate cartilage lined 'pseudo-joints' between the inferior articular process and the corticated ossicles. The ossicles show a degree of fibrocartilage bumper on their anterior surfaces that are separated from the opposing bony surface by a pseudo-joint between them and the bony inferior articular process of the L2 vertebra.

2. Transitional Lumbosacral Vertebrae Associated with Mechanical Low Back Pain (Figures 4.46 and 4.47)

Clinical Relevance: Sacralization or lumbarization anomalies at the lumbosacral junction between the spine and the sacrum can cause low back pain (Keim et al 1987) known as Bertolotti's syndrome (Bertolotti 1917). It is associated with the formation of a pseudo-articulation between the transverse process and the sacrum (Jancuska et al 2015). Also, it should be noted that it is an important cause of low back pain in young patients (Jain et al 2013) and that it is more common in males (Mahato 2011; Jancuska et al 2015).

Lumbosacral transitional vertebral (LSTV) anomalies are defined as either *sacralization* of the lowest lumbar segment or *lumbarization* of the most superior sacral segment of the spine. They are relatively common anomalies in the general population, with a reported prevalence of 4–30% (Konin et al 2010), with an average of approximately 25% (Gaillard et al 2021). The incidence of these two types of anomalies was found to be: lumbarization of S1–5.8%, and sacralization of L5–4.1% (French et al 2014).

The anomaly may be unilateral or bilateral. It can best be imaged on a Ferguson radiograph i.e. an anteroposterior radiograph obtained with the plain X-ray beam angled cranially at 30 degrees (Konin et al 2010).

LSTV anomalies are classified into four types (Castellvi et al 1984) and it is the Type IIb (bilateral lumbarization/sacralization with an enlarged transverse process that has a diarthrodial joint between itself and the sacrum) that may present with a herniated lumbar disc at the level of transition, while also presenting with a greater than normal incidence of herniations at the level just above the LSTV (Castellvi et al 1984).

Using skeletal *scintography* of the anomalous diarthrodial joints in patients with LSTV, Connolly et al (2003) showed an increased uptake at the anomalous articulation between the transverse process of the LSTV and the sacrum in 81% of patients.

Conservative non-surgical treatment of patients with mechanical pain from disturbance of the anomalous articulation is by local injection of anaesthetic and steroid into the pseudo-articulation and radiofrequency ablation (Konin et al 2010).

Two cases are briefly presented showing a radiographic example of *sacralization* (Figure 4.46A and B) and *lumbarization* (Figure 4.47A), respectively, in which both patients presented with localized lumbosacral pain, and the only clinical sign, in each case, was that of spinal flexion and extension aggravating the low back pain. Both patients complained of intermittent twinges of low back pain on left and right rotation of the torso.

Sacralization

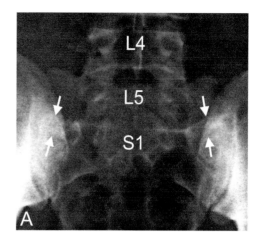

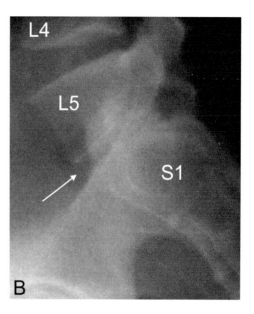

FIGURE 4.46 (A) Routine anteroposterior radiographic view of the lumbosacral area of a 38-year-old male who had been involved in a motor vehicle accident nine months before consultation. Note the bilateral *sacralization* with sclerotic changes (arrows) between the left and right dysplastic (i.e. exhibiting dysplasia; containing abnormal cells or showing abnormal development) transverse processes. This sclerosis indicates diarthrodial joints (Castellvi et al 1984) between the sacrum and the dysplastic transverse process on each side. **(B)** Lateral view radiograph of the sacralization of the L5 vertebra with the sacrum (S1). White arrow shows a rudimentary intervertebral disc space at the sacralization level that is much narrower than is the disc space at L4–5, which appears to be essentially normal, apart from slight retrolisthesis of the vertebral body of L4 on L5. The latter suggested that he may have an asymptomatic small posterior—or posterolateral—disc bulge or protrusion at this level (Giles et al 2006—see Figure 1.3).

Lumbarization

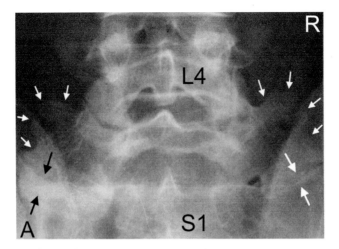

FIGURE 4.47 **(A)** Routine anteroposterior radiographic view of the lumbosacral area of a 27-year-old male with low back pain and a left leg length discrepancy of 31 mm. Note the bilateral *lumbarization* with sclerotic changes bilaterally (large arrows), especially on the left side, between the left and right dysplastic transverse processes and the sacrum. The small arrows outline the contour of the dysplastic transverse processes of the lumbarized segment bilaterally.

Source: **Reproduced with permission from Giles LGF, Anatomical Basis of Low Back Pain. Williams and Wilkins, Baltimore, © Wolters Kluwer, 1989.**

A cadaveric 'block' of trimmed osteoligamentous tissues X-rayed in the posteroanterior view from a 35-year-old male with *lumbarization* of the presacral segment is shown in Figure 4.47B. A histological section cut from the 'block' of lumbosacral tissue shown in Figure 4.47B is shown in Figure 4.47C.

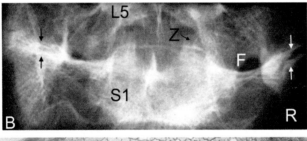

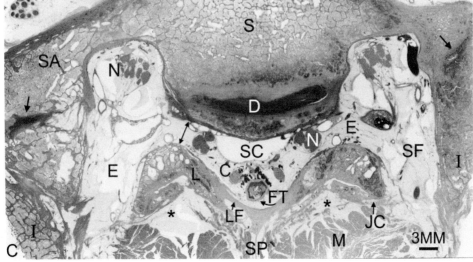

FIGURE 4.47 **(B)** Plain posteroanterior position X-ray of a trimmed block of osteoligamentous tissues from a 35-year-old male cadaver. Note the bilaterally enlarged transverse processes of the last presacral vertebra articulating

FIGURE 4.47 (Continued)

with the lateral mass of the sacrum, i.e. lumbarization of the presacral segment (arrows). Z = small anomalous diarthrodial zygapophysial 'facet' joints seen bilaterally. Osteoarthrotic changes are seen as sclerosis of the anomalous articulations. F = first sacral foramen; R = right side of specimen; S1 = first sacral segment. **(C)** A 200-μm-thick histological section, cut in not quite an axial/horizontal plane, through the level of the bilateral lumbarizations pseudo-articulation joints showing their staining characteristic for cartilage; this stain is also taken up by the rudimentary disc. The pseudo-joints have developed a type of fibrocartilage bumper due to mechanical forces across the pseudo-joints (arrows). C = cauda equina nerve roots; D = intervertebral disc (rudimentary) of the presacral joint; E = epidural fat; FT = filum terminale; I = ilium; JC = fibrous joint capsule of the right small zygapophysial joint of this anomalous presacral segment—both zygapophysial joints show osteoarthrotic hyaline articular cartilage degenerative changes; L = lamina; LF = ligamentum flavum; M = muscle; N = neural complex; S = sacrum; SA = sacral ala; SC = sacral canal; SF = sacral foramen (canal); SP = spinous process; asterisk = fibrofatty tissue replacing posterior muscle.

Source: **Reproduced with permission from Giles LGF Miscellaneous pathological and developmental (anomalous) conditions. In: Giles LGF, Singer KP (eds) Clinical anatomy and management of low back pain. Butterworth-Heinemann, Oxford, © Elsevier, 1997(c), p. 196–216.**

The importance of an initial plain X-ray investigation is illustrated by the two cases presented to demonstrate that correct identification of a LSTV is essential, because of clinical implications, as inaccurate identification may lead to surgical and procedural errors (Konin et al 2010). MRI and CT follow-up would provide greater detail.

Konin et al's (2010) extensive review of LSTV's concluded that they are associated with an increased incidence of disc pathology in the disc above the anomaly.

In conclusion, McCulloch et al (1980) proposed that the *functional L5 nerve root* always originates from the 'last mobile' segment of the spine, which is defined as the lowest level with a fully formed disc space, bilateral facet joints, and two free transverse processes that do not articulate with the ala of the sacrum or the pelvis; therefore, in the case of a sacralized L5 vertebra, the functional nerve root corresponds to the anatomical L4 nerve root, whereas in patients with a lumbarized S1, the last fully mobile level is usually L6-S2 and the *functional L5 nerve root* corresponds with the L6 nerve root (McCulloch et al 1980).

Finally, not only is it important to identify the correct level of the LSTV for clinical diagnosis and management of cases of Bertolotti's syndrome, but it has been helpful in the forensic identification of the deceased (Kanchan et al 2009)!

Summary

In the General Introduction it was stated that, in a large number of mechanical back pain cases, it may not be possible to identify the precise pain generator and that it is often impossible to reach a specific diagnosis (Deyo 2002; Finch 2006), as many spinal structures are involved in nociception. It is hoped that the aforementioned anatomical and histological/histopathological illustrations have provided the reader with insight into some of the possible anatomical causes of spinal pain syndromes that are often classified as being of mechanical or 'non-specific' origin.

Chapter 5
THREE CLINICAL EXAMPLES ASSOCIATED WITH
LUMBOSACRAL SPINE PAIN OF MECHANICAL ORIGIN

Abstract: 1. This chapter presents three examples of disorders that can cause spinal pain of mechanical origin. The effect of leg length inequality of 10 to 26 mm on the lumbosacral spine, pelvic obliquity, hip joints, and knee joints is described. Leg length inequality and its postural scoliosis in individuals up to the age of approximately 53 years can be corrected with a shoe raise; after that age a fixed curve with disc wedging and vertebral body osteophytosis occurs. Erect posture anteroposterior plain X-ray imaging of the pelvis and lumbar spine before and after shoe raise shows the effects on leg length inequality, pelvic obliquity, postural scoliosis, facet joint subluxation, hip joints, and the psoas major muscle shadows.

2. Mechanically induced degenerative spondylolisthesis due to facet joint tropism, with cartilage degeneration is illustrated.

3. Tethered cord occurs in infants, children and in adults and presents with a constellation of neurological signs and symptoms that result from mechanical traction/tension on the spinal cord between fixed points during growth. Its pathophysiology involves excessive mechanical tension of the spinal cord, vascular compromise, and hypoxia resulting in neurological impairment.

Key words: (1) leg length inequality, pelvic obliquity, postural scoliosis, hip joints, knee joints, shoe raise, erect posture imaging, facet joint subluxation, psoas major muscle

(2) degenerative spondylolisthesis, facet tropism, cartilage degeneration

(3) tethered cord, neurological signs, neurological symptoms, spinal cord traction, spinal cord tension, pathophysiology, vascular compromise, hypoxia, neurological impairment

Contents

Three examples follow to illustrate disorders that can cause spinal pain of mechanical origin. Although this text relates to degenerative anatomical conditions that may cause spinal pain of mechanical origin, this chapter has to include these three clinical examples in order to show the relevance of mechanical spinal joint dysfunction findings to clinical practice.

(1) Leg Length Inequality—Its Effect on the Lumbosacral Spine, Hip Joints, and Knee Joints ('Long Leg Arthropathy')

Introduction
Leg length discrepancy of 1–2 cm results in a 'short leg limp', which causes not only a change in the normal

DOI: 10.1201/9781003315964-5

gait pattern but also requires additional unphysiological muscle activity—it affects the spine and the hip joint and can result in serious disorders (Morscher 1977).

As clinical measurements for LLI are inaccurate, it is doubtful whether many clinicians would trust a measured difference of less than three-quarters of an inch (19 mm) (Gofton 1971), and (Eichler 1977) found an error of 15 mm, even in the hands of experienced examiners. Thus, the absolute leg length i.e. the distance from the acetabulum to the sole of the heel must be determined from X-ray images (Gofton et al 1971). Therefore, when LLI is suspected, carefully standardized radiographic erect posture examination for accurate LLI measurement is essential (Giles et al 1981).

It is important to note the types of leg lengths (Figure 5.1). The *absolute leg length*, i.e. from the femur head to the sole-floor contact, which includes the *sphyrion height* (the height of the medial malleolus of the tibia to the sole of the heel (two headed arrow)) is important as it relates to mechanical low back pain.

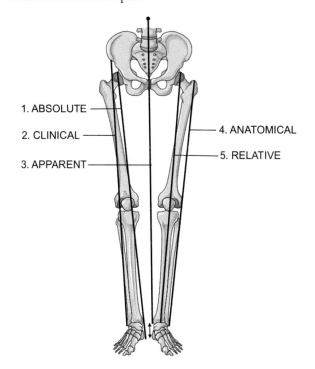

FIGURE 5.1 Diagram illustrating the types of leg length: 1= Absolute leg length (including the sphyrion height); 2 = Clinical leg length; 3 = Apparent leg length; 4 = Anatomical leg length; 5 = Relative leg length; Arrow = sphyrion height.

Eichler (1977) defined the various types of leg lengths as summarized in the following list, using imaging or tape measurement:

1. **Erect posture X-ray is used for** (i) an accurate *absolute leg length* measurement (1) i.e. the distance between the top of the femur head and the heel—floor contact, and (ii) *relative leg length* (5) i.e. the distance between the articular surface of the hip joint and the tibio-talar joint.

2. **Clinical tape measurement is used for:** (i) *clinical leg length* (2) i.e. the distance between the anterior superior iliac spine and the distal end of the lateral malleolus, (ii) *apparent leg length* (3) i.e. the distance between the umbilicus and the distal end of the medial malleolus, and (iii) *anatomical leg length* (4) i.e. the distance between the proximal end of the greater trochanter to the distal end of the lateral malleolus.

3. **Functional leg length discrepancy (LLD)**: leg shortening or lengthening caused by joint contractures or by axial malalignment (Eichler 1977) e.g. hip fixed deformity due to contracture of the joint capsule or of the muscles (Adams et al 2001).

Clinical measurements cannot take the place of an adequately controlled erect posture *radiologic study* of the pelvis and the lower extremities to determine the absolute LLD (Hughes et al 1977). Non-weightbearing imaging of the long bones in the lower extremity, such as scanography, can be inaccurate for measuring LLI as this method does not take into account the contribution of the sphyrion height as demonstrated by Giles (2009).

Erect Posture Plain X-Ray Imaging

Giles et al (1981) showed that carefully standardized erect posture radiography had a mean error of only 1.12 mm (± 0.92 mm) for *absolute leg length*. An erect posture pelvis and lumbar spine anteroposterior radiograph taken of a person with LLI, standing on a horizontal steel platform with the film in a horizontal X-ray bucky and touching the inside bottom of the X-ray cassette (Giles et al 1981) is shown in Figure 5.2A. This anteroposterior radiographic view shows a significant LLI of 26 mm on the right side. The lower (L3-S1) lumbosacral spine of this patient is shown enlarged in Figure 5.2B. The anteroposterior pelvis and lumbar spine radiograph was then repeated with the patient standing on a right foot raise of 26 mm that eliminated the pelvic obliquity and the postural scoliosis (Figure 5.2C).

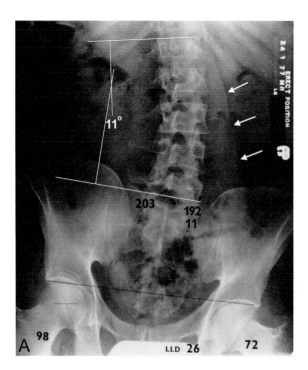

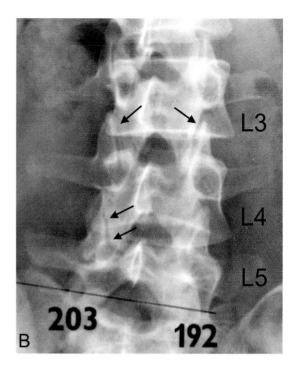

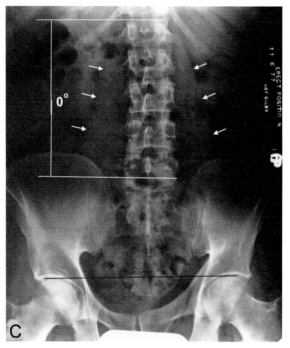

FIGURE 5.2   (A) An erect posture pelvis and lumbar spine anteroposterior X-ray image of a 37-year-old male. Note the right leg length deficiency of 26 mm, the sacral obliquity of 11 mm when measured across the left and right superior sacral notches, the lumbar postural scoliosis of 11 degrees (measured using the Cobb (1948) method), and the more prominently displayed lateral border of the psoas major muscle (arrows) on the convex side. (B) This enlargement of the lower part of (A) shows: (i) the L3–4 facets on the concave side of the postural scoliosis are more closely apposed superiorly than on the convex side (arrows); (ii) the L4–5 facets appear to be more closely apposed superiorly than inferiorly on the concave side (arrows), indicating misalignment (subluxation) of the paired facet joints, with reasonable apposition of the facets on the convex side. (C) An erect posture pelvis and lumbar spine anteroposterior image taken with the patient standing on a right foot raise of 26 mm; this raise virtually eliminated the pelvic obliquity and the scoliosis. The lateral borders of the left and right psoas major muscles now appear to be normal i.e. there is virtually no greater prominence on either side of the spine. The contact surface area between the femur head and the acetabulum on each side is now equal.

Source: **Reproduced with permission from Giles LGF, 100 Challenging Spinal Pain Syndrome Cases, Churchill Livingstone Elsevier, Edinburgh, © Elsevier, 2009.**

The misalignment between facet joints (Figure 5.2B) suggests asymmetrical pressure changes within a zygapophysial joint. As these joints are highly susceptible to degenerative changes and play a significant role in back-related morbidities (O'Leary et al 2017), physicians may suggest to patients that they should consider wearing a shoe raise on the short leg side in order to normalize paired facet joint biomechanical stresses on each side of the spine (Figure 5.2C).

In a histological study comparing (by measurement) cadaveric paired i.e. left and right facets from specimens with a LLI of greater than 9 mm, Giles et al (1984) showed that *mid-joint geometry* (i.e. at the area of *least wear* of the hyaline articular cartilage on opposing facets) demonstrated that there was asymmetrical change in the thickness of the joint cartilage and of the subchondral bone in the apical and lumbosacral zygapophysial joints of the postural scoliosis. In addition, in all likelihood, there will be *asymmetrical mechanical stresses* affecting anatomical structures such as the dural tube, nerve roots, and associated vascular structures with pathophysiological consequences. Using cadaveric spines Breig (1978) found that the pathodynamics owing to the shortening of the lateral wall of the spinal canal on the side toward which the vertebral column is flexed (concave) there is slackening of the lateral aspect of the dura, together with the root-sheaths and nerve roots as well as the sciatic nerve, together with the sacral plexus; the elongation of the opposite wall of the spinal canal results in stretching of all the structures on that side.

Furthermore, the effect of lateral flexion of the column on the spinal cord, nerve roots, dentate ligaments, sacral plexus, and sciatic nerve is that there will be *less tension* applied to the structures on the concave side (long leg side) than on the corresponding structures on the convex side (short leg side) (Breig 1978), which presumably will affect these structures and most likely affect the movement of spinal CSF between the two sides. Furthermore, when the spine is flexed to one side, the canal is elongated on its convex side and shortened on its concave side—as a consequence of these changes in length of the canal, there is a folding and unfolding of the cord, which involves most of its elements, the pia, axis cylinders, neuroglia, and blood vessels (Breig 1960). Above the lumbar cord, the dentate ligaments are especially concerned with the transmission of biomechanical forces (Breig 1960).

Moreover, significant LLI, i.e. greater than 9 mm, with postural scoliosis, causes the articulating facets at a given zygapophysial joint level to no longer be fully congruous, possibly resulting in increased friction at some point of their gliding movement (Cailliet 1968), resulting in osteoarthrosis (Huskisson et al 1978).

As a precaution, it should be noted that there may be a LLI but virtually no *pelvic* obliquity on comparing the left and right superior sacral notches on an erect posture anteroposterior X-ray film. Therefore, this should always be taken into account when measuring for LLI (see Figure 5.3).

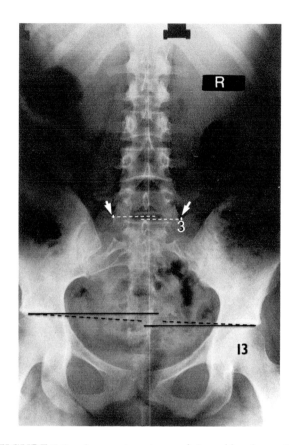

FIGURE 5.3   An erect posture pelvis and lumbar spine anteroposterior X-ray image of a 20-year-old female showing a right leg length deficiency of 13 mm by drawing a horizontal line at right angles to the plumb line and projecting it to each femur head to enable the difference between the two lines to be measured in millimetres. The broken line shows the inclination between the left and right femur heads. Note that there is no postural scoliosis as a line drawn at right angles to the plumb line to the left and right superior sacral notches (white arrows) are almost at the same height (within 3 mm). As there is no significant sacral base obliquity, this patient would not require a shoe-raise.

Source: **Modified from Giles LGF 1984(a) Letter to the Editor (re: Clinical symptoms and biomechanics of lumbar spine and hip joint in leg length inequality; Friberg O 1983 Spine 8: 643–651) Spine 9: 842, https://journals.lww.com/spinejournal/Citation/1984/11000/To_the_Editor.20.aspx.**

A further possibility is that there may be equal leg lengths but a presacral anomaly causes obliquity of the lumbosacral junction (Figure 5.4).

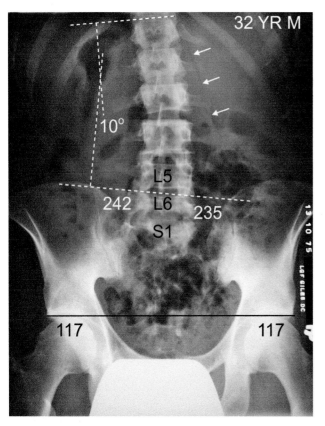

FIGURE 5.4 This erect posture X-ray image of a 34-year-old male shows that the leg lengths are equal. However, there is sacral base obliquity (lower on the right side by 7 mm) due to a pre-sacral L6 anomaly. This causes the lumbar spine postural scoliosis of 10 degrees, with a more prominent psoas major muscle shadow on the convex side of the spine (white arrows).

Leg length inequality is common (McCarthy et al 2001) with 15–18% of low back pain sufferers having a LLI of 1 cm or more (Rush et al 1946; Giles et al 1981), and in controls it was 4–8%, using erect posture imaging (Giles et al 1981). LLI may cause several different painful conditions. Many publications and daily clinical experience leave no doubt that *unequal leg lengths is a frequent cause of symptoms in the hip, pelvic or spinal areas* (Morscher 1977). Against this background, we now look at the issue of LLI, beginning with some definitions to clarify the issue of different types of weight bearing leg lengths.

The numerous causes of LLI can be divided into two broad categories—***acquired and congenital*** (McCarthy et al 2001). **Acquired** causes include anything that injures or slows the growth of the physis— e.g. trauma (long bone fracture with comminution), infection, paralysis, tumours, or any systemic condition resulting in asymmetric innervation or vascularization or radiation therapy damaging femoral or tibial epiphyseal plates (Taillard et al 1965; McCarthy et al 2001). Also, iatrogenic LLI following total hip arthroplasty can occur, but significant LLDs (defined as > 6 mm) can be minimized by using an intraoperative X-ray technique (Hofmann et al 2008).

The vast majority of patients with LLI of 1 cm or more have no known aetiology for this inequality (Ladermann 1976), which arises during growth without any apparent pathology. It is considered to be associated with 'out of phase' growth in the length of the long bone(s) of the lower limbs (Halliday 1976) prior to skeletal maturity at approximately 19 years of age for the femoral epiphyses.

It is important to remember that postural scoliosis and its correction in various age groups may be achieved by using a shoe raise up to the age of approximately 53 years; after that age, IVD wedging with associated vertebral body lipping occurs, resulting in a fixed curve (Giles et al 1981) (Figure 5.5 A to D).

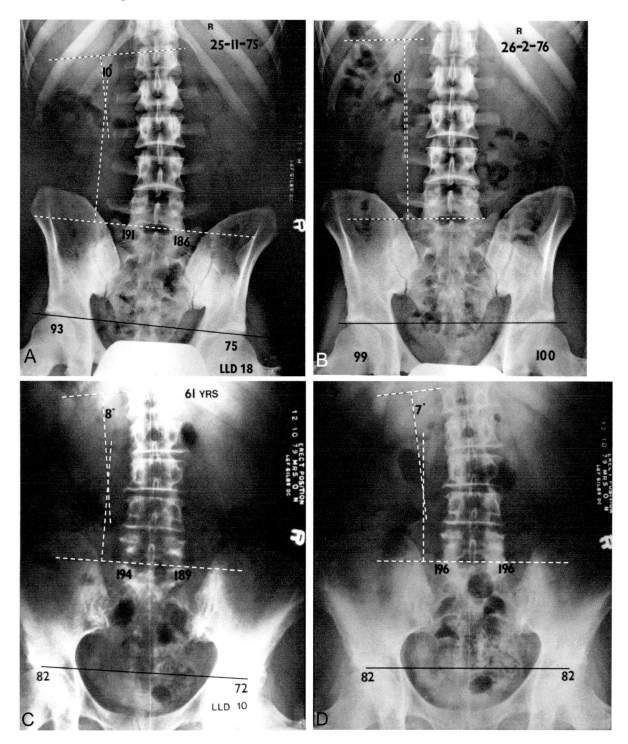

FIGURE 5.5 **(A)** A 27-year-old male with a right leg length deficiency of 18 mm and accompanying postural scoliosis of 10 degrees, measured using the Cobb method. **(B)** The scoliosis is corrected by the patient standing on a right foot raise of 18 mm. **(C)** A 61-year-old female with a right leg length deficiency of 10 mm and a postural scoliosis of 8 degrees that does not correct when she stands on a right foot raise of 10 mm **(D)**. Note the scoliosis has become fixed, with degenerative changes.

Source: (A) Giles LGF, Taylor JR 1981 Low-back pain associated with leg length inequality. Spine 6(5): 510–521, DOI: 10.1097/00007632–198109000–00014), (B) Giles LGF, Anatomical Basis of Low Back Pain. Williams and Wilkins, Baltimore, © Wolters Kluwer, 1989, p. 132.

Figure 5.5E is an enlargement of the lumbar spine (Figure 5.5C) in order to better visualize the degenerative changes that have occurred due to abnormal mechanical stresses acting on the spine over many years.

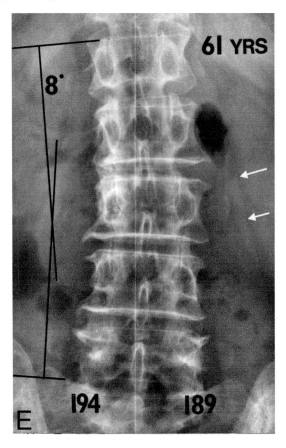

FIGURE 5.5 **(E)** Note the lateral wedging of the lumbar discs (wider on the convex side) with associated lipping of the vertebral bodies, various degrees of sclerotic changes of the zygapophysial joints indicating osteoarthrotic degenerative changes involving these joints and the more prominent psoas muscle major on the convex side (white arrows).

Source: **Giles LGF, Anatomical Basis of Low Back Pain. Baltimore, Williams and Wilkins, © Wolters Kluwer, 1989, p. 132.**

Hip Joint Femoral Head—Acetabulum Alignment Associated with Leg Length Inequality

The long leg may provoke the development of degenerative disease in the hip joint on the long leg side as a long leg imposes inordinate stress on its hip joint, whereas a short leg decreases the stress (Gofton et al 1971). Pauwels (1976) described altered weight-bearing between the left and right hip joints in cases of 'significant' LLI, with the hip joint on the *short leg* side having a greater incumbent load-bearing pressure transmitted through it as a result of the pelvic obliquity. However, the hip joint on the short leg side has an increase in the joint surface contact area between the femoral head and the acetabulum to better distribute

the greater incumbent body weight (Morscher 1977) (Figure 5.6A). Figure 5.6B illustrates the result achieved by equalizing LLD with a 26 mm raise under the right foot to eliminate the LLD.

Patients who have had LLI over the years show osteoarthrotic changes, particularly in the hip joint on the long leg side.

A correlation with hip joint degenerative changes (osteoarthrosis) (Gofton et al 1967; Pauwels 1976) due to the load on the hip joint of the longer leg being increased (Morscher 1977), not only by the diminution of the area of contact (Figure 5.6A) but also by an increase in tone of the abductor muscles, as shown by Merchant (1965).

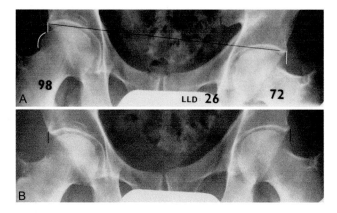

FIGURE 5.6 **(A)** This anteroposterior X-ray image shows greater coverage by the acetabular rim over the femur head on the *short leg* side (see perpendicular white line drawn from the acetabular rim to the femur head). On the *long leg* side (left), there is less area covered by the acetabular rim upon the femur head, as illustrated by the perpendicular white line. The curved white line represents the area of the femur head *not* covered by the acetabulum. **(B)** The same patient is now standing on a right foot raise of 26 mm to eliminate the leg length inequality, so the coverage of the left and right femur heads by the respective acetabular rims is equalized (see perpendicular black lines), so the incumbent body weight now passes equally through both the left and right femur heads.

Knee Joint Osteoarthrosis Associated with Leg Length Inequality

Harvey et al (2010) examined 3026 participants aged 50 to 79 years with or at high risk for knee osteoarthritis defined as Kellgren et al (1957) grade 2 or greater, and symptomatic osteoarthritis was defined as radiographic disease in a constantly painful knee. They found that, compared with LLI of less than 1 cm, LLI of 1 cm or more was associated with prevalent radiographic and symptomatic osteoarthritis in the shorter leg and in the longer leg and concluded that LLI was associated with increased symptomatic and progressive osteoarthritis in the knee. LLI is a potentially modifiable risk factor for knee osteoarthritis. The knee on the longer leg side is liable to earlier and more severe damage (Dixon et al 1969).

Zygapophysial Joints Associated with Leg Length Inequality

The zygapophysial joint facets contribute to load transmission in the motion segment (An et al 2006) and, as normal erect posture involves a permanent lordosis, lower lumbar joints are *always* subject to a *shearing force* (Farfan 1978). This force will be influenced by abnormal pelvic and spinal posture and any associated difference between paired left and right zygapophysial joint *plane angles* (Giles 1989). In cadaveric experiments, an intervertebral load cell at the L2–3 level estimated that the articular facets carry 20–40% of the total compressive spine load in the erect posture (Hakim et al 1976).

Davis (1961) proposed that the incumbent body weight above the lumbosacral joint would act as a vertical compression force that can be divided into two forces (Figure 5.7).

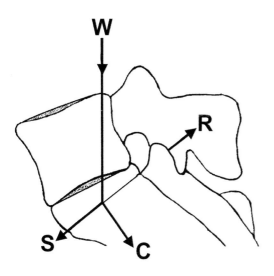

FIGURE 5.7 Schematic diagram illustrating the likely biomechanical forces at the lumbosacral junction for the incumbent body weight (W) above the lumbosacral joint and the compressive force (C) on the sacral base, with a shearing force (S) along the sacral base and a *counter reactive force* (R) to the shearing force S through the facets.

In the case of a person with equal leg lengths and no facet joint tropism, the shearing force through the paired facets should be equal on the left and right sides.

An erect posture pelvis and lumbar spine anteroposterior image of a 27-year-old male showing a left leg length deficiency of 12 mm and a 5-degree postural scoliosis is shown in Figure 5.8. In addition, using the plumb line for erect posture left and right 45-degree posterior oblique views, respectively, of this patient shows the method of measuring the plane of the joints (Figure 5.9). It can be seen from this figure that a comparison between the left and right lumbosacral zygapophysial facet joint 'angles' is associated with, in this case, an 8-degree difference between the two sides.

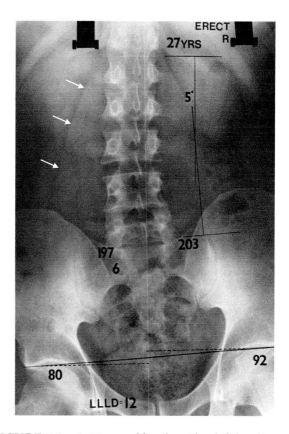

FIGURE 5.8 A 27-year-old male with a left-leg discrepancy of 12 mm and a postural scoliosis of 5 degrees. Note the more prominently displayed psoas muscle on the convex side (white arrows).

Source: **Reproduced with permission from Giles LGF and Taylor JR Low-back pain associated with leg length inequality Spine 6(5): 510–521, 1981, DOI: 10.1097/ 00007632–198109000–00014.**

A comparison between the left and right lumbosacral joint angles showed that, (i) in 100 cases with a mean leg length difference of 13 mm an 8.7-degree (± 4.5-degree) difference was present, and (2) in 100 cases with equal leg lengths i.e. (0–3 mm), only a 1.6-degree (± 1.5-degree) difference was present, representing a statistical value of p < 0.0005. The smaller angle with the horizontal is *always* on the short-leg side.

These findings suggest asymmetrical mechanical load bearing between the joint surfaces on the left and right sides.

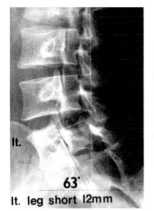
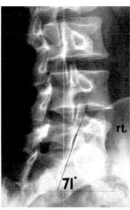

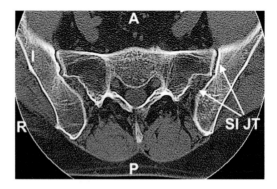

FIGURE 5.9 Measurement of left and right lumbosacral facet 'joint angle' in the 27-year-old male in Figure 5.8 with a left leg length discrepancy of 12 mm. A horizontal line was drawn at right angles to the vertical plumb-line, then a line was drawn through the plane of each facet joint to reach the horizontal line to enable the angles to be measured.

Source: **Reproduced with permission from Giles LGF, Lumbosacral facetal 'joint angles' associated with leg length inequality. Rheumatology and Rehabilitation 20: 233–238, 1981, Springer Nature.**

FIGURE 5.10 Axial CT scan slice of a 54-year-old male through the sacroiliac joints (SI JT) showing the *anterior* synovial cartilaginous part and the *posterior* ligamentous part. A = anterior; I = ilium; P = posterior; R = right.

When considering what structures may contribute to mechanical low back pain in cases of LLI and pelvic obliquity, apart from the difference in EMG muscle activity between the left and right sides of the spine that is known to occur with patients with a > 9 mm or more LLD (Vink et al 1989), there are other possible sources of low back pain arising from asymmetrical stresses affecting soft tissues of the spine. A postmortem histological section is shown in Figure 5.11, which shows

Clinical Importance of Leg Length Inequality

The clinical importance of LLI depends on the *degree of inequality* (Amstutz et al 1978; Nichols 1980) and relates to a number of possible consequences:

1. A possible correlation with low back pain (Rush et al 1946; Giles et al 1981).
2. Abnormal electromyographic examinations of paraspinal muscles with LLI of > 9 mm, resulting in abnormalities in the dynamics of the postural muscles with a remarkable increase in muscle activity of several muscle groups (Taillard et al 1965; Morscher 1977).
3. A possible correlation between the resulting pelvic obliquity and degenerative changes in the lumbar spine, for example: (i) zygapophysial facet joint osteoarthrosis, (ii) vertebral body spondylosis, and (iii) IVD wedging. Therefore, early correction of even minor degrees (1–2 cm) of LLI is recommended (Morscher 1977).
4. Excessive unilateral stress on the sacroiliac joint i.e. its capsule, ligaments, and articular cartilage (Dihlmann 1980) (Figure 5.10).
5. A correlation with knee joint osteoarthrosis i.e. '*long leg arthropathy*' (Dixon et al 1969) where the incumbent body weight passing through the left and right knee joints is not equal.
6. Trochanteric bursitis (Harvey et al 2010).
7. Psychological difficulties associated with the aesthetic consequences of postural deformity (Amstutz et al 1978).

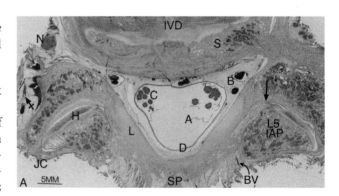

FIGURE 5.11 A 100-μm-thick slightly oblique axial histological section of the lumbosacral zygapophysial joints at the level of the inferior joint recesses from a 54-year-old male cadaver. This shows a highly vascular intra-articular synovial fold (black arrow) with a fibrotic tip. A = arachnoid mater; B = Batson's venous plexus (anterior internal vertebral (epidural) plexus); BV = blood vessel; C = cauda equina; D = dura mater; H = hyaline articular cartilage; L5 IAP = inferior articular process of L5 vertebra; IVD = intervertebral disc; JC = posterolateral fibrous joint capsule; L = ligamentum flavum; N = neural complex; S = sacrum; SP = spinous process. A neurovascular bundle close to the zygapophysial joint is shown by the tailed arrow.

Source: **Modified from Giles LGF, Taylor JR, Intra-articular synovial protrusion in the lower lumbar apophyseal joints. Bulletin of the Hospital for Joint Diseases Orthopaedic Institute 42(2): 248–255, 1982. With permission of the publisher.**

some soft tissue structures that may be affected in cases of pelvic obliquity and postural scoliosis. For example, the fibrous joint capsule may be subjected to different stresses between the left and right sides of the spine and the intra-articular synovial fold may become more vulnerable to pinching. In addition, it is possible that the outermost layers of the annulus fibrosus are subjected to abnormal stresses leading to disc injuries.

Patients who have LLD due to disorders in the lower extremities are at a greater risk of developing disabling spinal disorders due to exaggerated degenerative change; therefore, treatment for LLD may be helpful in preventing degenerative spinal changes (Kakushima et al 2003).

In spite of the foregoing, some clinicians still consider significant LLI to be 2 cm or more (Guichet et al 1991) and arbitrarily dismiss LLI of between 1 and 2 centimetres without any scientific basis (personal communication, J P

Gofton 1989), even though there is no universal agreement on what LLI is clinically significant (Krettek et al 1994). According to Hoffman et al (1994), levelling of the sacral base by shoe raise provides statistically significant relief from low back pain, often with spectacular reduction of symptoms (Williams 1974), and the lumbar pain may not be resolved until leg lengths are equalized (Mennell 1960).

With reference to larger LLDs, Tjernstrom et al (1994) found that correction of LLD of 3 cm and more improved patients' ability to work, walk, and perform recreational activities. This issue requires clarification as surgical prophylactic intervention can correct LLD before epiphyseal closure (Mattassi 1993; Harcke et al 1993), whereas leg lengthening in adult life entails potential risks of serious complications (Tjernstrom et al 1993) in a high percentage (72–84.8%) of cases (Dahl et al 1994; Zippel et al 1993).

(2) Degenerative Spondylolisthesis

Degenerative spondylolisthesis (Figure 5.12) is defined as "an acquired anterior displacement of one vertebra over the subjacent vertebra in the sagittal plane, associated with *degenerative* zygapophysial facet changes, without an associated disruption or defect in the vertebral ring" (arch) (Matz et al 2014) i.e. isthmus.

The anterolisthesis is due to zygapophysial joint hyaline articular cartilage degeneration and thinning across the facet surfaces, where the normal combined cartilage thickness at the *centre* of an L5-S1 zygapophysial joint is approximately 4.58 mm (Giles et al 1984).

As an example of degenerative spondylolisthesis (Grade 1) at the L4–5 level of a patient, a CT scout lateral and axial view are shown (Figure 5.13A and B).

With respect to degenerative spondylolisthesis, Gao (2017) compared the number of asymmetric joints in degenerative spondylolisthesis and found that there was a significant correlation between lumbar facet joint asymmetry and degenerative spondylolisthesis at the L4-L5 and L5-S1 spinal levels.

In the early stages of facet articular cartilage degeneration, lateral X-ray imaging views may not account for a patient's low back pain and even more sophisticated imaging such as CT or MRI would not show the origin of such mechanical low back pain, although tropism should be noted, particularly on a CT axial view. As the facet joint cartilage becomes thinner due to mechanical wear and tear, degenerative spondylolisthesis gradually begins to become noticeable on imaging.

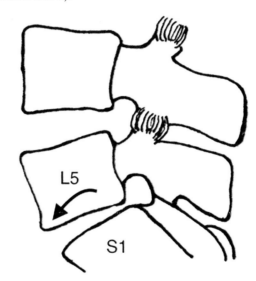

FIGURE 5.12   Note the anterolisthesis of L5 on S1 (arrow) without a pars interarticularis (isthmus) defect.

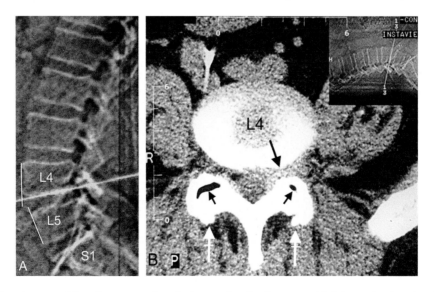

FIGURE 5.13   This 65-year-old male presented with chronic low back pain and left lower limb radiculopathy of unknow aetiology. His CT scan scout view **(A)** showed L4 anterolisthesis on L5 (represented by two lines drawn along the anterior margins of the L4 and L5 vertebral bodies, respectively). **(B)** shows bilateral zygapophysial joint lipping posteriorly (tailed arrows), as well as gas in the degenerating zygapophysial joint spaces (two short arrows) especially on the right side. There is localized spinal canal and intervertebral canal stenosis due to intervertebral disc bulging on the left side (arrow).

(3) Tethered Cord Syndrome

Introduction

Tethered cord syndrome (TCS) may well be over-looked unless clinicians are familiar with this condition.

The majority of patients with TCS are children and infants but TCS also occurs in adults (Nakashima et al 2016). There may be a history of *unusual growth spurt* perhaps causing *mechanical stretching* of the cord that grows more slowly than the spinal column, thus causing increased tension in the L-S cord between its tethered caudal part (coccyx) and the lowest pair of dentate ligaments (Yamada et al 1981). The dentate ligaments extend from the pia mater to the inner dural surface between anterior and posterior nerve roots down to T12—L1 (Yamada et al 2007). TCS occurs as a constellation of neurologic signs and symptoms resulting from longitudinal traction on the spinal cord between fixed points—this condition involves a tug-of-war between ascent and inhibition of ascent of intrathecal nervous tissue within the vertebral canal during growth (Theodore 2016).

Thus, the pathophysiology of TCS involves excessive mechanical tension of the spinal cord (Lew et al 2007), vascular compromise, and hypoxia resulting in metabolic derangements and neurological impairment (Filippidis et al 2010). The *stretch-induced neuronal dysfunction* is manifested by motor and sensory deficits of the lower limbs, incontinence, and musculoskeletal deformities—its underlying mechanism is the *impaired oxidative metabolism* and electrophysiologic activities in the grey matter (Yamada et al 2001).

The following TCS symptomatic approach is based on findings of Yamada et al (2004).

Symptoms

1. <u>Some common symptoms of TCS can be</u>: (i) pain in the lumbar region and legs; (ii) pain aggravation by postural changes, often by spinal flexion and extension; (iii) pain with positions that straighten the lumbosacral spine thus elongating the canal length i.e. the three 'B' signs: **B**udda pose i.e. sitting with legs crossed; **B**ending over the sink e.g. dish-washing or tooth-brushing; **B**aby holding (or equivalent weight) at waist level; (iv) lying supine.
2. <u>Other symptoms</u>: (i) increasing difficulty in urination or bowel control; (ii) increased difficulty with physical stress; (iii) decreased walking distance; (iv) leg numbness or urine dribbling after walking some distance; (v) progressive decrease in tolerance to driving—worse on bumpy roads; (vi) decreased standing tolerance for > 60 seconds.

Signs

<u>Common signs</u>:

1. *Weakness of some muscles*: (i) Weakness of small muscles: extensor hallucis longus (L5, S1); (ii) foot muscle weakness on tip-toeing (S1) or on heel walking (L5); (iii) weakness of peroneus longus (L5-S2), posterior tibialis (L4, 5), anterior tibialis (L4, 5), or gastrocnemius muscles (S1, 2).
2. *Musculoskeletal deformities* e.g: (i) Spinal—exaggerated lumbosacral lordosis, scoliosis; (ii) lower limb or foot e g. high-arched feet, hammer toes.
3. *Neurological Sensory deficits such as*: (i) Pinprick to: dorsum of the feet (L5)—diminished; lower limbs—*patchy* sensory distribution; perianal area (S4, S5, Co1)—diminished and decreased anal wink reflex; (ii) Anal sphincter tone reflex diminished on: digital insertion; voluntary contraction.

The preceding summary of symptoms and signs is not representative of a detailed differential diagnosis; however a differential diagnosis between lumbar herniated disc and TCS is shown in Table 5.1.

TABLE 5.1: A Summary Of Differential Diagnostic Findings Between Intervertebral Disc Herniation and Tethered Cord Syndrome. Modified from Ratliff et al 1999; Yamada et al 2001; Yamada et al 2004

		DISC HERNIA	TCS
1	RADIATING PAIN IN A DERMATOMAL PATTERN	+	−
2	PAIN MAY BE BILATERAL OR NON-DERMATOMAL	+	+
3	PAIN IN GROIN AND GENITO-RECTAL AREA	−	+
4	PAIN AGGRAVATED BY COUGHING OR SNEEZING (USUALLY TO PINPRICK)	+	−
5	PAIN WORSE IF SLOUCHING VERSUS SITTING UPRIGHT	−	+
6	PAIN WORSE ON LYING SUPINE	−	+
7	EFFECTS OF 3B POSTURES	−	+
8	SUBTLE, VAGUE DERMATOMAL OR MULTIPLE DERMATOMAL SENSORY DEFICIT E.G. *PATCHY* SENSORY CHANGES E.G. PERIANAL AND/OR LOWER LIMBS AND OFTEN ON DORSUM OF FOOT AND IN PERIANAL AREA	−	+
9	SUBTLE MYOTOMAL DYSFUNCTION	+	−
10	BLADDER DYSFUNCTION E.G. FROM URGENCY TO FREQUENCY TO ENURESIS OR INCONTINENCE	−	+
11	FREQUENT URINARY TRACT INFECTION	−	+
12	PARASPINAL MUSCLE SPASM	+	−
13	LOCAL LUMBOSACRAL SPINE TENDERNESS	+	−
14	PAIN ON STRAIGHT LEG RAISING TEST	+	−
15	MOTOR DYSFUNCTION IN 1 OR 2 MYOTOMES	+	−
16	BONY DEFORMATION MAY BE PRESENT E.G. HIGH ARCHED FEET, DIFFERENCE IN SIZE OF LEGS OR FEET	+	−

Source: Modified from Ratliff et al 1999; Yamada et al 2001; Yamada et al 2004.

In summary, note the importance of recognizing aggravation of—or initiation of—back and lower limb pain by any activities that cause spinal flexion and extension e.g. the typical three 'B' postures that straighten the lumbosacral spine, accentuating low back pain in all patients with adult TCS (Warder et al 1993). It is important to note that early teenagers may present with minimal prodromal symptoms and signs before developing adult TCS (Yamada et al 1996).

MR Imaging

Magnetic resonance imaging is currently the most useful imaging study, and some clues for diagnosis are an elongated spinal cord, a thick filum terminale (> 2 mm in diameter) or a fibroadipose tissue in the filum terminale, and a posteriorly displaced conus medullaris or filum—the latter is *not* a normal finding as the cauda equina fibres are usually separated by CSF from the posterior arachnoid membrane (Yamada et al 2001).

In patients clinically suspected of having TCS and in whom *supine* MRI depicted no abnormalities, *prone* MR imaging may provide additional information (Witkamp et al 2001).

Furthermore, symptomatic spinal cord tethering is often associated with caudal positioning of the conus medullaris; however, TCS can also occur in the presence of *structural filum abnormalities* despite a normally positioned conus medullaris (Selden 2006). There

is a subset of TCS patients in whom the tip of the conus lies at even liberally accepted normal levels, so clinicians treating patients with symptoms of tethered cord syndrome should not treat patients simply on imaging but use imaging coupled with clinical symptoms and physical examination signs (Tubbs et al 2004).

Physiological Diagnostic Studies

Studies such as urodynamics or electromyography of the lower extremities may be useful (Yamada et al 2001). For complete details, see the text *Tethered Cord Syndrome in Children and Adults* by Yamada (2010).

Factors Associated with the Onset of TCS Symptoms in Adolescents and Adults

Extrinsic factors such as sport, heavy labour, and low back trauma (e.g. motor vehicle accident) that may cause sudden stretching of the spinal cord in which there are already oxidative-metabolically impaired neurons; *intrinsic* factors such as cumulative effects of *impaired oxidative metabolism* after *repeated cord tractioning/ stretching* caused by flexion and extension activities leading to a progressive increase in filum terminale fibrous tissue (Yamada et al 2010(a)).

Part of the extensive vascular supply of nerve roots and spinal nerves that may be subjected to tractioning and stretching is shown in Figure 5.14A and B.

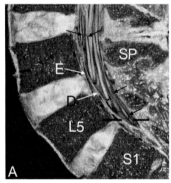 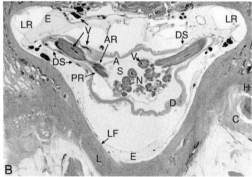

FIGURE 5.14 **(A)** Lower lumbosacral spine bisected in the sagittal plane. Cauda equina nerve roots descend with their small diameter blood vessels i.e. vasa radiculorum (black arrows) within the dural tube (D) that is surrounded by epidural fat (E), then pass out of the dural tube, enveloped within *root sleeves*, as shown in (B). SP = spinous process. **(B)** This 100-μm-thick axial histological section has been cut approximately at the lumbosacral level represented by the broken black line in (A) from a 55-year-old male cadaver. The dural tube (D) surrounds the arachnoid mater (A) that contains the *cerebrospinal fluid* and the cauda equina nerve roots (N) with their small diameter blood vessels (V). In this section, the left dural sleeve (DS) illustrates how blood vessels are normally seen in these structures. Within the subarachnoid space, the *sacral* roots occupy a more posterior position than do the *lumbar* roots that are more anterior (see Figure 2.9 B); E = epidural fat within the spinal canal that surrounds the dural tube and the nerve root sleeves. The anterior nerve root (AR) and the posterior nerve root (PR) pass from the dural tube, within the dural sleeve (DS), to the *lateral recess* (LR) of the vertebral foramen before entering the IVF. C = fibrous capsule of the L5-S1 zygapophysial joint; H = hyaline articular cartilage on the sacral superior articular process; L = lamina; LF = ligamentum flavum. Some blood vessels are seen in various regions of the epidural fat. (Please see an enlargement of this figure in the Atlas section Figure 4.27).

Source: **Reproduced with permission from Giles LGF, 100 Challenging Spinal Pain Syndrome Cases, Edinburgh, Churchill Livingstone Elsevier, © Elsevier, 2009.**

Summary

Adult presentation of tethered cord syndrome is unusual and it is difficult to diagnose and evaluate truly adult-onset tethered cord syndrome in patients with no history of spinal dysraphism, previous spinal procedure, or evidence of cutaneous manifestations (Ratliff et al 1999).

Clinical awareness of the possible association between TCS and bladder dysfunction is essential as bladder dysfunction can be: (i) associated with tethered cord syndrome in 40–72% of adult cases (Yamada et al 2000), (ii) the exclusive complaint in 4% of TCS cases (French 1990), and (iii) representative of the earliest sign of tethered cord syndrome (Hadley et al 1996).

1. The following signs should alert a clinician to the possibility of late teenage and adult tethered cord syndrome in the absence of neural spinal dysraphism: (i) no paravertebral muscle spasm; (ii) no lumbosacral spine tenderness; (iii) exaggerated lumbar lordosis; (iv) scoliosis; (v) deformity of foot or leg; (vi) weakness of (a) extensor hallucis longus, (b) peroneus longus, (c) posterior tibialis, (d) anterior tibialis, or (e) gastrocnemius; (vii) flabby or atrophic muscles in the lower extremities; (viii) ankle joint instability on toe or heel walking; (ix) diminished pinprick sensation (a) on the dorsum of the foot, (b) perianal area and groin, and (c) patchy sensation in the lower limbs; (x) diminished or lost anal wink reflex; (xi) diminished sphincter tone reflex on voluntary contraction during digital insertion; (xii) hypoactive deep tendon reflexes; (xiii) painless straight leg raising test; (xiv) post-void residual urine (Yamada et al 2010(a)).

2. It has been suggested that location of the caudal end of the spinal cord *above* L1–2 (Warder et al 1993) or *above* L2–3 IVD level (Yamada et al 2001) *may* occur in some adult TCS patients.

3. For a detailed understanding of tethered cord syndrome with its various presentations see the textbook edited by Yamada (1996).

4. For a diagnostic work-up, see Yamada et al (2010(a)).

Key Point

Cases of unexplained patchy sensation to pin prick in the lower extremities, as well as urinary bladder dysfunction, should alert the clinician to the possibility of adolescent and adult TCS due to spinal cord dysfunction resulting from mechanical tethering.

Research into the pathophysiology of TCS indicates that its symptoms and signs are associated with characteristic impairments in oxidative metabolic and electrophysiological activities within the spinal cord, rather than with histological damage; this may explain why untethering of the cord reverses the symptoms of TCS (Yamada et al 2010(b)).

Prompt diagnosis and treatment of adult TCS is essential to prevent the progression and irreversibility of symptoms and deficits (Yamada et al 2001).

CONCLUSION

The fundamental rule that clinicians should 'abstain from doing harm' links to the Hippocratic Oath (Luxford 2016) and the principle of *primum non nocere*, meaning 'first, do no harm' (Giles 2014; Luxford 2016; Travers 2018) while caring for the *whole* patient i.e. applies to *physical* and *psychological* aspects of patient care.

Before treatment commences, it is imperative that it should be based on an appropriate history being recorded, followed by an appropriate diagnostic work-up. In a large number of mechanical back pain cases it may not be possible to identify the precise pain generator, and it is often impossible to reach a specific diagnosis (Deyo 2002; Finch 2006), as many spinal structures are involved in nociception. This is a significant challenge that may lead to inappropriate treatment.

The Preface discussed the serious issues that may occur with treatment relying upon prescription of opioid drugs in particular that are known to have significant consequences such as dependence, which, in turn, exacerbate the overall presenting condition of such spinal pain syndrome sufferers—in fact, the literature states that first-line therapy should involve non-drug therapy (Tello 2017). Furthermore, clinical data showed that the use of anti-inflammatory drugs was associated with increased risk of persistent pain, suggesting that anti-inflammatory treatments might have negative effects on pain duration (Parisien et al 2022).

The General Introduction raised the issue of the cost burden of low back pain syndromes to societies worldwide and the necessity for appropriate assessment in the management of acute and chronic spinal pain, while acknowledging the contributions of a patient's physical, psychological, and social factors. Also, attention was drawn to the subject of imaging for mechanical spinal pain syndromes and the importance of *erect posture* imaging of the lumbosacral spine and pelvis, versus recumbent imaging. With regard to plain X-ray imaging, erect posture images have been shown to be far more useful to aid in radiological diagnosis for mechanical spinal pain syndromes than are recumbent images (Giles 1981; Giles et al 1981, 2006). This principle also applies to MR imaging as championed by the late radiology professor J. R. Jinkins, who published a great deal of literature on the topic of *weight-bearing kinetic MR imaging*. For example, Figure 1.5 illustrates the importance of this MRI procedure and its relationship to making an appropriate diagnosis to aid the clinician, in conjunction with detailed patient history and clinical examination findings, to make an appropriate diagnosis. This figure also highlights the importance of weight-bearing kinetic MRI for surgical decision making as, when instability exists at a given level of the spine, it will be missed on recumbent MRI, probably leading to unsuccessful treatment. This

is obviously of fundamental importance to the clinician and to the patient. Treatment options should be based on a sound scientific clinical basis with the use of *appropriate* imaging.

This approach to clinical evaluation, diagnosis, and treatment of mechanical lumbosacral spine disorders is important, otherwise a patient who has a genuine complaint of pain may well be relegated to a 'neurotic' or 'malingerer' category. This leads to misery for the patient and to frustration for the clinician and may well result in *psychiatric sequelae* for the patient that add to the burgeoning healthcare costs for the management of mechanical spinal pain syndromes.

Unfortunately, imaging may only provide "shadows of the truth" (Giles et al 1997(a)). Thus, it is not possible to identify all the possible causes of lumbosacral pain syndromes, so it is important for the clinician to be aware of various probable causes of such pain syndromes, based on knowledge gleaned from anatomical and histological examples showing some likely causes of *radiologically unidentifiable* lumbosacral spine mechanical dysfunction or failure.

Thus, following a brief gross anatomy and histology presentation of the lumbosacral spine in Chapter 3, a greater number of examples of possible spinal pain generators are provided in the anatomical Atlas section in Chapter 4, which illustrates some likely causes of mechanical lumbosacral spine pain that may *not* be discerned on MR imaging, depending on the stage of the condition and yet underlie a diagnostic label of 'non-specific' or 'idiopathic' pain being made, much to the frustration of patients.

It has been my experience over many years that very few patients are malingerers. In fact, I can only recall seeing two, out of many thousands of patients, who were malingerers. In addition, a number of patients with spinal pain syndromes were seen following referral from a psychiatrist who had been asked to see patients who were thought to be malingerers. The psychiatrist was also a qualified specialist physician and wanted some patients to obtain a second opinion as to whether their pain actually had a mechanical or dysfunctional spinal joint origin for their pain and previous diagnosis of 'malingering', as the psychiatrist believed that some patients did have a genuine, hitherto unexplained, cause for their low back pain and that their psychological distress was due to being told that there was 'nothing wrong' with their spine.

In the Atlas section, Figure 4.34C illustrates posterior migration and leakage of nuclear material causing chemical radiculopathy due to a full thickness disc tear in the annulus fibrosus and is a stark reminder that every patient must be treated as genuine, unless proven otherwise, as serious *iatrogenic psychiatric conditions* may

DOI: 10.1201/9781003315964-6

result from misdiagnosis, causing complete misery for a patient experiencing genuine pain.

The aim of the research presented in this text was to look for 'mechanical' causes of lumbosacral spine pain, including pain arising in the sacroiliac joints, that may be responsible for generating low back pain syndromes resulting in the 'enigma' of such pain syndromes. The contribution of scientific knowledge presented in this text was obtained by using human cadaveric lumbosacral spines for anatomical dissection and fresh human material (from patients undergoing routine laminectomy and discectomy) that was used for histological examination by light microscopy. These approaches have provided some insight into the enigma of mechanical low back pain syndromes.

The author concurs with the opinion of many others that, for patients with chronic low back pain, conservative treatment should first be used i.e. priority should be given to non-drug treatments combined with exercise (Traeger et al 2021) or non-drug therapy such as superficial heat, massage, acupuncture, or spinal manipulation (Tello 2017; Knezevic et al 2021) and aquatic exercises (Peng et al 2022). In this regard, patients are best served by a collaborative clinical multidisciplinary team approach (Giles et al 2006; Knezevic et al 2021) where clinicians from different healthcare disciplines co-operate in order to help the patient, as not one profession is trained in all clinical skills. For example, spinal manipulative therapy (SMT) to increase or restore spinal motion (Haldeman 1986) should be performed by clinicians trained in this procedure. Spinal manipulation has been practised as a healing activity for centuries, and one such clinical activity employs a relatively high velocity, low amplitude force applied to the vertebral column with therapeutic intent (Pickar et al 2012). Such treatment, used short term, is beneficial (Wong et al 2007). Although the mechanism responsible for the therapeutic effects of SMT remain unclear, it is likely that, for example, SMT may release a trapped synovial fold, break down facet joint adhesions, or generally improve spinal joint movement in the case of limited joint movement, resulting in relief from pain. In addition, Pickar et al (2012) propose, based upon the experimental literature, that SMT may produce a sustained change in the synaptic efficacy of central neurons by evoking a high frequency, bursting discharge from several types of dynamically sensitive, mechanosensitive paraspinal primary afferent neurons.

There is no therapy that does not present some risk (Maigne 1972), but the general consensus is that SMT, applied appropriately to the correct spinal level performed to diminish pain, does decrease stiffness and diminish muscle spasm (Kenna et al 1989). It is well documented that appropriate SMT is a safe procedure (Kenna et al 1989; Maigne 1972; Waddell et al 2004) provided that appropriate indications and safety guidelines are followed (Kenna et al 1989), and serious complications are rare (Berman 2006). There exist indications that SMT can shorten the painful exacerbation of functional locomotor disturbances, which, in turn, significantly diminishes work absenteeism (Schneider et al 1988).

Aerobic exercise increases blood flow and nutrients to the soft tissues of the back, improving the healing process and reducing stiffness that can result in back pain (Gordon et al 2016), thus promoting good health. It appears that patients suffering from idiopathic low back pain should be encouraged to remain active in order to promote better circulation around the neural structures within the vertebral canal and the intervertebral foramina, just as it has been suggested that frequently changing body positions is important to promote flow of fluid (nutrition) to the disc (Wilke et al 1999). This principle of frequently changing body positions may also apply to the CSF that does not have a 'circulatory system', so its movement depends upon the downward pull of gravity and a person's *physical activity* to move it around within the subarachnoid spaces of the spine and brain. The suggested frequent physical activity may promote spinal cord health by ensuring that the optimal CSF functions of *supplying nutrients* to the spinal cord (Yoshizawa 2002) and *elimination of metabolic wastes* (Spector et al 2015) caused by the considerable metabolic activity of the CNS take place. The elimination of such metabolic waste requires efficient drainage and detoxification (Thomas et al 2019), for example via the spinal cord's arachnoid villi in the spinal dural nerve sleeves and adjacent radicular veins that have been illustrated by Tubbs et al (2007b) and Sakka et al (2011).

Basic neurovascular anatomical principles of the human spinal cord's nerve and vascular systems, including its intricate blood supply and vascular drainage and the relationship between the spinal nerves and the CSF, have been presented. These anatomical relationships may suggest that spinal movement exercises should be a component of daily health activities, as is the case with activities to promote cardiovascular health.

In addition, it is thought that regular physical activity may also keep one's thinking, learning, and judgement skills sharp as one ages, reducing the risk of depression and anxiety, while also improving sleep (CDC 2021).

It must be remembered that it is a privilege to care for patients and that every endeavour should be made to make an appropriate diagnosis, based on best practice principles, to alleviate physical pain and any psychological distress that many patients endure.

Once treatment options and risks have been discussed, patient management should include obtaining a signed informed 'Consent Form' indicating possible risks. Patient cooperation should be sought regarding their involvement in, for example, a healthy lifestyle including taking part in appropriate exercises and adhering to a proper diet for their particular needs.

In order to clearly inform patients about possible causes of the origins of spinal mechanical pain, plastic models and spinal anatomy figures are useful to illustrate basic spinal anatomy to patients, as well as to explain the important principle that not all causes of mechanical spine pain can be demonstrated for a given patient, in view of the limitations of imaging procedures that simply cannot show all such possible causes of spinal pain.

It is important to ask the patient if they have any queries or concerns that they wish to have explained. This builds up a good rapport with the patient who then realizes that the clinician has taken the necessary steps to determine what is the likely cause of their pain, and this, in turn, underpins their confidence in what the clinician proposes as treatment options for them.

Finally, it behooves clinicians to remember what are some words of wisdom that our predecessors have bestowed upon us over the generations since Hippocrates (460–370 BC) stated: "First do no harm". For example, the physician, surgeon, and philosopher, Galen of Pergamon (130–210 AD), stated in his *Methodus Medendi*: "The magnitude of a disease is in proportion to its deviation from the healthy state; and the extent of this deviation can be ascertained by him only who is perfectly acquainted with the healthy state" (Blumenbach et al 1817). Therefore, it is essential for clinicians to be well versed in the basics of the normal healthy state of the spine with respect to its anatomy and physiology so the clinician is able to understand its functions in the presence of mechanical dysfunction. In this regard, Vesalius (1543) wrote: "*Anatomy . . . should rightly be regarded as the firm foundation of the whole art of medicine*". It is hoped that this text has helped to expand the knowledge base of anatomy and physiology with respect to the function of the spine with all its associated soft tissue structures.

DEFINITIONS

Adhesion: A band of scar tissue that binds two parts of the body tissue that are not normally joined together.

Antalgic posture: A posture assumed by patients experiencing acute low back pain, with or without leg pain, in which they lean away from the painful area.

Anteroposterior (A-P): The *position* of patients when an X-ray beam is directed to their anterior surface and an X-ray plate is positioned behind them. In this text, the A-P radiographs are *viewed* from behind the patient; the patient's right side is indicated by a right marker (R).

Axial, horizontal, or transverse plane: This plane divides the body into superior and inferior parts—it is perpendicular to the coronal and sagittal planes.

Cobb's method (1948): A method for measuring the angle of scoliotic spinal curvature. The angle of curvature is measured by drawing lines parallel to the superior surface of the most upper vertebral body of the curvature and to the inferior surface of the lowest vertebra of the curvature (Figure D.1).

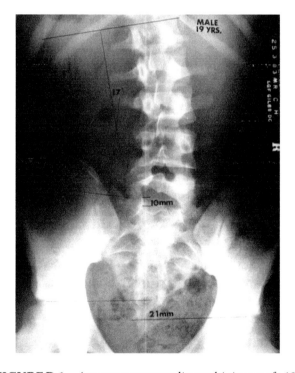

FIGURE D.1 An erect posture radiographic image of a 19-year-old male showing a right leg length deficiency of 21 mm, sacral base obliquity and postural scoliosis with a 17-degree angle of curvature. R = right side of the patient. Note the vertical plumb-line shadow that is used for measuring leg lengths by drawing a horizontal line from the top of each femur head to meet the plumb-line at right angles. The vertical difference between paired horizontal lines gives

FIGURE D.1 (Continued)

the difference in leg lengths. Similarly, sacral base obliquity is measured by drawing a horizontal line from each superior sacral notch to meet the plumb-line at right angles.

Source: Reproduced with permission from Giles L G F 1989 Anatomical basis of low back pain. Williams and Wilkins, Baltimore.

Degenerative spondylolisthesis (Pseudospondylolisthesis): Is secondary to longstanding degenerative arthrosis of the lumbar zygapophysial joints and discovertebral articulations, without a pars separation (Yochum et al 1996).

Disability: According to The World Health Organization (2001), a **disability** has three dimensions: (i) **Impairment** in a person's body structure or function, or mental functioning; examples of impairments include loss of a limb, loss of vision, or memory loss; (ii) **Activity limitation**, such as difficulty seeing, hearing, walking, or problem solving; and (iii) **Participation restrictions** in normal daily activities, such as working, engaging in social and recreational activities, and obtaining healthcare and preventive services.

Dura mater: Also known as dura or dural membrane.

Dural tube: Also known as dural sac or thecal sac. The dura mater forms the spinal dural tube, a long tubular sheath within the vertebral canal (Moore et al 2006). The dura is the outermost of three spinal meninges, i.e. dura mater, arachnoid mater, and pia mater.

Dysaesthesia: An unpleasant abnormal sensation produced by normal stimuli (*Dorland's Illustrated Medical Dictionary* 1994).

EMG *Electromyography*: An electrodiagnostic technique for recording the extracellular activity (action potentials and evoked potentials) of skeletal muscles at rest, during voluntary contractions and during electrical stimulation, performed using any of a variety of surface electrodes, needle electrodes, and devices for amplifying, transmitting, and recording the signals (*Dorland's Illustrated Medical Dictionary* 1994).

Intervertebral canal (intervertebral foramen, lateral canal, nerve root tunnel, radicular canal, root canal, interpedicular canal): A clinically very important structure (Dorwart et al 1983). Some authors use the term *intervertebral foramen* to describe both the osseous nerve root canal and the medial and lateral 'openings'; however, Dommisse (1975) correctly suggests that the term 'foramen' should only be used to describe the inner and outer boundaries of intervertebral canals. The term intervertebral foramen is used in this text unless reference is specifically being made to the canal.

155

Intervertebral disc conditions:

Annular bulge refers to a concentric extension of the margins of the disc circumferentially beyond the vertebral margins (Hodges et al 1999).

Broad-based protrusion refers to protrusion of disc material extending beyond the outer edges of the vertebral body apophyses over an area greater than 25% and less than 50% of the circumference of the disc (Fardon et al 2001).

Contained herniation is when nuclear material does not escape from the confines of the annular fibres.

Extrusion is the extension of the nucleus completely through the outer annulus into the epidural space (Hodges et al 1999).

Fissuring of the disc refers to annular tearing (Tenny et al 2021).

Herniation is defined as a localized displacement of disc material beyond the limits of the IVD space (Fardon et al 2001).

Herniation sites (Postacchini et al 1999(a)), unless shown otherwise):

Anterior—nucleus pulposus bulges or herniates anteriorly (Cloward 1952).

Midline (or central)—occurs in the midportion of the disc.

Paramedian—occurs in the centrolateral portion of the disc.

Posterior epidural—intervertebral disc material migration extends around one side of the dural tube and *posterior* to the dural tube (Palmisciano et al 2022).

Posterolateral—disc material protrudes posteriorly and laterally towards the foramen. A posterolateral disc herniation occurs where the annulus fibrosus is thinner and lacks structural support from the posterior longitudinal ligament (Dydyk et al 2022).

Intraforaminal—within the limits of the intervertebral foramen.

Extraforaminal—occurs entirely or mainly outside the neuroforamen.

Intervertebral (Schmorl's nodes)—through a fracture of the vertebral endplate and subchondral bones (Schmorl 1927).

Protrusion is a focal area of extension of the nucleus beyond the vertebral margin that remains beneath the outer annular and posterior longitudinal ligament complex (Hodges et al 1999).

Sequestration is a specific type of extrusion in which there is a free disc fragment (Hodges et al 1999).

Intra-articular synovial fold: A fibrous or highly vascular fat-filled zygapophysial joint synovial fold which is covered by a synovial lining membrane.

Intranuclear cleft: A hypointense linear signal seen on a T2-weighted sagittal MR image as a continuous smooth band within the centre of the intervertebral disc.

The intranuclear cleft represents normal appearance of central fibres inside the nucleus (Yrjämä et al 1997).

'Leg length' inequality: The absolute inequality in length of the lower limbs. In this text a 'significant leg length inequality' is referred to when an inequality of 9 mm or more is found using an accurate method for erect posture radiography (Figure D.1).

Manipulation (Sandoz 1976, 1981): A manipulation or lumbar intervertebral joint 'adjustment' is a passive manual manoeuvre during which the three-joint complex is suddenly carried beyond the normal physiological range of movement without exceeding the boundaries of anatomical integrity. The usual characteristic is a thrust—a brief, sudden, and carefully administered 'impulsion' that is given at the end of the normal passive range of movement. It is usually accompanied by a 'cracking' noise.

Metachromasia: The staining of tissue or tissue components such that the colour of the tissue-bound dye complex differs significantly from the colour of the original dye complex to give a marked contrast in colour (Pearse 1968).

Motion Segment of Junghanns: All the space between two vertebrae where movement occurs: the intervertebral disc with its cartilaginous plates, the anterior and posterior longitudinal ligaments, the zygapophysial joints with their fibrous joint capsules and the ligamenta flava, the contents of the spinal canal and the left and right intervertebral foramen, and the supraspinous and interspinous ligaments (see Figure 3.1).

Neuron figures showing neurons with their cell body, dendrites and axon (Figure D.2).

Micron (μm): 1 μm = 1,000 millimetres.

Obliquity:

Pelvic obliquity—this is a lateral inclination of the pelvis which is tilted downward to the short leg side.

Sacral base obliquity—a lateral inclination of the sacral base (Figure D.1).

Osteoarthritis (degenerative joint disease, degenerative arthritis, hypertrophic arthritis): characterized by degeneration of articular cartilage, hypertrophy of bone at joint margins, and synovial membrane changes; usually associated with pain and stiffness (Hellmann 1992).

Osteoarthrosis: Chronic non-inflammatory arthritis.

Osteophytes: Result from ossification of the articular cartilage, the joint capsule and/or the ligamenta flava where they are attached to bone (Postacchini et al 1999(b)).

Posterior (dorsal) nerve root: Contains sensory fibres from a limb to the spinal cord.

Posterior nerve root ganglion (spinal root ganglion): Located on the posterior nerve root and contains nerve cell bodies.

Radiculopathy: Irritation of or injury to a nerve root (as from being compressed) that typically causes pain, numbness, or weakness in the part of the body that is supplied with nerves from that root (Merriam-Webster dictionary 2022), for example, sciatica.

Recumbent: Lying down.

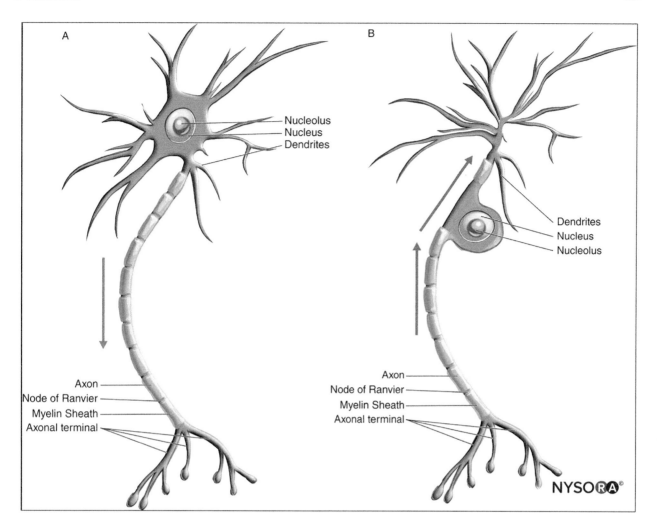

FIGURE D.2 Diagram illustrating multipolar (A) and a unipolar or pseudo-unipolar (B) neuron. **(A)** The *multipolar motor* neuron with its cell body and its associated anatomical parts. The arrow illustrates the direction of conduction. **(B)** The *sensory* neuron with its cell body and its associated anatomical parts. The arrows illustrate the direction of conduction with regard to the cell body, which is located in sensory ganglia.

Source: Reproduced with permission from Cvetko E, Meznarič M, Stopar Pintaric T 2022 Histology of the peripheral nerves and light microscopy, New York School of Regional Anesthesia (NYSORA), www.nysora.com/foundations-of-regional-anesthesia/anatomy/histology-peripheral-nerves-light-microscopy/.

Recurrent meningeal nerve: German anatomist Hubert von Luschka first described the sinuvertebral nerve in 1850, and it has acquired many other names, including (i) the recurrent nerve of Luschka, (ii) recurrent meningeal nerve, and (iii) meningeal branch of the spinal nerve (Shayota et al 2019). In this text the term *recurrent meningeal nerve* is used.

Scoliosis:

Angle of curvature—the angle between lines drawn parallel to the superior surface of the upper vertebra of the curvature and to the inferior surface of the lowest vertebra of the curvature.

Postural compensatory—this is a lumbar or thoracolumbar scoliosis (lateral curvature), which is an adaptation of the vertebral column to pelvic obliquity and which is convex on the short leg side. The intervertebral discs are wedged from the concave to the convex sides on the A-P radiograph with the discs being wider on the convex side of the scoliosis (Figure D.1).

Shoe-raise therapy: The provision of a shoe-raise on the sole and heel on the side of the short leg.

Spinal pain (Skouen et al 2002):

Acute spinal pain refers to severe pain of recent onset (less than four weeks) with marked limitation of spinal movements

Sub-acute spinal pain refers to pain of greater than 4 weeks and less than 13 weeks.

Chronic spinal pain refers to pain of long duration (12 weeks or more) without marked limitation of spinal movements.

Spondylosis: Osteophytosis secondary to degenerative intervertebral disc disease (Weinstein et al 1977).

Subluxation: In this text, the term is used when opposing facet surfaces of the zygapophysial joint are no longer congruous, as demonstrated by imbrication (telescoping) of the zygapophysial joint facet surfaces (Hadley 1964; Macnab 1977) (Figure D.3).

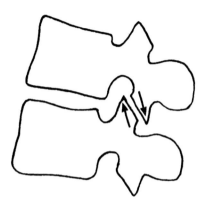

FIGURE D.3   Note the subluxation (imbrication, telescoping) of the zygapophysial joint facet surfaces as indicated by the arrows.

Source: **Reproduced with permission from Giles L G F 1989 Anatomical basis of low back pain. Williams and Wilkins, Baltimore.**

Supine: Lying face upward.

Syndrome: A group of signs and symptoms that occur together and characterize a particular abnormality or condition (Merriam-Webster dictionary), for example, low back pain with radiculopathy.

Tropism: Asymmetry in the horizontal plane of paired left and right zygapophysial joints. A difference *of 5 degrees or more* between the horizontal planes of the left and right zygapophysial joints represents tropism (Cihák 1970).

Vasa radiculorum: Refers to the blood supply of spinal nerve roots, for example of the human lumbosacral nerve roots (Parke et al 1985).

Zygapophysial joint: The diarthrodial synovial joint between adjacent vertebral arches (apophysial joint, 'facet' joint, interlaminar joint).

Zyga pophysial joint cartilage: This is of the hyaline articular cartilage variety and it lines the facet surfaces; extension of cartilage beyond the facet surface, known as 'fibrocartilage bumper', is not composed of hyaline cartilage (Hadley 1964).

REFERENCES

AANS (American Association of Neurological Surgeons) (2020). www.aans.org/en/Patients/Neurosurgical-Conditions-and-Treatments/Anatomy-of-the-Spine-and-Peripheral-Nervous-System

Ackerley R, Curr Opin Behav Sci (2022). DOI: 10.1016/j.cobeha.2021.08.012

Ackerley R, et al., J Neurophysiol (2018). PMID: 30256737 DOI: 10.1152/jn.00109.2018

Adams JC, et al., Outline of Orthopaedics, 13th edn (Churchill Livingstone, London, 2001).

Adams MA, et al., J Bone Joint Surg (1986). PMID: 3941139 DOI: 10.1302/0301-620X.68B1.3941139

Adeeb N, et al., Child's Nerv Syst (2013). PMID: 23381008 DOI: 10.1007/s00381-013-2044-5

Ahimsadasan N, et al., StatPearls [Internet]. Treasure Island (FL): StatPearls Publishing (2021). PMID: 30335324 Bookshelf ID: NBK532291

Akdemir G, J Neurosurg Spine (2010). DOI: 10.3171/2010.3.SPINE09799

Akinrodoye MA, et al., StatPearls [Internet]. Treasure Island (FL): StatPearls Publishing (2021). www.ncbi.nlm.nih.gov/books/NBK556027/

Albert HB, et al., Modic changes following lumbar disc herniation. Euro Spine J (2007). DOI: 10.1007/s00586-007-0336-8

Al-Chalabi M, et al., StatPearls [Internet]. Treasure Island (FL): StatPearls Publishing (2021). www.ncbi.nlm.nih.gov/books/NBK507824/

Allan DB, et al., Acta Orthop Scand Supp (1989). PMID: 2533783 DOI: 10.3109/17453678909153916

Allison JM, et al., The FASEB Journal (2018). DOI: 10.1096/fasebj.31.1_supplement.748.6

Alshak M, et al., StatPearls [Internet]. Treasure Island (FL): StatPearls Publishing (2021). www.ncbi.nlm.nih.gov/books/NBK542195/

American Society of Anesthesiologists (2019). www.asahq.org/whensecondscount/pain-management/opioid-treatment/what-are-opioids/?_sf_s=What+are+opioids

Amonoo-Kuofi HS, et al., J Anat (1988). PMID: 3417545

Amonoo-Kuofi HS, et al., In: Clinical Anatomy and Management of Low Back Pain, Chapter 7 (Butterworth Heinemann, Edinburgh, 1997).

Amstutz HC, et al., Clin Orthop (1978). PMID: 729287

An HS, et al., J Orthop Sci (2006). PMID: 17013747 DOI: 10.1007/s00776-006-1055-4

Antonacci MD, et al., J Spinal Disord (1998). PMID: 9884299

Aprill, CN, In: First Interdisciplinary World Congress on Low Back Pain and its Relation to the Sacroiliac Joint (ECO, Rotterdam, 1992).

Arey LB, Developmental Anatomy. A Textbook and Laboratory Manual of Embryology (WB Saunders Co, Philadelphia, 1965).

Arnoldi CC, Clin Orthop 115: 30–34 (1976).

Arnoldi CC, Acta Orthopaedica Scand (1994). DOI: 10:3109/174536794091552266

Ashaye T, et al., BMJ Open (2018). DOI: 10.1136/bmjopen-2017-019491

Atlas of Normal Anatomy, Medical Student Edition, Lumbar and Sacral Regions of the Spinal Cord, Plate 2 and 48, 1956. Lederle Laboratories, American Cyanamid International, Pearl River, NY.

Australian Institute of Health and Welfare. Alcohol, Tobacco and other Drugs in Australia [web report]. Canberra: AIHW (2021). www.aihw.gov.au/reports/alcohol/alcohol-tobacco-other-drugs-australia/contents/introduction (viewed May 2021).

Avins AL, JAMA (2010). PMID: 20606157 DOI: 10.1001/jama.2010.922

Bae WC, et al., Radiology (2013). PMID: 23192776 DOI: 10.1148/radiol.12121181

Bailey JF, et al., J Anat (2011). PMC3058212 DOI: 10.1111/j.1469-7580.2010.01332.x

Baker DR, et al., Spondyloschisis and spondylolisthesis in children. J Bone Joint Surg, 38-A:933–934 (1956).

Bannister LH, et al., Gray's Anatomy, 38th edn (Churchill Livingstone, New York, 1996).

Barr ML, et al., The Human Nervous System. An Anatomical Viewpoint, 4th edn (Harper and Row, Philadelphia, 1983).

Barros G, et al., Fed Pract (2019). PMID: 31456628

Bartynski WS, et al., Magn Reson Imaging Clin N Am (2007). PMID: 17599636 DOI: 10.1016/j.mric.2007.01.010

Basara I, et al., Acta Orthop Traumatol Turc (2015). PMID: 26200415 DOI: 10.3944/AOTT.2015.3224

Beaman DN, et al., Spine (1993). PMID: 7690159 DOI: 10.1097/00007632-199306150-00014

Becker I, et al., J Anat (2010). PMID: 20840351 PMCID: PMC3035856 DOI: 10.1111/j.1469-7580.2010.01300.x

Beckworth WJ, et al., PM&R (2018). PMID: 28918116 DOI: 10.1016/j.pmrj.2017.09.004

Bednar DA, et al., Spine (2021). PMID: 34474448 DOI: 10.1097/BRS.0000000000004110

Beers MH, et al. (eds) The Merck Manual of Diagnosis and Therapy, 18th edn (Merck Research Laboratories, Whitehouse Station NJ, 2006).

Berg EJ, et al., StatPearls [Internet]. Treasure Island (FL): StatPearls Publishing (2020). www.ncbi.nlm.nih.gov/books/NBK513251/

Berman BM, The Merck Manual of Diagnosis and Therapy, 18th edn, Chapter 330 (Merck Research Laboratories, Whitehouse Station NJ, 2006).

Bernard TN, et al., Clin Orthop Rel Res (1987). PMID: 2951048

Bernard TN, et al., In: The Adult Spine Principles and Practice, 2nd edn, Chapter 109 (Lippincott-Raven, New York, 1997).

Bernard TN, et al., In: Managing Low Back Pain, 4th edn, Chapter 11 (Churchill Livingstone, Philadelphia, 1999).

Bernick S, et al., Spine (1982). PMID: 7089697 DOI: 10.1097/00007632-198203000-00002

Berry M, et al., Nervous system. In: Gray's Anatomy, 38th edn (Churchill Livingstone, London, 1995).

Bertolotti M, Contributo alla conoscenza dei vizi di differenziazione regionale del rachide con speciale raguardo all assimilazione sacrale della v. lombare. Radiologiqu medica, 4: 113–144 (1917).

Betts JG, et al., The cardiovascular system: blood vessels and circulation. In: Anatomy and Physiology (OpenStax, Rice University, TX, 2019). https://openstax.org/books/anatomy-and-physiology/pages/20-1-structure-and-function-of-blood-vessels

Binch ALA, et al., Nat Rev Rheumatol (2021). DOI: 10.1038/s41584-020-00568-w

Binokay F, et al., Acta Radiol (2006). PMID: 16739700 DOI: 10.1080/02841850600557158

Bishop GH, Physiol Rev (1946). PMID: 21012601 DOI: 10.1152/physrev.1946.26.1.77

Blakemore L, et al., J Pediatr Orthop (2018). PMID: 27137907 DOI: 10.1097/BPO.0000000000000781

Bland JH, Am J Med (1983). PMID: 6344622 DOI: 10.1016/0002-9343(83)90524-7

Bland JH, Disorders of the Cervical Spine. Diagnosis and Medical Management (WB Saunders, Philadelphia, 1987).

Blom AW, et al., BMJ (2021). DOI: 10.1136/bmj.n1511

Blumenbach JF, et al., The Institution of Physiology, 2nd edn (E Cox and Son, London, 1817, p xiv).

Boden SD, et al., J Bone Joint Surg Am (1990). PMID: 2312537

Bogduk N, Clinical Anatomy of the Lumbar Spine and Sacrum, 3rd edn (Churchill Livingstone, Edinburgh, 1997).

Bogduk N, Evidence-based Clinical Guidelines for the Management of Acute Low Back Pain (National Medical Research Council, Canberra, Australia, November 1999).

Bonica JJ, JAMA (1957). PMID: 13428545 DOI: 10.1001/jama.1957.02980070014003

Boos N, et al., Spine (1995). PMID: 8747239 DOI: 10.1097/00007632-199512150-00002

Boos N, et al., Spine (2000). PMID: 10851096 DOI: 10.1097/00007632-200006150-00006

Bordoni B, et al., StatPearls [Internet]. Treasure Island (FL): StatPearls Publishing (2021). www.ncbi.nlm.nih.gov/books/NBK535407/

Borenstein D, Curr Rheumatol Rep (2004). PMID: 15509467 DOI: 10.1007/s11916-004-0075-z

Bothwell SW, et al., Fluids Barriers CNS (2019). DOI: 10.1186/s12987-019-0129-6

Bowen V, et al., Spine (1991). PMID: 7336283 DOI: 10.1097/00007632-198111000-00015

Bradley KC, Aust NZ J Surg, 2 (1974). PMID: 4282245 DOI: 10.1111/j.1445-2197.1974.tb04409.x

Brailsford JF, Br J Surg, 1 (1929). DOI: 10.1002/bjs.1800166405

Breig A, Biomechanics of the Central Nervous System (Upsalla, Almqvist and Wiksells, Stockholm, 1960).

Breig A, Adverse Mechanical Tension in the Central Nervous System (Almqvist and Wiksell International, Stockholm, 1978).

Breig A, et al., Acta Radiol (Stockh.) (1963). PMID: 14086403 DOI: 10.1177/028418516300100603

Bridwell K (2021). www.spineuniverse.com/anatomy/ligaments

Brisby H, et al., Spine (1999). PMID: 10222523 DOI: 10.1097/00007632-199904150-00003

Brown MF, et al., Bone Joint J (1997). PMID: 9020464 DOI: 10.1302/0301-620x.79b1.6814

Buchbinder R, et al., Lancet (2018). PMID: 29573871 DOI: 10.1016/S0140-6736(18)30488-4

Buirski G, et al., Spine (1993). PMID: 8235866 DOI: 10.1097/00007632-199310000-00016

Burgess PR, et al., In: Handbook of Sensory Physiology, Vol 2 (Springer-Verlag, Berlin, 1973, pp. 29–78).

Butler D, et al., Spine (1990). PMID: 2326704 DOI: 10.1097/00007632-199002000-00012

Butler P, et al., Applied Radiological Anatomy (Cambridge University Press, Cambridge, 2012).

Bydder GM, Spine (2002). PMID: 12065972 DOI: 10.1097/00007632-200206150-00005

Bydder GM, et al., In American Society of Neuroradiology, 39th Annual Meeting, Boston, April (2001).

Byun WM, et al., Am J Neuroradiol (2012). PMCID: PMC7966457 DOI: 10.3174/ajnr.A2813

Cailliet R, Low Back Pain Syndrome, 2nd edn (F.A. Davis Company, Philadelphia, 1968).

Cailliet R, Low Back Pain Syndrome, 5th edn (F.A. Davis Company, Philadelphia, 1995).

Cailliet R, Low Back Disorders. A Medical Enigma (Lippincott Williams and Wilkins, Philadelphia, 2003).

Carpenter MB, Neuroanatomy, 3rd ed. (Williams and Wilkins, Baltimore, 1985).

Carr RB, et al., AJR (2012). PMID: 23169709 DOI: 10.2214/AJR.12.9083

Carrera A, et al (2020). www.nysora.com/foundations-of-regional-anesthesia/anatomy/functional-regional-anesthesia-anatomy/

Cashin AG, et al., BMJ (2021). DOI: 10.1136/bmj.n1446

Cassel CK, Ann Intern Med (1995). PMID: 8998907

Cassidy JD, J Manipulative Physiol Ther (1992). PMID: 1531489

Cassidy JD, et al., In: Principles and Practice of Chiropractic (Appleton and Lange, Norwalk, 1992, pp. 211–224).

Castellvi AE, et al., Spine (1984). PMID: 6495013 DOI: 10.1097/00007632-198407000-00014

Cavanaugh JM, et al., J Biomech (1996). PMID: 8872268 DOI: 10.1016/0021-9290(96)00023-1

CDC. (2021). Benefits of Physical Activity. www.cdc.gov/physicalactivity/basics/pa-health/index.htm

Cervero F, et al., Pain Foru (1996). DOI: 10.1016/S1082-3174(96)80020-1

Ceylan D, et al., Acta Neurochir (Wien) (2012). PMID: 22555553 DOI: 10.1007/s00701-012-1361-x

Chaudhry A, et al AJNR Am J Neuroradiol (2018). DOI: 10.3174/ajnr.A5698

Chen X, et al., J Healthc Eng (2021). DOI: 10.1155/2021/5534227

Chila AG, et al., Patient Care (1990). https://go.gale.com/ps/i.do?p=AONE&u=googlescholar&id=GALE|A9035911&v=2.1&it=r&sid=bookmark-AONE&asid=b21eb987

Choi YK, Korean J Pain (2019). PMCID: PMC6615450 DOI: 10.3344/kjp.2019.32.3.147

Chusid JG, Correlative Neuroanatomy and Functional Neurology, 19th edn (Lange Medical Publications, California, 1985).

Cihák R, Acta Univ Carol [Med Monogr] [Praha] (1970). PMID: 5432709

Clifford JR, Lumbar discography: An outdated procedure (letter). J Neurosurg, 64: 686 (1986).

Cloward RB, AMA Arch Surg (1952). DOI: 10.1001/archsurg.1952.01260010473005

Cobb JR, Outline for the study of scoliosis. Instructional course lectures. J Am Acad Orthop Surg, 5: 261–275 (1948).

Connolly LP, et al., J Nucl Med (2003). PMID: 12791818

Connor MJ, et al., ISRN Anatomy (2013). DOI: 10.5402/2013/424058

Cooke PM, et al., Phys Med Rehabil Clin North Am (2000). PMID: 11092021

Coulter ID, et al., J Manipulative Physiol Ther (2018). PMCID: PMC6420353 DOI: 10.1016/j.jmpt.2018.11.002

Coventry MB, et al., The intervertebral disc: its microscopic anatomy and pathology. Part I: Anatomy, development, and physiology. J Bone Joint Surg, 27: 105–112 (1945).

Cramer GD, et al., J Manipulative Physiol Ther (2002). PMID: 12021738 DOI: 10.1067/mmt.2002.123174

Cramer GD, et al., J Manipulative Physiol Ther (2013). PMCID: PMC3756802 DOI: 10.1016/j.jmpt.2013.04.003

Crock HV, Clin Orthop (1976). PMID: 1253473

Crock HV, J Bone Joint (1981). PMID: 7298672 DOI: 10.1302/0301-620X.63B4.7298672

Crock HV, et al., J Bone Joint Surg Br (1973). PMID: 4729020

Crock HV, et al., Clin Orthop (1976). PMID: 1253499

Crock HV, et al., The Blood Supply of the Vertebral Column and Spinal Cord in Man (Springer-Verlag, New York, 1977).

Crown S, Clin Rheum Dis (1980). DOI: 10.1016/S0307-742X(21)00281-2

Cuello AC, In: Neuroimmunology (Raven Press, New York, 1984, pp. 37–45).

Cyriax J, Lancet (1945). DOI: 10.1016/S0140-6736(45)91686-2

Cyron B, et al., Spine (1980). PMID: 7384910 DOI: 10.1097/00007632-198003000-00011

Dafny N (2020). https://nba.uth.tmc.edu/neuroscience/m/s2/chapter03.html

Dahl MT, et al., Clin Orthop Relat Res (1994). PMID: 8156659

Dahm MR, et al., Diagnosis (2021). DOI: 10.1515/dx-2021-0086

Danielson BI, et al., Acta Radiol (1998). PMID: 9817029 DOI: 10.3109/02841859809175484

Dao DPD, et al., StatPearls [Internet]. Treasure Island (FL): StatPearls Publishing (2021). www.ncbi.nlm.nih.gov/books/NBK554574/

Daube JR, et al., An Approach to Anatomy Pathology and Physiology by Systems and Levels, 2nd edn (Little, Brown and Co., Boston, 1986).

Dauleac C, et al., JNS (2019). PMID: 31299646 DOI: 10.3171/2019.4.SPINE19404

Davis PR, J Anat (1961). PMID: 17105124 PMCID: PMC1244489

Dawodu ST (2018). https://emedicine.medscape.com/article/1148690-overview?src=emailthis

Deepak HR, et al., Int J Res Orthop (2020). DOI: 10.18203/issn.2455-4510.IntJResOrthop20200474

Degmetich S, et al., Eur Spine J (2016). DOI: 10.1007/s00586-015-4037-4

DeLucca JF, et al., J Biomech (2016). PMCID: PMC4779374 DOI: 10.1016/j.jbiomech.2016.01.007

DeSai C, et al., StatPearls [Internet]. Treasure Island (FL): StatPearls Publishing (2020). www.ncbi.nlm.nih.gov/books/NBK526133/

Deyo RA, N Engl J Med (1994). PMID: 8208253 DOI: 10.1056/NEJM199407143310209

Deyo RA, Arch Intern Med (2002). PMID: 12090877 DOI: 10.1001/archinte.162.13.1444

Deyo RA, et al., J Gen Intern Med (1986). PMID: 2945915 DOI: 10.1007/BF02596320

Deyo RA, et al., JAMA (1992). PMID: 1386391

Deyo RA, et al., J Manipulative Physiol Ther (2014). PMID: 25127996 DOI: 10.1016/j.jmpt.2014.07.006

Dick WC, An Introduction to Clinical Rheumatology (Churchill Livingstone, Edinburgh, 1972).

DiFiore MSH, An Atlas of Human Histology, 3rd edn (Lea and Fibiger, Philadelphia, 1967).

Dihlmann W, Diagnostic Radiology of the Sacroiliac Joints (Year Book Medical Publishers, Chicago, 1980).

Dijkstra PF, In: Movement, Stability and lumbopelvic Pain. Integration of Research and Therapy, 2nd edn, Chapter 20 (Churchill Livingston Elsevier, Edinburgh, 2007).

Divi S, et al., Spine (2020). DOI: 10.1097/BRS.0000000000003322

Dixon AST, et al., Ann Rheum Dis (1969). DOI: 10.1136/ard.28.4.359

DiZerega GS, et al., Materials (2010). DOI: 10.3390/ma3053331

Djenoune L, et al., J Neurogenet (2017). PMID: 28789587 DOI: 10.1080/01677063.2017.1359833

Dommisse GF, Orthop Clin North Am (1975). PMID: 1113965

Dorland's Illustrated Medical Dictionary, 25th edn (WB Saunders, Philadelphia, 1974).

Dorland's Illustrated Medical Dictionary, 28th edn (WB Saunders, Philadelphia, 1994).

Dörr W, Archiv fur Orthopädische und Unfallchirurgie (1958). PMID: 13606803 DOI: 10.1007/BF00416096

Dorwart RH, Radiol Clin North Am (1983). PMID: 6867310

Dreyer SJ, et al., Arch Phys Med Rehabil (1996). PMID: 8600875 DOI: 10.1016/s0003-9993(96)90115-x

Dreyfuss P, et al., Spine (1994). PMID: 8059269 DOI: 10.1097/00007632-199405001-00007

Duarte MP, et al., StatPearls [Internet]. Treasure Island (FL): StatPearls Publishing (2021). www.ncbi.nlm.nih.gov/books/NBK545191/

Dubin AE, et al., 2010 J Clin Invest (2010). DOI: 10.1172/JCI42843

Dupont G, et al., Clin Anat (2019). PMID: 30362622 DOI: 10.1002/ca.23308

Dupuis PR, In: Managing Low Back Pain, 4th edn, Chapter 2 (Churchill Livingstone, New York, 1999).

Dyck P, Spine (1985). PMID: 2931832

Dydyk AM, et al., StatPearls [Internet]. Treasure Island (FL): StatPearls Publishing (2020). www.ncbi.nlm.nih.gov/books/NBK546593/

Dydyk AM, et al., StatPearls [Internet]. Treasure Island (FL): StatPearls Publishing (2022). www.ncbi.nlm.nih.gov/books/NBK441822/

The Economist (2020(a)). www.economist.com/leaders/2020/01/16/vast-sums-are-wasted-on-treatments-for-back-pain-that-make-it-worse

The Economist (2020(b)). www.economist.com/briefing/2020/01/18/back-pain-is-a-massive-problem-which-is-badly-treated

Editorial, Br J Pain (2020). DOI: 10.1177/2049463720905209

Egund, N., et al., Acta Rad Diagn (1978). PMID: 717034 DOI: 10.1177/028418517801900513

Eichler J, In: Leg Length Discrepancy the Injured Knee (Springer-Verlag, Berlin, 1977, pp. 29–39).

Eidelson SG, Lumbar Spine (2021). www.spineuniverse.com/anatomy/lumbar-spine.

Ellis H, Reg Anaesth (2006). DOI: 10.1053/j.mpaic.2006.08.006

Elsig JPJ, et al., Minim Invasive Ther (2006). PMID: 17062399 DOI: 10.1080/13645700600958457

Encyclopaedia Britannica, Cerebrospinal Fluid (Encyclopaedia Britannica, Inc, 2018). www.britannica.com/science/cerevrospinal-fluid.

Epstein BS, AJR (1966). www.ajronline.org/doi/pdf/10.2214/ajr.98.3.704

Epstein BS, The Spine: A Radiological Text and Atlas, 4th edn (Lea and Febiger, Philadelphia, 1976).

Eriksson S, et al., Spine (2022). PMID: 34265808 DOI: 10.1097/BRS.0000000000004160

Eubanks JD, et al., Clin Orthop Relat Res (2007(a)). PMID: 17767079 DOI: 10.1097/BLO.0b013e3181583d4e

Eubanks JD, et al., Spine (2007(b)). PMID: 17762805 DOI: 10.1097/BRS.0b013e318145a3a9

Fardon DF, et al., Spine (2001). PMID: 11242399 DOI: 10.1097/00007632-200103010-00006

Farfan HF, Mechanical Disorders of the Low Back (Lea and Febiger, Philadelphia, 1973).

Farfan HF, Spine (1978). PMID: 741240 DOI: 10.1097/00007632-197812000-00006

Farfan HF, Clin Rheum Dis (1980). DOI: 10.1016/S0307-742X(21)00285-X

Farrell M (2019). National Drug and Alcohol Research Centre, University of New South Wales. Powerful Opioid Fentanyl Poses Serious Risk of Fatal Overdose. https://ndarc.med.unsw.edu.au/blog/powerful-opioid-fentanyl-poses-serious-risk-fatal-overdose.

Fatemi P, et al., Spine (2020). PMID: 32833930 DOI: 10.1097/BRS.0000000000003663

Fields AJ, et al., Radiology (2015). PMCID: PMC4314292 DOI: 10.1148/radiol.14141082

Fields AJ, et al., Curr Mol Biol Rep (2018). DOI: 10.1007/s40610-018-0105-y

Filippidis AS, et al., Neurosurg Focus (2010). PMID: 20594007 DOI: 10.3171/2010.3.FOCUS1085

Finch P, Nat Clin Pract Rheumatol (2006). DOI: 10.1038/ncprheum0293

Findlay DM, Rheumatology (2007). PMID: 17693442 DOI: 10.1093/rheumatology/kem191

Fischgrund JS, et al., Int J Spine Surg (2019). DOI: 10.14444/6015

FMP Global, The Back-breaking Cost of Back Pain in the US (2018). https://fmpglobal.com/blog/the-back-breaking-cost-of-back-pain-in-the-us/.

Fordyce WE, Behavioral Methods for Chronic Pain and Illness (CV Mosby, Saint Louis, 1976).

Forst SL, et al., Pain Physician (2006). PMID: 16700283

Foster NE, et al., Lancet (2018). PMID: 29573872 DOI: 10.1016/S0140-6736(18)30489-6

Fraser RD, et al., In: The Adult Spine: Principles and Practice, 2nd edn, Chapter 37 (Lippincott-Raven, Philadelphia, 1997).

French BN, In: Neurological Surgery (WB Saunders, Philadelphia, 1990, pp. 1183–1185).

French HD, et al., Global Spine J (2014). PMCID: PMC4229381 DOI: 10.1055/s-0034-1387808

Frymoyer JW, Forward. In: Clinical Anatomy and Management of Low Back Pain (Preface) (Butterworth-Heinemann, Edinburgh, 1997).

Frymoyer JW, et al., New Perspectives on Low Back Pain (American Academy of Orthopaedic Surgeons, Park Ridge, IL, 1989).

Fujiwara A, et al., Eur Spine J (1999). PMCID: PMC3611192 DOI: 10.1007/s005860050193

Fulton WS, et al., Arch Surg (1934). DOI: 10.1001/archsurg.1934.01180010045005

Funke M, et al., Fortschritte auf dem Gebiete der Rontgenstrahlen und der Nuklearmedizin (1992). PMID: 1638004 DOI: 10.1055/s-2008-1032963

Gaillard F, et al., Radiopaedia.org (2021) (accessed on 23 Jan 2022) DOI: 10.53347/rID-13624.

Ganapathy MK, et al., StatPearls [Internet]. Treasure Island (FL): StatPearls Publishing (2020). PMCID: PMC2913007 DOI: 10.1111/j.1469-7580.2010.01227.x

Gandhi JS, BMJ (2000). DOI: 10.1136/bmj.321.7268.1087/a

Gao T, et al., BMC Musculoskelet Disord (2017). DOI: 10.1186/s12891-017-1849-x

Garcia-Cosamalón J, et al., J Anat (2010). PMCID: PMC2913007 DOI: 10.1111/j.1469-7580.2010.01227.x

Garfin SR, et al., Spine (1995). PMID: 7502139 DOI: 10.1097/00007632-199508150-00012

Garg K, et al., World Neurosurg (2021). PMID: 33309642 DOI: 10.1016/j.wneu.2020.11.171

Garland EL Prim Care (2012). PMID: 22958566 DOI: 10.1016/j.pop.2012.06.013

Gasser HC, et al., Am J Physiol (1927). DOI: 10.1152/ajplegacy.1927.80.3.522

Gautam D (2021). https://emedicine.medscape.com/article/1263961-overview (assessed article Nov 2021).

Gellhorn AC, et al., Nat Rev Rheumatol (2013). PMCID: PMC4012322 DOI: 10.1038/nrrheum.2012.199

Gharries H, J Anes Criti Care (2018). DOI: 10.15406/jaccoa.2018.10.00378

Ghormley RK, JAMA (1933). DOI: 10.1001/jama.1933.02740480005002

Ghuman MS, et al., Neurol India (2014). DOI: 10.4103/0028-3886.144513

Gilbert JW, et al., J Manipulative Physiol Ther (2011). PMID: 21907413 DOI: 10.1016/j.jmpt.2011.08.002

Giles LGF, Rheumatol Rehabil (1981). PMID: 6458081 DOI: 10.1093/rheumatology/20.4.233

Giles LGF, Spine (1984(a)). https://journals.lww.com/spinejournal/Citation/1984/11000/To_the_Editor.20.aspx

Giles LGF, JMPT (1984(b)). PMID: 6716015

Giles LGF, Lumbo-sacral and cervical zygapophysial joint inclusions. Man Med, 2: 89–92 (1986(a)).

Giles LGF, Pressure related changes in human lumbo-sacral zygapophyseal joint articular cartilage. J Rheumatol, 13: 1093–1095 (1986(b)).

Giles LGF, Lancet (letter) (1987(a)). DOI: 10.1016/S0140-6736(87)92485-8

Giles LGF, Clin Biomech (1987(b)). DOI: 10.1016/0268-0033(87)90038-6

Giles LGF, Anat Rec (1988). PMID: 2451453 DOI: 10.1002/ar.1092200202

Giles LGF, Anatomical Basis of Low Back Pain (Williams & Wilkins, Baltimore, 1989).

Giles LGF, J Manipulative Physiol Ther (1991(a)). PMID: 1828493

Giles LGF, A review and description of some possible causes of low back pain of mechanical origin in homo sapiens. Proc Aust Soc Hum Biol, 4: 193–212 (1991(b)).

Giles LGF, Anat Rec (1992(a)) 233: 350–356. PMID: 1609968 DOI: 10.1002/ar.1092330303

Giles LGF, Ligaments traversing the intervertebral canals of the human lower lumbosacral spine. Neuro-Orthopedics, 13: 25–38 (1992(b)).

Giles LGF, In: Clinical Anatomy and Management of Low Back Pain, Chapter 3 (Butterworth-Heinemann, Oxford, 1997(a)).

Giles LGF, In: Clinical Anatomy and Management of Low Back Pain, Chapter 14 (Butterworth-Heinemann, Edinburgh, 1997(b)).

Giles LGF, In: Clinical Anatomy and Management of Low Back Pain, Chapter 13 (Butterworth-Heinemann, Oxford, 1997(c)).

Giles LGF, In: Clinical Anatomy and Management of Low Back Pain, Chapter 5 (Butterworth-Heinemann, Edinburgh, 1997(d)).

Giles LGF, BMJ (2003(a)). DOI: 10.1136/bmj.327.7416.681-a

Giles LGF, 50 Challenging Spinal Pain Syndrome Cases (Butterworth-Heinemann, Oxford, 2003(b)).

Giles LGF, Spine (2005). DOI: 10.1097/01.brs.0000150479.25854.6e

Giles LGF, 100 Challenging Spinal Pain Syndrome Cases (Churchill Livingstone Elsevier, Edinburgh, 2009).

Giles LGF, Med J Aust (2014). DOI: 10.5694/mja13.11172

Giles LGF, Back Off! Memoir of the Vicissitudes of a Complementary Health Practitioner (Blurb Publishing, Blurb.com, Australia, 2017).

Giles LGF, et al., Spine (1981). PMID: 6458101 DOI: 10.1097/00007632-198109000-00014

Giles LGF, et al., Bull Hosp Joint Dis Orthop Inst (1982). PMID: 6309300

Giles LGF, et al., Stain Technol (1983). PMID: 6192553 DOI: 10.3109/10520298309066748

Giles LGF, et al., Scand J Rheumatol (1984). PMID: 6484537 DOI: 10.3109/03009748409100389

Giles LGF, et al., J Manipulative Physiol Ther (1985). PMID: 4078503

Giles LGF, et al., Br J Rheumatol (1987(a)). PMID: 2444304 DOI: 10.1093/rheumatology/26.5.362

Giles LGF, et al., Br J Rheumatol (1987(b)). PMID: 2435355 DOI: 10.1093/rheumatology/26.2.93

Giles LGF, et al., J Rheumatol (1990). PMID: 2273488

Giles LGF, et al., Lumbosacral intervertebral disc degeneration revisited: a radiological ad histological correlation. Manual Med, 6: 62–66 (1991).

Giles LGF, et al., Can J Psychiatry (1997(a)). PMID: 9040922 DOI: 10.1177/070674379704200106

Giles LGF, et al., In: Clinical Anatomy and Management of Low Back Pain, Chapter 11 (Butterworth-Heinemann, Oxford, 1997(b)).

Giles LGF, et al., J Manipulative Physiol Ther (2003). DOI: 10.1016/S0161-4754(03)00045-9

Giles LGF, et al., J Bone Joint Surg (Br) (2006). https://online.boneandjoint.org.uk/doi/abs/10.1302/0301-620X.88BSUPP_III.0880450

Gliedt JA, et al., Spine (2021). DOI: 10.1097/BRS.0000000000004047

Glynn LE, Lancet (1977). DOI: 10.1016/S0140-6736(77)92003-7

Gofton JP, Can Med Assoc J (1971). PMID: 5576039 PMCID: PMC1930940

Gofton JP, et al., Can Med Assoc J (1967). PMID: 6057132 PMCID: PMC1923539

Gofton JP, et al., Can Med Assoc J (1971). PMID: 5089638 PMCID: PMC1931011

Gofur EM, et al., StatPearls [Internet]. Treasure Island (FL): StatPearls Publishing (2020). www.ncbi.nlm.nih.gov/books/NBK541083/

Goldthwait JE, et al., Boston Med Surg J (1905). www.nejm.org/doi/full/10.1056/NEJM190506011522204

Goodman BP, Continuum (Minneap Minn) (2018). PMID: 29613901 DOI: 10.1212/CON.0000000000000584

Goodman CW, et al., N Engl J Med (2017). DOI: 10.1056/NEJMp1704633

Gordon R, et al., Healthcare (2016). DOI: 10.3390/healthcare4020022

Goupille P, et al., Semin Arthritis Rheum (1998). PMID: 9726337 DOI: 10.1016/s0049-0172(98)80029-2

Goupille P, et al., Ann Rheum Dis (2006). DOI: 10.1136/ard.2005.039669

Govind J, Aust Fam Physician (2004). https://search.informit.org/doi/abs/10.3316/informit.373038752393319

Grant JCB, Grant's Atlas of Anatomy, 5th edn (The Williams and Wilkins Co., Baltimore, 1962).

Grant MP, et al., Eur Cell Mater (2016). PMID: 27452962, DOI: 10.22203/ecm.v032a09

Gray H, Anatomy of the Human Body (Lea and Febiger, Philadelphia, 1858).

Greenman PE, 1st Interdisciplinary World Congress on Low Back Pain and its Relation to the Sacroiliac Joint (San Diego, 1992).

Gregory NS, et al., Curr Top Behav Neurosci (2014). PMCID: PMC4294469 DOI: 10.1007/7854_2014_294

Groen GJ, et al., Acta Neurochir (Wien) (1988). PMID: 3407473 DOI: 10.1007/BF01401971

Groen GJ, et al., Am J Anatomy (1990). PMID: 2371968 DOI: 10.1002/aja.1001880307

Groen GJ, et al., In: Clinical Anatomy and Management of Thoracic Spine Pain, Chapter 8 (Butterworth-Heinemann, Edinburgh, 2000).

Grönblad M, et al., Spine (1991(a)). PMID: 1825893 DOI: 10.1097/00007632-199101000-00006

Grönblad M, et al., Acta Orthop Scand (1991(b)). PMID: 1837417 DOI: 10.3109/17453679108994512

Grönblad M, et al., In: Clinical Anatomy and Management of Low Back Pain, Chapter 15 (Butterworth-Heinemann, Oxford, 1997).

Gross D, In: Advances in Pain Research and Therapy, Vol 3 (Raven Press, New York, 1979, pp. 671–683).

Grunhagen T, et al., Orthop Clin North Am (2011). PMID: 21944584 DOI: 10.1016/j.ocl.2011.07.010

Guichet JM, et al., Clin Orthop Relat Res (1991). PMID: 1934739

Gumina S, et al., In: Lumbar Disc Herniation, Chapter 3 (Springer-Verlag, New York, 1999).

Guyton S, et al., Textbook of Medical Physiology, 10th edn (WB Saunders, Philadelphia, 2000).

Haberberger RV, et al., Front Cell Neurosci (2019). PMCID: PMC6598622 DOI: 10.3389/fncel.2019.00271

Habsi SA, et al., Orthop Res (2020). DOI: 10.1159/000506179

Hadley LA, Apophyseal subluxation. Disturbances in and about the intervertebral foramen causing back pain. JBJS, 18(2): 428–433 (1936).

Hadley LA, J Neurosurg (1950). PMID: 15422401 DOI: 10.3171/jns.1950.7.4.0347

Hadley LA, Am J Roentgenol Radium Ther (1951). PMID: 14819421

Hadley LA, Anatomico-roentgenographic Studies of the Spine (Charles C Thomas, Springfield, 1964).

Hadley R, et al., In: Tethered Cord Syndrome (The American Association of Neurological Surgeons, Chicago, 1996, pp. 79–88).

Haijiao W, et al., J Spinal Disord (2001). PMID: 11285427 DOI: 10.1097/00002517-200104000-00009

Hakim NS, et al., Proceedings, 20th STAPP Car Crash Conference (1976). DOI: 10.4271/760819.

Haldeman S, In: Approaches to the Validation of Manipulation Therapy, Chapter 10 (Charles C Thomas, Springfield, IL, 1977).

Haldeman S, In: Modern Developments in the Principles and Practice of Chiropractic, Chapter 7 (Appleton-Century-Crofts, New York, 1980).

Haldeman S, Clin Sport Med (1986). DOI: 10.1016/S0278-5919(20)31132-7

Haldeman S, In: Managing Low Back Pain, 4th edn, Chapter 12 (Churchill Livingstone, New York, 1999).

Haldeman S, et al., An Atlas of Back Pain (Parthenon Publishing Group, London, 2002).

Hall JE, et al., Guyton and Hall Textbook of Medical Physiology, 14th edn (Elsevier, Philadelphia, PA, 2020).

Halliday M, Limb length asymmetry and scoliosis. Bachelor of Science Honours Thesis. Department of Anatomy and Human Biology, University of Western Australia, Perth (1976).

Hamanishi C, et al., Spine (1994). PMID: 8178234 DOI: 10.1097/00007632-199402001-00012

Hanson P, et al., Arch Phys Med Rehabil (1994). PMID: 7979937 DOI: 10.1016/0003-9993(94)90013-2

Hansson T, et al., Spine (1981). PMID: 7280815 DOI: 10.1097/00007632-198103000-00007

Haouimi A, et al., Radiopaedia.org (2021). https://radiopaedia.org/articles/eos-imaging-systems

Harcke HT, et al., Semin Nucl Med (1993). DOI: 10.1016/S0001-2998(05)80108-4

Harshavardhana NS, et al., Orthop Rev (Pavia) (2014). PMCID: PMC4195988 DOI: 10.4081/or.2014.5428

Hartvigsen J, et al., Lancet (2018). DOI: 10.1016/S0140-6736(18)30480-X

Harvard Health Publishing (2018). www.health.harvard.edu/pain/babying-your-back-may-delay-healing?utm_content=buffer2d613&utm_medium=social&utm_source=facebook&utm_campaign=buffer&fbclid=IwAR0-XkduXOQerVMC393BJJCInRjNjlanuAAC5zzVL7E2jJj6ESNtE0G8VSk

Harvey WF, et al., Ann Intern Med (2010). DOI: 10.1059/0003-4819-152-5-201003020-00006

Hasan S, et al., StatPearls [Internet]. Treasure Island (FL): StatPearls Publishing (2021). www.ncbi.nlm.nih.gov/books/NBK539889/

Hasegawa K, et al., BMC Musculoskelet Disord (2018). PMCID: PMC6284293 DOI: 10.1186/s12891-018-2355-5

Hassin GB, Arch Neurol Psychiat (Chicago) (1930). DOI: 10.1001/archneurpsyc.1930.02220070068003

He S-C, et al., Pain Physician (2017). PMID: 28158154

Hellmann DB, In: Current Medical Diagnosis and Treatment (Appleton & Lange, Norwalk, CT, 1992, pp. 659–671).

Henderson D, et al., J Can Chiropr Assoc (suppl) (1994).

Henry JL, Brain Res (1976). PMID: 953765 DOI: 10.1016/0006-8993(76)90965-3

Henry JL, In: Substance P in the Nervous System (Ciba Foundation Symposium, London and Pitman, CO, 1982, pp. 206–224).

Henson B, et al., StatPearls [Internet]. Treasure Island (FL): StatPearls Publishing (2021). www.ncbi.nlm.nih.gov/books/NBK537074/

Herman AO (2018). www.jwatch.org/fw114424/2018/08/01/more-patients-getting-risky-steroid-injections-back-pain

Hermann K-GA, et al., Fortschr Röntgenstr (2014). DOI: 10.1055/s-0033-1350411

Herregods N, et al., J Belg Soc Radiol (2016). DOI: 10.5334/jbr-btr.1198

Hilton RC, et al., Ann Rheum Dis (1976). PMCID: PMC1006522 DOI: 10.1136/ard.35.2.127

Hippocrates, Epidemics, Bk 1, Sect. XI, 400 BCE.

Hipps HE, J Bone Joint Surg (1939). https://journals.lww.com/jbjsjournal/abstract/1939/21020/fissure_formation_in_articular_facets_of_the.2.aspx

Ho WM, et al., In: Primer on Cerebrovascular Diseases, 2nd edn, Chapter 6 (Academic Press, London, UK, 2017).

Hodges SD, et al., J South Orthop Assoc (1999). PMID: 12132869

Hoffman KS, et al., J Am Osteopath Assoc (1994). PMID: 8200825

Hofmann AA, et al., Am J Orthop (2008). PMID: 18309380

Hofmann M, Die Befestigung der Dura mater im Wirbelkanal. Arch Anat Physio (Anat Abt), 403 (1899).

Holm S, et al., Conn Tissue Res (1981). DOI: 10.3109/03008208109152130

Hooten WM, et al., Mayo Clin Proc (2015). PMID: 26653300 DOI: 10.1016/j.mayocp.2015.10.009

Hoppenfeld S, Orthopaedic Neurology: A Diagnostic Guide to Neurologic Levels (JB Lippincott, Philadelphia, 1977).

Hoyland JA, et al., Spine (1989). PMID: 2749370 DOI: 10.1097/00007632-198906000-00002

Hsu KY, et al., Spine (1995). PMID: 7709284 DOI: 10.1097/00007632-199501000-00015

Hughes JL, et al., In: Leg Length Discrepancy the Injured Knee (Springer-Verlag, Berlin, 1977, pp. 3–8).

Hunt SP, et al., Philos Trans R Soc Lond B Biol Sci (1985). PMID: 2580323 DOI: 10.1098/rstb.1985.0028

Huskisson EC, et al., Joint Disease: All the Arthropathies, 3rd ed. (John Wright and Sons, Bristol, 1978).

Ido K, et al., Spinal Cord (2001). PMID: 11438843 DOI: 10.1038/sj.sc.3101157

Idriss HT, et al., Microsc Res Tech (2000). PMID: 10891884 DOI: 10.1002/1097-0029(20000801)50:3<184::AID-JEMT2>3.0.CO;2-H

Iggo A, In: Recent Advances in Pain. Pathophysiology and Clinical Aspects (CC Thomas, Springfield, 1974, pp. 3–35).

Iggo A, et al., In: Nociception and Pain (Cambridge University Press, Cambridge, 1985, pp. 17–34).

Illés T, et al., Int Orthop (SICOT) (2012). PMID: 22371113 DOI: 10.1007/s00264-012-1512-y

Imhof H, et al., Skeletal Radiol (1997). PMID: 9259096 DOI: 10.1007/s002560050254

Imhof H, et al., Top Magn Reson Imaging (1999). PMID: 10565710 DOI: 10.1097/00002142-199906000-00002

Inman VT, et al., J Bone Joint Surg (1947). PMID: 20240207

Inoue N, et al., Spine Surg Relat (2020). PMID: 32039290 DOI: 10.22603/ssrr.2019-0017

Institute for Chronic Pain (2019). www.instituteforchronicpain.org/understandng-chronic-pain/complications/opioid-dependence-and-addition

Institute for Health Metrics and Evaluation (IHME). Findings from the Global Burden of Disease Study (IHME, Seattle, WA, 2017). www.healthdata.org/policy-report/findings-global-burden-disease-study-2017

Ito K, et al., In: Lumbar Disc Herniation, Chapter 8 (Lippincott Williams and Wilkins, Philadelphia, 2002).

Iwanaga J, et al., Asian J Neurosurg (2019). PMCID: PMC6896651 DOI: 10.4103/ajns.AJNS_87_19

Izci Y, et al., Turk Neurosurg (2005). DOI: 10.7860/IJARS/2021/47110:2613

Jackson DW, Am J Sports Med (1979). PMID: 159628 DOI: 10.1177/036354657900700614

Jackson R, Cervical Syndrome (Charles C Thomas, Springfield, IL, 1956).

Jadon A, Gen Med (Los Angeles) (2016). DOI: 10.4172/2327-5146.1000252

Jain A, et al., Korean J Pain (2013). PMID: 24156003 DOI: 10.3344/kjp.2013.26.4.368

James B, et al., In: Clinical Anatomy and Management of Low Back Pain, Chapter 19 (Butterworth-Heinemann, Edinburgh, 1997).

Jancuska JM, et al., Int J Spine Surg (2015). PMCID: PMC4603258 DOI: 10.14444/2042

Jansen NW, et al., Arthritis Rheum (2007). PMID: 17195222 DOI: 10.1002/art.22304

Jarvik JG, et al., Ann Intern Med (2002). PMID: 12353946 DOI: 10.7326/0003-4819-137-7-200210010-00010

Jarvik JJ, et al., Spine (2001). PMID: 11413431 DOI: 10.1097/00007632-200105150-00014

Jaumard NV, et al., J Biomech Eng (2011). PMID: 21823749 DOI: 10.1115/1.4004493

Jayson MI, Clin Orthop Relat Res (1992). PMID: 1534723

Jayson MIV, Spine (1997). PMID: 9160461 DOI: 10.1097/00007632-199705150-00001

Jensen MC, et al., NEJM (1994). DOI: 10.1056/NEJM199407143310201

Jessell TM, Lancet (1982). DOI: 10.1016/S0140-6736(82)90014-9

Jessell TM, et al., Nature (Lond) (1977). PMID: 18681 DOI: 10.1038/268549a0

Jinkins JR, Neuroimaging Clin N Am (1993). DOI: 10.1177/19714009950080S106

Jinkins JR, In: Clinical Anatomy and Management of Low Back Pain, Chapter 17 (Butterworth-Heinemann, Oxford, 1997).

Jinkins JR, Eur J Radiol (2004(a)). PMID: 15081129 DOI: 10.1016/j.ejrad.2003.10.014

Jinkins JR, J Neuroradiol (2004(b)). PMID: 15356442 DOI: 10.1016/s0150-9861(04)96988-x

Jinkins JR, et al., Am J Roentgenol (1989). www.ajronline.org/doi/abs/10.2214/ajr.152.6.1277

Jinkins JR, et al., JBR-BTR (2003(a)). PMID: 14651085

Jinkins JR, et al., J HK Coll Radiol (2003(b)). http://fonar.com/pdf/jhk.pdf

Joe E, et al., AJR (2015). www.ajronline.org/doi/full/10.2214/AJR.14.13319

Johnson EF, et al., J Anat (1982). PMID: 7174505 PMCID: PMC1168235

Jones J, et al. Radiopaedia.org (2021(a)). (accessed on 30 Oct 2021) DOI: 10.53347/rID-10569.

Jones L, et al., In: Lumbar Spine Textbook. Section 1, Chapter 2 (2021(b)). www.wheelessonline.com/ISSLS/lumbar-vertebrae-ligaments/

Julin M, et al., Spine (2021). PMID: 33692323 DOI: 10.1097/BRS.0000000000003797

Kakushima M, et al., Spine (2003). PMID: 14595166 DOI: 10.1097/01.BRS.0000090829.82231.4A

Kampen WU, et al., Anat embryol (1998). PMID: 9833689 DOI: 10.1007/s004290050200

Kanchan T, et al., Singapore Med J (2009). PMID: 19296021

Karabulut O, et al., Int J Morphol (2016). DOI: 10.4067/S0717-95022016000400029

Karacan I, et al., Spine (2004). PMID: 15131443 DOI: 10.1097/00007632-200405150-00016

Karppinen J, et al., Spine (2001). PMID: 11295915 DOI: 10.1097/00007632-200104010-00015

Kasch R, et al., Spine (2021). PMID: 34405825 DOI: 10.1097/BRS.0000000000004198

Kauppila LI, Eur J Vasc Endovasc Surg (2009). PMID: 19328027 DOI: 10.1016/j.ejvs.2009.02.006

Kauppila LI, et al., Spine (1997). PMID: 9253101 DOI: 10.1097/00007632-199707150-00023

Kayalioglu G, In: The Spinal Cord, Chapter 4 (Elsevier Ltd, London, UK, 2008).

Keats TE, et al., Atlas of Normal Roentgen Variants That May Simulate Disease, 8th edn (Mosby, St. Louis, MO, 2007).

Keefe FJ, et al., Assessment of pain behaviours. In: Encyclopedia of Pain (Springer-Verlag, Berlin, 2007). DOI: 10.1007/978-3-642-28753-4_302

Keele CA, Proc Royal Soc Med (1967). PMID: 6021673

Keim HA, et al., Clinical Symposia. Low Back Pain, vol. 39 (Ciba-Geigy, Jersey, 1987).

Kellgren JH, On the distribution of pain arising from deep somatic structures with charts of segmental pain areas. Clin Sci, 4: 35–46 (1939).

Kellgren JH, et al., Ann Rheum Dis (1957). PMCID: PMC1006995 DOI: 10.1136/ard.16.4.494

Kenna C, et al., Back Pain and Spinal Manipulation (Butterworth-Heinemann, Oxford, 1989).

Kido DK, et al., Neuroradiology (1976). PMID: 980235 DOI: 10.1007/BF00328377

Kikuchi S, et al., Spine (1986). PMID: 3033836 DOI: 10.1097/00007632-198612000-00006

Kim K-H, et al., In: Minimally Invasive Percutaneous Spinal Techniques, Chapter 2 (Saunders Elsevier, Philadelphia, 2011).

Kim HS, et al., Int J Mol Sci (2020). PMCID: PMC7073116 DOI: 10.3390/ijms21041483

Kim S, et al., Rev Bras Anestesiol (2018). PMID: 28987417 DOI: 10.1016/j.bjan.2017.07.007

Kimmell KT, et al., Surg Neurol Int (2011). PMCID: PMC3144594 DOI: 10.4103/2152-7806.82990

Kirkaldy-Willis, WH, In: Managing Low Back Pain (Churchill Livingstone, New York, 1988, pp. 133–154).

Kirkaldy-Willis WH, Managing Low Back Pain (Churchill Livingstone, New York, 1999).

Kirkaldy-Willis WH, et al., In: Managing Low Back Pain, 4th edn, Chapter 13 (Churchill Livingstone, New York, 1999).

Kirkpatrick DR, et al., Clin Trans Sci (2015). PMCID: PMC4641846 DOI: 10.1111/cts.12282

Kleinstück F, et al., Spine (2006). PMID: 16946663 DOI: 10.1097/01.brs.0000232802.95773.89

Knezevic NN, et al., Lancet (2021). DOI: 10.1016/S0140-6736(21)00733-9

Knipe H, et al., Radiopaedia.org (2021). DOI: 10.53347/rID-24695

Kobayashi S, et al., Spine (2005). PMID: 15682006 DOI: 10.1097/01.brs.0000152377.72468.f4

Konin GP, et al., AJNR (2010). PMCID: PMC7964015 DOI: 10.3174/ajnr.A2036

Konttinen YT, et al., Spine (1990). PMID: 1694599 DOI: 10.1097/00007632-199005000-00008

Koop L, et al., StatPearls [Internet]. Treasure Island (FL): StatPearls Publishing (2021). www.ncbi.nlm.nih.gov/books/NBK539846/

Korkala O, et al., Spine (1985). PMID: 2408343 DOI: 10.1097/00007632-198503000-00009

Kraan GA, et al., Eur Spine J (2009). PMCID: PMC2899458 DOI: 10.1007/s00586-009-0881-4

Krames ES, Pain Med (2014). PMID: 24641192 DOI: 10.1111/pme.12413

Krettek C, et al., Unfallchirurg (1994). PMID: 8153650

Kumar A, et al., QJM (2019). DOI: 10.1093/qjmed/hcy241

Kumar DS, et al., Skeletal Radiol (2012). PMID: 22639203 DOI: 10.1007/s00256-012-1428-z

Kuntz A, The Autonomic Nervous System, 4th edn (Lea and Febiger, Philadelphia, 1953).

Kushchayev SV, et al., Insights Imaging (2018). PMID: 29569215 DOI: 10.1007/s13244-017-0584-z

Ladermann JP, About inequalities of the lower extremities. Ann Swiss Chiropr Assoc, 6: 37–57 (1976).

Lam KHS, et al., J Pain Res (2020). PMID: 32801851 DOI: 10.2147/JPR.S247208

Lama P, et al., J Anat (2018). PMCID: PMC5987834 DOI: 10.1111/joa.12817

Lang J, Vertebral Nerve in Clinical Anatomy of the Cervical Spine (Thieme, New York, 1993).

Lavignolle B, et al., Anat Clin (1983). PMID: 6671062 DOI: 10.1007/BF01799002

Le-Breton C, et al., Sarcomes pagetiques rechidiens. A propos de huit observations. Revue du Rhumatisme (ed Francaise), 60: 16–22 (1993).

Lee CK, et al., Spine (1988). PMID: 3388117 DOI: 10.1097/00007632-198803000-00015

Leung M, Wilson Institute, Canada Institute (2019). www.wilsoncenter.org/article/the-opioid-crisis-the-united-states-and-canadas-fentanyl-epidemic

Lew SM, et al., Pediatr Neurosurg (2007). PMID: 17409793 DOI: 10.1159/000098836

Li G, et al., Arthritis Res Ther (2013). DOI: 10.1186/ar4405

Li J, et al., J Orthop Res (2011). PMCID: PMC3115475 DOI: 10.1002/jor.21387

Li Z, et al., Eur J Radiol Open (2019). DOI: 10.1016/j.ejro.2019.06.001

Liang T, et al., Spine (2017). PMID: 28146016 DOI: 10.1097/BRS.0000000002085

Liesi P, et al., Lancet 1 (1983). DOI: 10.1016/S0140-6736(83)92435-2

Lin W, et al., Orthop Surg (2020). PMCID: PMC7454223 DOI: 10.1111/os.12747

Lipton S, In: Recent Advances in Anaesthesia and Analgesia, 12th edn, Chapter 16 (Little Brown, Boston, 1978).

Little JS, et al., J Biomech Eng (2005). PMID: 15868784 DOI: 10.1115/1.1835348

Liu Y-JJ, et al., AJR (2009). PMID: 19304703 DOI: 10.2214/AJR.08.1597

Lloyd DPC, J Neurophysiol (1943). DOI: 10.1152/jn.1943.6.4.293

Loeser JD, Spine (1985). PMID: 2986297 DOI: 10.1097/00007632-198504000-00007

Lotz JC, et al., Global Spine J (2013). PMCID: PMC3854605 DOI: 10.1055/s-0033-1347298

Louvet A, et al., Hepatology (2020). PMID: 33306215 DOI: 10.1002/hep.31678

Lowis CGT, et al., BMJ Open Sport Exerc Med (2018). DOI: 10.1136/bmjsem-2017-000338

Luoma K, et al., Spine (2000). PMID: 10707396 DOI: 10.1097/00007632-200002150-00016

Lurie JD, In: Lumbar Spine Textbook, Section 4, Chapter 2 (2021). www.wheelessonline.com/ISSLS/section-4-chapter-2-epidemiology-and-use-of-opioids-in-back-pain/

Luxford K, Patient Exp J (2016). DOI: 10.35680/2372-0247.1189

Maatman RC, et al., J Pain Res (2019). PMCID: PMC6388752 DOI: 10.2147/JPR.S178492

Machado G C, et al., BMJ (2015). PMCID: PMC4381278 DOI: 10.1136/bmj.h1225

Mackinnon SE, Hand Clin (2002). PMID: 1613031

MacMillan J, et al., Spine (1991). PMID: 2011770

Macnab I, Backache (Williams & Wilkins, Baltimore, 1977).

Madry H, et al., Knee Surg Sports Traumatol Arthrosc (2010). PMID: 20119671 DOI: 10.1007/s00167-010-1054-z

Madsen KB, et al., J Rheumatol (2010). DOI: 10.3899/jrheum.090519

Mahato NK, Spine (2011). PMID: 21924685 DOI: 10.1016/j.spinee.2011.08.007

Maigne J-Y (1996). www.sofmmoo.org/thoracolumbar_junction_aus tralie.htm

Maigne J-Y, In: Clinical Anatomy and Management of Thoracic Spine Pain, Chapter 10 (Butterworth-Heinemann, Oxford, 2000).

Maigne J-Y, et al., Surg Radiol Anat (1989). PMID: 2533408 DOI: 10.1007/BF02098698

Maigne J-Y, et al., Arch Phys Med Rehabil (1991). PMID: 1834038

Maigne J-Y, et al., Spine (1997). PMID: 9160476 DOI: 10.1097/00007632-199705150-00017

Maigne R, Orthopedic Medicine. A New Approach to Vertebral Manipulations (Charles C Thomas, Springfield, 1972).

Maigne R, Rev Rhum (1974). PMID: 4281928

Maigne R, Arch Phys Med Rehabil (1980). PMID: 6448030

Maigne R, Phys Med Reh Clin N Am (1997). DOI: 10.1016/S1047-9651(18)30345-0

Main CJ, et al., In: Clinical Psychology and Medicine: A Behavioural Perspective (Plenum Publishing, New York, 1982, pp. 1–62).

Main CJ, et al., Spine (1998). PMID: 9820920 DOI: 10.1097/00007632-199811010-00025

Manchikanti L, et al., Pain Physician (2002). PMID: 16896355

Manchikanti L, et al., Neuromodulation Suppl (2014). PMID: 25395111 DOI: 10.1111/ner.12018

Maniadakis N, et al., Pain (2000). PMID: 10601677 DOI: 10.1016/S0304-3959(99)00187-6

Manniche C, Clin Pract (2014). DOI: 10.2217/cpr.14.69

Marshall LL, et al., Lancet (letter) (1973). PMID: 4124797 DOI: 10.1016/s0140-6736(73)90818-0

Marshall LL, et al., Clin Orthop (1977). PMID: 608297

Martinez-Santos JL, et al., Surg Neurol Int (2021). DOI: 10.25259/SNI_894_2020

Matesan M, et al., J Orthop Surg and Res (2016). PMCID: PMC4936246 DOI: 10.1186/s13018-016-0402-1

Matsumae M, et al., Neurol Med Chir (Tokyo) (2016). PMCID: PMC4945600 DOI: 10.2176/nmc.ra.2016-0020

Mattassi R, Semin Vasc Surg (1993). PMID: 8305978

Matz P, et al., Diagnosis and Treatment of Degenerative Lumbar Spondylolisthesis, 2nd edn (NASS, 2014). www.researchgate.net/publication/301219891

May R, et al., Physiology (2019). DOI: 10.1016/j.mpaic.2019.10.017

McCarthy JJ, et al., J South Orthop Assoc (2001). PMID: 12132831

McCorry LK, Am J Pharm Educ (2007). PMCID: PMC1959222 DOI: 10.5688/aj710478

McCulloch JA, et al., JBJS(Br) (1980). DOI: 10.1302/0301-620X.62B4.7430228

McGeer PL, et al., Molecular Neurobiology of the Mammalian Brain (Plenum Press, New York, 1979).

McLarnon A, Bone Marrow. British Society for Immunology (2021). www.immunology.org/public-information/bitesized-immunology/organs-and-tissues/bone-marrow

Melhem E, et al., J Child Orthop (2016). PMID: 26883033 DOI: 10.1007/s11832-016-0713-0

Mellado JM, et al., AJR (2011(a)). PMID: 21700970 DOI: 10.2214/AJR.10.5803

Mellado JM, et al., AJR (2011(b)). PMID: 21700971 DOI: 10.2214/AJR.10.5811

Mendelson G, Med J Aust (1982). DOI: 10.5694/j.1326-5377.1982.tb124267.x

Menetrey J, et al., Knee Surg Sports Traumatol Arthrosc (2010). PMID: 20148327 DOI: 10.1007/s00167-010-1053-0

Mennell J McM, Back Pain. Diagnosis and Treatment Using Manipulative Techniques (Little, Brown and Co, Boston, 1960).

Mercadante AA, et al., StatPearls [Internet]. Treasure Island (FL): StatPearls Publishing (2021). www.ncbi.nlm.nih.gov/books/NBK547743/

Merchant AC, J Bone Joint Surg (1965). PMID: 14275166

Merriam-Webster Dictionary (2022) https://www.merriam-webster.com/dictionary/radiculopathy

Merz B, JAMA-J Am Med Assoc (1986). PMID: 3723718

Meschan I, An Atlas of Normal Radiographic Anatomy (WB Saunders Company, Philadelphia, 1959).

Meschan I, Synopsis of Roentgen Signs (WB Saunders Company, Philadelphia, 1962).

Michel BA, et al., J Rheumatol (1990). PMID: 2189996

Min J-H, et al., Neurosurgery 57 Oper Neurosurg Suppl (2005). PMID: 15987568 DOI: 10.1227/01.neu.0000163481.58673.1a

Mixter WJ, et al., 1934 N Engl J Med (1934). www.nejm.org/doi/full/10.1056/NEJM193408022110506

Mixter WJ, et al., N Engl J Med (1935). www.nejm.org/doi/full/10.1056/NEJM193508292130901

Modic MT, et al., Radiology (1988(a)). PMID: 3336678 DOI: 10.1148/radiology.166.1.3336678

Modic MT, et al., Radiology (1988(b)). PMID: 3289089 DOI: 10.1148/radiology.168.1.3289089

Moini J, et al., Functional and Clinical Neuroanatomy, Chapter 4 (Academic Press, Elsevier, London, UK, 2020).

Monash University Medicine, Nursing and Health Sciences (2018). www.monash.edu/medicine/news/latest/2018-articles/global-burden-of-low-back-pain-a-consequence-of-medical-negligence-and-misinformation

Monnier M, Functions of the Nervous System, Vol 3 (Elsevier Pub Co, Amsterdam, 1975).

Moon SM, et al., Eur Spine J (2013). PMID: 23674162 DOI: 10.1007/s00586-013-2798-1

Mooney V, In: First Interdisciplinary World Congress on Low Back Pain and its Relation to the Sacroiliac Joint (ECO, Rotterdam, 1992).

Mooney V, et al., Clin Orthop Relat Res (1976). PMID: 130216

Moore KL, Clinically Oriented Anatomy, 3rd edn (Williams & Wilkins, Baltimore, 1992).

Moore KL, In: Clinical Anatomy and Management of Low Back Pain, Chapter 9 (Butterworth-Heinemann, Oxford, 1997).

Moore KL, et al., Clinically Oriented Anatomy, 5th edn (Williams & Wilkins, Baltimore, 2006).

Moore KL, et al., Clinically Oriented Anatomy, 8th edn (Lippincott, Williams and Wilkins, Baltimore, 2018).

Moore RJ, Eur Spine J (2006). PMCID: PMC2335377 DOI: 10.1007/s00586-006-0170-4

Morimoto M, et al., Spine Surg Relat Res (2019). PMID: 31435551 DOI: 10.22603/ssrr.2017-0099

Morscher E, In: Leg Length Discrepancy. The Injured Knee (Progress in Orthopaedic Surgery, Vol 1). (Springer-Verlag, New York, 1977, pp. 9–19).

Murakami E, In: Sacroiliac Joint Disorder (Springer, Singapore, 2019). DOI: 10.1007/978-981-13-1807-8_2

Murray MR, et al., Euro Spine J, 21 (2012). PMCID: PMC3463701 DOI: 10.1007/s00586-012-2303-2

Nachemson AL, Acta Orth Scan (1969). PMID: 4312806 DOI: 10.3109/17453676908989482

Nachemson AL, Acta Orthop Scand (1991). PMID: 2014737

Nakashima H, et al., Global Spine J (2016). PMCID: PMC4993609 DOI: 10.1055/s-0035-1569004

Namba K, Neurol Med Chir (Tokyo) (2016). PMCID: PMC4908074 DOI: 10.2176/nmc.ra.2016-0006

Natarajan R N, et al., Spine (2004). PMID: 15564922 DOI: 10.1097/01.brs.0000146471.59052.e6

Nathan H, J Bone Joint Surg (1962). https://citeseerx.ist.psu.edu/viewdoc/download?doi=10.1.1.851.9465&rep=rep1&type=pdf

Nathan H, Surgery (1968). PMID: 5645381

Nathan H, Spine (1987). PMID: 3660077 DOI: 10.1097/00007632-198707000-00003

National Institute on Drug Abuse (2019). www.drugabuse.gov/drugs-abuse/opioids/opioid-overdose-crisis

Nencini S, et al., Front Physiol (2016). PMCID: PMC4844598 DOI: 10.3389/fphys.2016.00157

Newell RLM, In: Gray's Anatomy: The Anatomical Basis of Clinical Practice, 40th edn, anniversary edn, Section 5 (Churchill Livingstone/Elsevier, Edinburgh, 2008).

Nichols PJR, Rehabilitation Medicine. The Management of Physical Disabilities, 2nd edn (Butterworths, London, 1980).

Niharika R, et al., Health and Medicine Anaesthetists (2017). www.slideshare.net/KarthavyaSL/anatomy-of-epidural-space.

Nomizo A, et al., Anat Sci Int (2005). PMID: 16333917 DOI: 10.1111/j.1447-073X.2005.00115.x

Noren R, et al., Spine (1991). PMID: 2052995 DOI: 10.1097/00007632-199105000-00008

Nowogrodzki A, Nature (2018). https://media.nature.com/original/magazine-assets/d41586-018-07182-7/d41586-018-07182-7.pdf

O'Leary SA, et al., Acta Biomater (2017). PMID: 28300721 DOI: 10.1016/j.actbio.2017.03.017

Oliveira CB, et al., Eur Spine J (2018). PMID: 29971708 DOI: 10.1007/s00586-018-5673-2

Olmarker K, Acta Orthop Scand (1991). PMID: 1645923

Olmarker K, et al., J Orthop Res (1989). PMID: 2795321 DOI: 10.1002/jor.1100070607

Oppenheimer A, Radiology (1942). DOI: 10.1148/39.1.98

Oreskovic D, et al., CNS (2014). PMID: 25089184 DOI: 10.1186/2045-8118-11-16

Osti OL, et al., J Bone Joint Surg (1992). PMID: 1587896 DOI: 10.1302/0301-620X.74B3.1587896

Paajanen H, et al., Arch Orthop Trauma Surg (1997). PMID: 9006777 DOI: 10.1007/BF00434112

Page RL (II), et al., Circulation (2016). PMID: 27400984 DOI: 10.1161/CIR.0000000000000426

Paksoy Y, et al., Spine (2004). PMID: 15507805 DOI: 10.1097/01.brs.0000144354.36449.2f

Pallure L (2017). http://un-medecin-vous-informe.blogspot.com/2017_01_20_archive.html

Palmgren T, et al., Spine (1999). PMID: 10543001 DOI: 10.1097/00007632-199910150-00002

Palmisciano P, et al., J Clin Neurosci (2022). PMID: 35152147 DOI: 10.1016/j.jocn.2022.01.039

Pang H, et al., Spine (2018). PMCID: PMC5794660 DOI: 10.1097/BRS.0000000000002369

Panteliadis P, et al., Global Spine J (2016). PMCID: PMC4993622 DOI: 10.1055/s-0036-1586743

Parisien M, et al., Sci Transl Med (2022). DOI: 10.1126/scitranslmed.abj9954

Parke WW, et al., Spine (1985). PMID: 4081865 DOI: 10.1097/00007632-198507000-00004

Parke WW, et al., Spine (1990). PMID: 2141188 DOI: 10.1097/00007632-199004000-00010

Parkkola R, et al., Spine (1993). PMID: 8316880 DOI: 10.1097/00007632-199306000-00004

Pauchet B, et al., Pocket Atlas of Anatomy, 3rd edn (Oxford University Press, London, 1937).

Pauwels F, Biomechanics of the Normal and Diseased Hip (translation of German 1973 edition) (Springer-Verlag, Berlin, 1976).

Pearse AG, Histochemistry, Theoretical and Applied, 3rd edn (Churchill Livingstone, London, 1968).

Pech P, et al., AJNR (1985). PMID: 3927681 PMCID: PMC8335176

Peng B, et al., Pain (2007). PMID: 16963186 DOI: 10.1016/j.pain.2006.06.034

Peng M-S, et al., JAMA Network Open (2022). DOI: 10.1001/jamanetworkopen.2021.42069

Penington Institute, Australia's Annual Overdose Report 2021 (2021). www.penington.org.au/publications/australias-annual-overdose-report-2021/

Perez AF, et al., Eur J Radiol (2007). PMID: 17412542 DOI: 10.1016/j.ejrad.2006.12.007

Perina DG, Mechanical Back Pain (2020). https://emedicine.medscape.com/article/822462-overview

Perolat R, et al., Insights Imaging (2018). PMCID: PMC6206372 DOI: 10.1007/s13244-018-0638-x

Perry W, BMJ (1995). DOI: 10.1136/bmj.311.7010.952b

Peterson CK, et al., Spine (2000). PMID: 10685487 DOI: 10.1097/00007632-200001150-00013

Pfirrmann CWA, et al., Spine (2001). PMID: 11568697 DOI: 10.1097/00007632-200109010-00011

Philipp LR, et al., Cureus (2016). PMCID: PMC4762769 DOI: 10.7759/cureus.465

Pickar JG, et al., J Electromyogr Kenesiol (2012). PMCID: PMC3399029 DOI: 10.1016/j.jelekin.2012.01.015

Poilliot A, et al., Sci Rep (2019). DOI: 10.1038/s41598-019-51300-y

Pope JE, et al., Pain Med (2013). PMID: 23802747 DOI: 10.1111/pme.12171

Pope MH, et al. (eds) Occupational Low Back Pain (Praeger Scientific, New York, 1984).

Pope MH, et al., J Biomech Eng (1993). DOI: 10.1115/1.2895542

Porter RW, The Spine and Medical Negligence (Bios Scientific Publishers, Oxford, 1998).

Postacchini F, et al., In: Lumbar Disc Herniation, Chapter 8 (Springer-Verlag, New York, 1999(a)).

Postacchini F, et al., In: Lumbar Disc Herniation, Chapter 5 (Springer-Verlag, New York, 1999(b)).

Prakash LV, et al., Osteoporos Int (2007). PMID: 17404781 DOI: 10.1007/s00198-007-0373-5

Puhakka KB, et al., Skelet Radiol (2004). PMID: 14614576 DOI: 10.1007/s00256-003-0691-4

Quiring DP, et al., The Head, Neck and Trunk. Muscles and Motor Points (Henry Kimpton, London, 1960).

Quon JA, et al., In: Managing Low Back Pain, 4th edn, Chapter 8 (Churchill Livingstone, London, 1999).

Radanov BP, et al., Br J Rheumatol (1994). PMID: 8173848 DOI: 10.1093/rheumatology/33.5.442

Rade M, et al., Spine (2018). PMCID: PMC5756623 DOI: 10.1097/BRS.0000000000002352

Rahman M, et al., StatPearls [Internet]. Treasure Island (FL): StatPearls Publishing (2021). www.ncbi.nlm.nih.gov/books/NBK555921/

Raj PP, Pain Pract (2008). PMID: 18211591 DOI: 10.1111/j.1533-2500.2007.00171.x

Raja SN, et al., Pain (2020). PMCID: PMC7680716 DOI: 10.1097/j.pain.0000000000001939

Rajwani T, et al., Sud Health Technol Inform (2002). PMID: 15457728

Ramirez N, et al., J Bone Joint Surg Am (1997). PMID: 9070524 DOI: 10.2106/00004623-199703000-00007

Ramos-Matos CF, et al. StatPearls [Internet]. Treasure Island (FL): StatPearls (2021). www.ncbi.nlm.nih.gov/books/NBK459275/ PMID: 29083586, Bookshelf ID: NBK459275

Ratcliffe JF, J Anat (1980). PMCID: PMC1233287

Ratliff J, et al., South Med J (1999). PMID: 10624914 DOI: 10.1097/00007611-199912000-00013

Rauschning W, Spine (1987). PMID: 3441815 DOI: 10.1097/00007632-198712000-00012

Rauschning W, In: The Adult Spine Principles and Practice, 2nd edn, Chapter 77 (Lippincott-Raven, New York, 1997).

Rauschning W, Spine (2016). PMID: 27015075 DOI: 10.1097/BRS.0000000000001420

Redberg RF, JAMA Intern Med (2013). DOI: 10.1001/jamainternmed.2013.6621

Reina MA, et al., Acta Anaesth Belg (2009). PMID: 19459550

Reinhardt K, Dtsch Med Wochensch (1951). DOI: 10.1055/s-0028-1116670

Rhodin JAG, Histology: A Text and Atlas (Oxford University Press, London, 1974).

Richardson J, et al., Contin Ed Anaesth Crit Care Pain (2005). DOI: 10.1093/bjaceaccp/mki026

Rickenbacher J, et al., Applied Anatomy of the Back (Springer-Verlag, Berlin, 1985).

Rimmer CT, et al., Folio Morphol (2018). PMID: 29569699 DOI: 10.5603/FM.a2018.0024

Roberts S, et al., Spine (1989). PMID: 2922637 DOI: 10.1097/00007632-198902000-00005

Roberts S, et al., Spine (1995). PMID: 8747242 DOI: 10.1097/00007632-199512150-00005

Rosatelli AL, et al., J Orthop Sports Phys Ther (2006). PMID: 16676869 DOI: 10.2519/jospt.2006.36.4.200

Rosenberg NJ, et al., Spine (1981). PMID: 7209672 DOI: 10.1097/00007632-198101000-00005

Ross MH, et al., Histology: A Text and Atlas (Harper and Row Publishers, JB Lippincott Company, New York, 1985).

Rosse C, et al., Hollinshead's Textbook of Anatomy (Lippincott Williams & Wilkins, Baltimore, 1997).

Rossell S, In: Substance P in the Nervous System. Ciba Foundation Symposium 91 (Pitman, London, 1982, p. 219).

Rothman RH, et al., The Spine, 3rd edn, Vol. 1 (WB Saunders Company, Philadelphia, 1992).

Roudsari B, et al., AJR (2010). PMID: 20729428 DOI: 10.2214/AJR. 10.4367

Rudert M, et al., Acta Orthop Scand (1993). PMID: 8451943 DOI: 10. 3109/17453679308994524

Rush WA, et al., AJR (1946). PMID: 20275162

Ruta DA, et al., Spine (1994). PMID: 7997920 DOI: 10.1097/000 07632-199409000-00004

Rydevik B, Acta Orthop Scand Suppl (1993). PMID: 8451986 DOI: 10. 3109/17453679309160117

Rydevik B, et al., Spine (1984). PMID: 6372124 DOI: 10.1097/ 00007632-198401000-00004

Rydevik B, et al., Acta Physiol Scand (1990). PMID: 2316385 DOI: 10. 1111/j.1748-1716.1990.tb08843.x

Sääksjärvi S, et al., Spine (2020). PMID: 32453239 DOI: 10.1097/ BRS.0000000000003548

Saito T, et al., Anesthesiology (2013). PMID: 23165471 DOI: 10.1097/ ALN.0b013e318272f40a

Sakka L, et al., Eur Ann Otorhinolary (2011). PMID: 22100360 DOI: 10.1016/j.anorl.2011.03.002

Salt TE, et al., Neuroscience (1982). PMID: 6180350 DOI: 10.1016/ 0306-4522(82)91121-6

Sandoz R, Some physical mechanisms and effects of spinal adjustments. Ann Swiss Chiropr Assoc, 6: 91 (1976).

Sandoz R, Some reflex phenomena associated with spinal derangements and adjustments. Ann Swiss Chiropr Assoc, 7: 45 (1981).

Sato S, et al., Okajimas Folia Anat. JPN (2002). PMID: 12199537 DOI: 10.2535/ofaj.79.43

Savvopoulou V, et al., J Magn Reson Imaging (2011). PMID: 21274980 DOI: 10.1002/jmri.22444

Schaumburg HH, et al., In: The Research Status of Spinal Manipulative Therapy. US Department of Health, Education, and Welfare, Public Health Service, National Institutes of Health, National Institute of Neurological and Communicative Disorders and Stroke, Bethesda, Maryland. NINCDS Monograph No 15 (1975).

Schellhas KP, et al., Spine (1996). PMID: 8742205 DOI: 10.1097/ 00007632-199602010-00009

Schiotz EH, et al., Manipulation Past and Present (William Heinemann Medical Books, London, 1975).

Schleich C, et al., Osteoarthr Cartil (2016). PMID: 27163444 DOI: 10.1016/j.joca.2016.05.004

Schlösser TPC, et al., Spine J (2013). DOI: 10.1016/j.spinee.2012.11.057

Schmid, H, Das Iliosakralgelenk in einer Untersuchung mit Rontgenstereophotogrammetrie und einer klinischen Studie. Act Rheumatol, 5: 163 (1980).

Schmorl G, Uber die an den wirbelbandscheiben vorkommenden ausdehnungs—und zerreisungsvorgange und die dadurch an ihnen und der wirbelspongiosa hervorgerufenen veranderun-gen. Verh Dtsch Path Ges, 22: 250 (1927).

Schmorl G, et al., The Human Spine in Health and Disease, 2nd edn (Grune and Stratton, New York, 1971).

Schneider W, et al., Manual Medicine Therapy (Thieme Medical Publishers, Inc., New York, 1988).

Schug SA, et al., In: Mechanisms of Vascular Disease: A Reference Book for Vascular Specialists [Internet], Chapter 20 (University of Adelaide Press, Adelaide, AU, 2011). www.ncbi.nlm.nih.gov/ books/NBK534269/

Schwartz JH, In: Principles of Neural Science, Chapter 10 (Elsevier/ North-Holland, New York, 1981).

Schwarzer AC, et al., Spine (1995). PMID: 7709277 DOI: 10.1097/ 00007632-199501000-00007

Selden NR, J Neurosurg (5 Suppl Pediatrics) (2006). PMID: 16848085 DOI: 10.3171/ped.2006.104.5.302

Serafini-Fracassini A, et al., The Structure and Biochemistry of Cartilage (Churchill Livingstone, Edinburgh, 1974).

Shalen PR, Radiological techniques for diagnosis of lumbar disc degen-eration. SPINE: State Art Rev, 3: 27–48 (1989).

Shapiro R, Radiology (letter) (1986). DOI: 10.1148/radiology.159. 3.3704164

Shaw JL, In: First Interdisciplinary World Congress on Low Back Pain and its Relation to the Sacroiliac Joint (ECO, Rotterdam, 1992).

Shayota B, et al., Anat Cell Biol (2019). PMCID: PMC6624329 DOI: 10.5115/acb.2019.52.2.128

Sherrington CS, The Integrative Action of the Nervous System (Yale University Press, New Haven, 1906).

Siccardi MA, et al., StatPearls [Internet]. Treasure Island (FL): StatPearls Publishing (2021). www.ncbi.nlm.nih.gov/books/NBK535418/

Sicuteri F, et al., In: Recent Advances on Pain (Charles C. Thomas, Springfield, 1974, pp. 148–167).

Sinnatamby CS, Last's Anatomy: Regional and Applied, 12th edn (Churchill Livingstone/Elsevier, Edinburgh, 2011).

Skouen JS, et al., Spine (1993). PMID: 8434328 DOI: 10.1097/000 07632-199301000-00012

Skouen JS, et al., J Spinal Disord (1994). PMID: 8186584 DOI: 10.1097/ 00002517-199407010-00002

Skouen JS, et al., J Spinal Disord (1997). PMID: 9438816

Skouen JS, et al., Spine (2002). PMID: 11979157 DOI: 10.1097/000 07632-200205010-00002

Sleeman K, et al. (2018). www.bbc.com/news/health-44797545.

Slipman CW, et al., Spine (1998). PMID: 9802168 DOI: 10.1097/ 00007632-199810150-00019

Slipman CW, et al., Pain Physician (2002). PMID: 16902651

Smith FW, et al., European Society of Skeletal Radiology (EESR)— Augsburg, Germany (2004). http://fonar.com/research_essr_ 2004.htm

Soames RW, In: Gray's Anatomy, 38th edn, Chapter 6 (Churchill Livingstone, New York, 1995).

Sokolowski W, et al., Biologia (Bratisl) (2018). PMCID: PMC6097054 DOI: 10.2478/s11756-018-0074-x

Solonen KA, Acta Orthop Scand (1957). DOI: 10.3109/ort.1957.28. suppl-27.01

Song Q, et al., Medicine (2019). PMCID: PMC6783151 DOI: 10.1097/ MD.0000000000017336

Spector R, et al., Exp Neurol (2015). PMID: 26247808 DOI: 10.1016/j. expneurol.2015.07.027

Spratt KF, et al., Spine (1990). PMID: 2139245 DOI: 10.1097/0000 7632-199002000-00009

Stefanakis M, et al., Spine (2012). PMID: 22706090 DOI: 10.1097/ BRS.0b013e318263ba59

Steinke H, et al., Spine (2010). PMID: 20075779 DOI: 10.1097/ BRS.0b013e3181b7c675

Stockwell RA, Biology of Cartilage Cells (Cambridge University Press, Cambridge, 1979).

Stoddard A, Manual of Osteopathic Practice (Hutchinson, London, 1969).

Stokes IAF, et al., Spine (2004). PMCID: PMC7173624 DOI: 10.1097/01. brs.0000146049.52152.da

Stöppler MC (2021). www.medicinenet.com/multidetector_computed_ tomography/definition.htm

Sturesson B, et al., Spine (1989). PMID: 2922636 DOI: 10.1097/ 00007632-198902000-00004

Summers B, et al., Spine (2005). PMID: 15682017 DOI: 10.1097/01. brs.0000152378.93868.c8

Sunderland S, Nerves and Nerve Injuries (ES Livingstone, Edinburgh, 1968).

Sunderland S, J Neurosurg (1974). PMID: 4826601 DOI: 10.3171/ jns.1974.40.6.0756

Sunderland S, In: The research status of spinal manipulative therapy. US Department of Health, Education, and Welfare, Public Health Service, National Institutes of Health, National Institute of Neurological and Communicative Disorders and Stroke, Bethesda, Maryland. NINCDS Monograph No 15 (1975). https:// centerforinquiry.org/wp-content/uploads/sites/33/quackwatch/ ninds_1975pdf.pdf

Sunderland S, In: The Neurobiologic Mechanisms in Manipulative Therapy (Plenum Press, New York, 1978, pp. 137–166).

Sunderland S, In: Modern Developments in the Principles and Practice of Chiropractic, Chapter 3 (Appleton-Century-Crofts, New York, 1980).

Suri P, et al., PLoS Genet (2018). PMCID: PMC6159857 DOI: 10.1371/journal.pgen.1007601

Sutton NG, Injuries of the Spinal Cord. The Management of Paraplegia and Tetraplegia (Butterworth and Co, Ltd, London, 1973).

Syrmou E, et al., Spondylolysis: A review and reappraisal. Hippokratia, 14: 17–21 (2010). PMID: 20411054 PMCID: PMC2843565

Taillard W, et al., Die Beinlängenunterschiede (S. Karger, Basel, 1965).

Takahashi K, et al., Eur Spine J (1995). PMID: 7749909 DOI: 10.1007/BF00298420

Tanenbaum LN, Appl Radiol (2006). PMID: 16530631 DOI: 10.1016/j.mric.2005.12.004

Tardieu GG, et al., Cureus (2016). DOI 10.7759/cureus.779. PMCID: PMC5063636 DOI: 10.7759/cureus.779

Taylor JR, et al., In: Clinical Anatomy and Management of Low Back Pain, Chapter 4 (Butterworth-Heinemann, Oxford, 1997).

Teasell RW, Pain Research Management (1997). http://citeseerx.ist.psu.edu/viewdoc/download?doi=10.1.1.667.2181&rep=rep1&type=pdf

Tegeder I, et al., J Cell Mol Med (2009). PMCID: PMC6529970 DOI: 10.1111/j.1582-4934.2009.00703.x

Telano LN, et al., StatPearls [Internet]. Treasure Island (FL): StatPearls Publishing (2020). www.ncbi.nlm.nih.gov/books/NBK519007/

Tello M (Harvard Health Publishing, 2017). www.health.harvard.edu/blog/what-to-do-low-back-pain-2017120712839.

Tenny S, et al. StatPearls [Internet]. Treasure Island (FL): StatPearls Publishing (2021). www.ncbi.nlm.nih.gov/books/NBK459235/

Teodorczyk-Injeyan J, et al., The Clin J Pain (2019). PMCID: PMC6735949 DOI: 10.1097/AJP.0000000000000745

Theodore N, Spine (2016). PMID: 27015066 DOI: 10.1097/BRS.0000000000001433

Theodorou DJ, et al., AJR (2020). PMID: 32069076 DOI: 10.2214/AJR.19.22081

Thomas GD, Adv Physiol Educ (2011). PMID: 21385998 DOI: 10.1152/advan.00114.2010

Thomas J-L, et al., Med Sci (Paris) (2019). PMID: 30672459 DOI: 10.1051/medsci/2018309

Tirgari M, J Am Vet Radiol (1978). DOI: 10.1111/j.1740-8261.1978.tb01146.x

Tisot RA, et al., Coluna/Columna (2018). DOI: 10.1590/S1808-185120181701179264

Tjernstrom B, et al., J Orthop Trauma (1993). PMID: 8308608 DOI: 10.1097/00005131-199312000-00010

Tjernstrom B, et al., Acta Orthop Scand (1994). PMID: 8042488 DOI: 10.3109/17453679408995463

Tobita T, et al., Spine (2003). DOI: 10.1097/01.BRS.0000083595.10862.98

Todd TW, et al., Am J Phys Anthropol (1928). DOI: 10.1002/ajpa.1330120211

Tomaszewski KA, et al., Folia Morphol (Warsz) (2015). PMID: 26050801 DOI: 10.5603/FM.2015.0026

Tondury G, Anatomie fonctionelle des petites articulations de rachis. Ann Med Phys, 15: 173–191 (1972).

Torebjork E, In: Nociception and Pain (University Press, Cambridge, 1985, pp. 9–16).

Traeger AC, et al., JAMA (2021). PMID: 34283182 DOI: 10.1001/jama.2020.19715

Travell J, et al., Postgrad Med (1952). DOI: 10.1080/00325481.1952.11694280

Travers H, J South Dakota State Med Assoc (2018). PMID: 29990413

Tsujimoto R, et al., BMC Musculoskelet Disord (2016). DOI: 10.1186/s12891-016-1343-x

Tubbs RS, et al., Neurol Res (2004). PMID: 15494112 DOI: 10.1179/016164104225017910

Tubbs RS, et al., J Neurosurg Spine (2007). PMID: 17877268 DOI: 10.3171/SPI-07/09/328

Tucker WD, et al., StatPearls [Internet]. Treasure Island (FL): StatPearls Publishing (2021). www.ncbi.nlm.nih.gov/books/NBK470401/

Turner JA, et al., Spine (1998). PMID: 9516702 DOI: 10.1097/00007632-199802150-00011

Twomey L, et al., Spinal Cord (1988). DOI: 10.1038/sc.1988.37

Tzika, M., et al., Surg Radiol Anat (2021). DOI: 10.1007/s00276-021-02690-0

Urban JPG, et al., Spine (2004). PMID: 15564919 DOI: 10.1097/01.brs.0000146499.97948.52

Urban JPG, et al., J Magn Reson Imaging (2007). PMID: 17260404 DOI: 10.1002/jmri.20874

Urits I, et al., Pain Ther (2021). PMCID: PMC8119576 DOI: 10.1007/s40122-020-00211-2

Vallbo AB, J Neurophysiol (2018). PMID: 29924706 DOI: 10.1152/jn.00933.2017

Van Dieën JH, et al., Med Hypotheses (1999). PMID: 10580532 DOI: 10.1054/mehy.1998.0754

van Norel GJ, et al., J Bone Joint Surg (1996). PMID: 8636195

van Tulder MW, et al., Spine (1997). PMID: 9055372 DOI: 10.1097/00007632-199702150-00015

Vernon-Roberts B, In: The Lumbar Spine and Back Pain, Chapter 4 (Pitman Medical, Tunbridge Wells, 1980).

Vernon-Roberts B, et al., Spine (2008). PMID: 19050583 DOI: 10.1097/BRS.0b013e31817bb989

Vesalius A, De Fabrica Corporis Humani, Preface (translated by B Farrington) (1543). https://journals.sagepub.com/doi/pdf/10.1177/003591573202500901

Videman T, et al., Spine (1998). PMID: 9854746 DOI: 10.1097/00007632-199812010-00002

Videman T, et al., Spine (2003). PMID: 12642766 DOI: 10.1097/01.BRS.0000049905.44466.73

Videman T, et al., Spine (2004). PMID: 15564915 DOI: 10.1097/01.brs.0000146461.27105.2b

Vilensky JA, et al., Spine (2002). PMID: 12045518 DOI: 10.1097/00007632-200206010-00012

Vink P, et al., Clin Biomech (1989). DOI: 10.1016/0268-0033(89)90049-1

Vleeming A, et al., Spine (1990). PMID: 2326707 DOI: 10.1097/00007632-199002000-00017

Vleeming A, et al., In: First Interdisciplinary World Congress on Low Back Pain and its Relation to the Sacroiliac Joint (Rotterdam, ECO, 1992(a)).

Vleeming A, et al., Clin Biomech (Bristol, Avon). (1992(b)). PMID: 23915725 DOI: 10.1016/0268-0033(92)90032-Y

Vleeming A, et al., Spine (1996). PMID: 8852309 DOI: 10.1097/00007632-199603010-00005

Vleeming A, et al., J Anat (2012). PMCID: PMC3512279 DOI: 10.1111/j.1469-7580.2012.01564.x

Von Hagens G, et al., The Visible Human Body: An Atlas of Sectional Anatomy (Lea and Febiger, London, 1991).

Von Luschka H, Die Nerven des menschlichen Wirbelkanales (Laupp, Tubingen, 1850).

Vukicevic S., et al., Spine (1991). PMID: 2011779

Waddell G, The Backpain Revolution, 2nd edn (Churchill Livingstone, Edinburgh, 2004).

Waddell G, et al., The Backpain Revolution, 2nd edn, Chapter 17 (Churchill Livingstone, Edinburgh, 2004).

Wadhwani S, et al., Spine (2004). PMID: 15014271 DOI: 10.1097/01.brs.0000115129.59484.24

Waljee JF, et al., JAMA Network Open (2018). DOI: 10.1001/jamanetworkopen.2018.0236

Walker JM, J Orthop Sports Phys Ther (1986). PMID: 18802258 DOI: 10.2519/jospt.1986.7.6.325

Wall PD, In: Recent Advances in Pain: Pathophysiology and Clinical Aspects (CC Thomas, Springfield, 1974, pp. 36–63).

Wang M, et al., Neural Function (Little, Brown and Co., Boston, 1987).

Warder DE, et al., Neurosurgery (1993). PMID: 8413866 DOI: 10.1227/00006123-199309000-00004

Watts C, et al., Surg Neurol (1986). DOI: 10.1016/0090-3019(86)90155-2

Waxenbaum JA, et al., StatPearls [Internet]. Treasure Island (FL): StatPearls Publishing (2021). www.ncbi.nlm.nih.gov/books/NBK539845/

Weeks WB, et al., J Manipulative Physiol Ther (2018). PMID: 29456094 DOI: 10.1016/j.jmpt.2017.12.003

Weinstein PR, et al., In: Lumbar Spondylosis, Diagnosis, Management and Surgical Treatment (Year Book Medical Publishers, Chicago, 1977, pp. 115–133).

Weir J, et al., Imaging Atlas of Human Anatomy, 3rd edn (Mosby, Edinburgh, 2003).

Weis EB, Jr, In: The research status of spinal manipulative therapy. US Department of Health, Education, and Welfare, Public Health Service, National Institutes of Health, National Institute of Neurological and Communicative Disorders and Stroke, Bethesda, Maryland. NINCDS Monograph No 15 (1975). https://centerforinquiry.org/wp-content/uploads/sites/33/quackwatch/ninds_1975pdf.pdf

Weisel H, Acta Anat (1955). PMID: 14349535

Weitz EM, Spine (1981). PMID: 7280828 DOI: 10.1097/00007632-198107000-00010

Weitz EM, J Bone Joint Surg Am (1984). PMID: 6384222

Whedon JM, et al., Spine (2021). DOI: 10.1097/BRS.0000000000004078

Whelan MA, et al., AJR (1982). PMID: 6983265 DOI: 10.2214/ajr.139.6.1183

White AA, et al., Spine (1982). PMID: 6211779 DOI: 10.1097/00007632-198203000-00009

Wiley JJ, et al., Can J Surg (1968). PMID: 5694965

Wilke H-J, Spine (2016). DOI: 10.1097/BRS.0000000000001419

Wilke H-J, et al., Spine (1999). PMID: 10222525 DOI: 10.1097/00007632-199904150-00005

Wilkinson JL, Neuroanatomy for Medical Students (John Wright & Sons, Bristol, 1986).

Willen JH, et al., Spine (1997). PMID: 9431634 DOI: 10.1097/00007632-199712150-00021

Williams PC, Low Back and Neck Pain (Charles C Thomas, Springfield, 1974).

Williams PL, et al., Gray's Anatomy, 36th edn (Churchill Livingstone, London, 1980).

Willis TA, J Bone Joint Surg (1959). https://journals.lww.com/jbjsjournal/Citation/1959/41050/Lumbosacral_Anomalies.12.aspx

Willis WD, In: Nociception and Pain (Cambridge University Press, Cambridge, 1985, pp. 35–50).

Wills CR, et al., Front Physio (2018). PMCID: PMC6156535 DOI: 10.3389/fphys.2018.01210

Wiltse LL, et al., J Bone Joint Surg Am (1975). PMID: 1123367

Wiltse LL, et al., Spine (1993). PMID: 8367771 DOI: 10.1097/00007632-199306150-00013

Witkamp TD, et al., Radiology (2001). PMID: 11425999 DOI: 10.1148/radiology.220.1.r01jl06208

Wong DA, et al., Macnab's Backache, 4th edn (Lippincott Williams and Wilkins, Philadelphia, 2007).

Wong J, et al., Osteoarthr Cartil (2019). PMCID: PMC6536352 DOI: 10.1016/j.joca.2019.01.013

Wong M, et al., StatPearls [Internet]. Treasure Island (FL): StatPearls Publishing (2020). www.ncbi.nlm.nih.gov/books/NBK507801/.

Wood PHN, In: The Lumbar Spine and Back Pain, 2nd edn, Chapter 1 (Pitman Medical, Kent, 1980).

Woolf AD, et al., Nat Clin Pract Rheumatol (2008). PMID: 18172446 DOI: 10.1038/ncprheum0673

Woolf CJ, et al., Neuron (2007). PMID: 17678850 DOI: 10.1016/j.neuron.2007.07.016

World Health Organization, International Classification of Functioning, Disability and Health (ICF) (2001). www.cdc.gov/ncbddd/disabilityandhealth/disability.html

World Medical Association Declaration of Geneva (2017). www.wma.net/policies-post/wma-declaration-of-geneva/#:~:text=I%20WILL%20ATTEND%20TO%20my,freely%2C%20and%20upon%20my%20honour.

Wu Y, et al., Spine (2017). PMCID: PMC5509527 DOI: 10.1097/BRS.0000000000002061

Wyke BD, Neurological mechanisms in the experience of pain. Acupunct Electrother Res Int J, 4: 27–35 (1979).

Wyke BD, In: The Lumbar Spine and Back Pain, 2nd edn, Chapter 11 (Pitman Medical, Tunbridge Wells, 1980).

Yahia L, et al., Ann Anat (1993). PMID: 8489030 DOI: 10.1016/s0940-9602(11)80162-7

Yahia LH, et al., Acta Orthop Scand (1988). PMID: 2461043 DOI: 10.3109/17453678809148773

Yahia LH, et al., Z Mikrosk Anat Forsch (1989). PMID: 2815931

Yahia LH, et al., Z Mikrosk Anat Forsch (1990). PMID: 2349823

Yam MF, et al., Int J Mol Sci (2018). PMCID: PMC6121522 DOI: 10.3390/ijms19082164

Yamada S, Tethered Cord Syndrome (The American Association of Neurological Surgeons, Chicago, IL, 1996).

Yamada S, Tethered Cord Syndrome in Children and Adults, 2nd edn (Thieme Medical Publishers, Inc., and The American Association of Neurological Surgeons, New York, 2010).

Yamada S, et al., J Neurosurg (1981). PMID: 6259301 DOI: 10.3171/jns.1981.54.4.0494

Yamada S, et al., In: Tethered Cord Syndrome, Chapter 15 (The American Association of Neurological Surgeons, Chicago, IL, 1996).

Yamada S, et al., J Spinal Disord (2000). PMID: 10941891 DOI: 10.1097/00002517-200008000-00008

Yamada S, et al., Neurosurg Q (2001). https://oce.ovid.com/article/00013414-200112000-00003?sequence=1&clickthrough=y

Yamada S, et al., Neurol Res (2004). PMID: 15494115 DOI: 10.1179/016164104225017965

Yamada, S, et al., Neurosurg Focus (2007). DOI: 10.3171/FOC-07/08/E6

Yamada, S, et al., Tethered Cord Syndrome in Children and Adults, 2nd edn, Chapter 15 (Thieme Medical Publishers, Inc., and The American Association of Neurological Surgeons, New York, 2010(a)).

Yamada, S, et al., Tethered Cord Syndrome in Children and Adults, 2nd edn, Chapter 3 (Thieme Medical Publishers, Inc., and The American Association of Neurological Surgeons, New York, 2010(b)).

Yamashita T, et al., Spine (1993). PMID: 8278841 DOI: 10.1097/00007632-199311000-00018

Yamashita T, et al., N Engl J Med (2009). PMID: 19641218 DOI: 10.1056/NEJMc0902318

Yang G, et al., J Int Med Res (2018). PMCID: PMC6259376 DOI: 10.1177/0300060518799902

Yang M, et al., J Orthop Surg Res (2020). DOI: 10.1186/s13018-020-01706-6

Yochum TR, et al., In: Essentials of Skeletal Radiology, 2nd edn, Chapter 6 (Williams & Wilkins, Baltimore, 1996).

Yoshizawa H, Spine (2002). PMID: 12065971

Yoshizawa H, et al., Orthop Clin N Am (1991). PMID: 2014118

Yrjämä M, et al., Spine (1997). PMID: 9106323 DOI: 10.1097/00007632-199704010-00020

Yu S, et al., AJNR (1989). PMID: 2505527 PMCID: PMC8335281

Zeng C, et al., JAMA (2019). PMCID: PMC6439672 DOI: 10.1001/jama.2019.1347

Zhang H, et al., Spine (2010). PMID: 20042959 DOI: 10.1097/BRS.0b013e3181b790a0

Zhang Y, et al., Spine (2014). PMCID: PMC4086915 DOI: 10.1097/BRS.0000000000000174

Zhao Q, et al., Spine (2016). PMID: 27060710 DOI: 10.1016/j.spinee.2016.03.048

Zhao C, et al., Sci Rep (2020(a)). DOI: 10.1038/s41598-020-60714-y

Zhao X, et al., Font Cell Dev Biol (2020(b)). DOI: 10.3389/fcell.2020.595969

Zhao Q, et al., Spine (2020(c)). PMID: 31415472 DOI: 10.1097/BRS.0000000000003190

Zhong E, et al., Spine (2017). PMID: 28187067 DOI: 10.1097/BRS.0000000000002120

Zinn DJ, et al., Stain Technol (1962). PMID: 14003755

Zippel H, et al., Zentralbl Chir (1993). PMID: 8303957

Zou J, et al., Spine (2008). PMID: 18317181 DOI: 10.1097/BRS.0b013e3181657f7e

INDEX

Note: Page numbers in italics indicate a figure on the corresponding page.